Human Anatomy

Publisher: Richard Furn
Project Development Manager: Janice Urquhart
Project Manager: Frances Affleck
Designer: George Ajayi
New illustrations: Richard Tibbitts

Human Anatomy

COLOR ATLAS AND TEXT

FOURTH EDITION

J.A. Gosling MD, MB ChB, FRCS
Professor of Anatomy
Stanford University
USA

P.F. Harris MD, MB ChB, MSc
Emeritus Professor of Anatomy
University of Manchester
UK

I. Whitmore MD, MB BS, LRCP, MRCS
Professor of Anatomy
Stanford University
USA

P.L.T. Willan MB ChB, FRCS
Formerly Professor of Anatomy
University of UAE,
Al-Ain
United Arab Emirates

Photography by:
A.L. Bentley ABIPP, AIMBI, MBKS
Medical Photographer,
School of Biological Sciences,
University of Manchester, UK

Embalming and section cutting by:
J.T. Davies LIAS
Senior Anatomical Technician,
School of Biological Sciences,
University of Manchester, UK

Contributors to previous editions:
J.R. Humpherson MB ChB
Senior Lecturer in Anatomy
School of Biological Sciences
University of Manchester, UK

J.L. Hargreaves BA(Hons)
Medical Photographer

EDINBURGH • LONDON • NEW YORK • PHILADELPHIA • ST LOUIS • SYDNEY • TORONTO 2002

M Mosby

An imprint of Elsevier Science Limited

Fourth edition 2002

ISBN 0 7234 3195 7
International edition ISBN 0 7234 3296 1

British Library Cataloguing in Publication Data
A catalogue record for this book is available from the British Library

Library of Congress Cataloging in Publication Data
A catalog record for this book is available from the Library of Congress

Note
Medical knowledge is constantly changing. As new information becomes available, changes in treatment, procedures, equipment and the use of drugs become necessary. The authors and the publishers have taken care to ensure that the information given in this text is accurate and up to date. However, readers are strongly advised to confirm that the information, especially with regard to drug usage, complies with the latest legislation and standards of practice.

The
publisher's
policy is to use
paper manufactured
from sustainable forests

Printed in Spain

Preface to Fourth Edition

This new edition retains the unique mixture of comprehensive concise text with photographs of dissections each designed to illustrate points from the text on specific pages. This very close relationship between text and illustrations makes for easy cross reference. The font size has been increased to improve the readability and the terminology updated to conform with the recent internationally agreed *Terminologia Anatomica*, which has rendered redundant the glossary of English and Nomina Anatomica terms. We have continued to improve the text by remedying omissions and removing errors and ambiguities. The clinical skills pages have been simplified and the content of the exam skills pages has been rewritten in the most commonly used MCQ format.

The opportunity has been taken to replace many cross-sections with new sections viewed from below in accordance with modern practice for viewing radiological images. A very few sections from the Third Edition were able to be inverted. The self-assessment aspects of the book, previously available by covering labels to drawings, have been enhanced by expansion of several chapters to include observation skills pages based on cadaver cross-sections, MR images and CT scans. The identity of each labelled item is provided at the foot of the page to facilitate their use in both learning and assessment.

The additional content introduced in the previous two editions has been retained. This includes a section on the back, introductions to each section and clinical and exam skills pages. Additional osteology, radiographs and illustrations of the surface features of the brain and spinal cord were also added.

We regret that Dr Humpherson was unable to participate in this edition and we wish to record our great appreciation for his equal contribution to previous editions.

J.A.G., P.F.H., I.W., P.L.T.W.

Preface to First Edition

Despite the many anatomical atlases and textbooks currently available, there appeared to be a need for a book which combined the advantages of each of these forms of presentation. This book was conceived with the intention of filling that need. With a unique combination of photographs of dissections, accompanying diagrams and concise text, this volume aims to provide the student with a better understanding of human anatomy.

The basis of this work is the cadaver as seen in the dissecting room; therefore, reference to surface and radiological anatomy is minimal. Likewise, comments on the clinical and functional significance of selected anatomical structures are brief. However, comparison is made where appropriate between the anatomy of the living and that of the cadaver.

Each dissection was specially prepared and photographed to display only a few important features. However, since photographs of dissections are inherently difficult to interpret, each is accompanied by a guide in the form of a drawing. Each drawing is coloured and labelled to highlight the salient features of the dissection and is accompanied by axes to indicate the orientation of the specimen. Adjacent photographs often depict different stages of the same dissection to help the student construct a three-dimensional image.

The first chapter introduces anatomical terminology, provides general information about the basic tissues of the body, and includes overall views of selected systems. Because the six subsequent chapters describe anatomy primarily through dissection, a regional approach has been employed. Features of bones are described only when considering their related structures, especially muscles and joints; osteology is not considered in its own right. The internal structure of the ear and eye are beyond the scope of this book since the study of these topics requires microscopy; the anatomy of the brain and spinal cord are also excluded as they are usually taught in special courses.

The level of detail contained in this book is appropriate for current courses in topographical anatomy for medical and dental undergraduates. In addition, it will be of value to postgraduates and to students entering those professions allied to medicine in which anatomy is part of the curriculum.

The terminology employed is that which is most frequently used in clinical practice. Where appropriate, alternatives (such as those recommended in *Nomina Anatomica*) are appended in brackets.

Preparation of the dissections and the text has occupied the authors for nearly five years. Our objective was to create a high quality and visually attractive anatomical work and we hope that the time and effort spent in its preparation is reflected in the finished product.

J.A.G., P.F.H., J.R.H., I.W., P.L.T.W.
Manchester, 1985

Acknowledgements for all editions

The authors are indebted to the Department of Radiology at Manchester University for the provision of radiographs and to Professors R.S. Harris and A.R. Moody for CT and MR scans.

The staff at the various publishing firms that have owned the imprint under which this book has been published have always been helpful and, where necessary, have applied gentle pressure. With their stimulus we met the various deadlines.

Our families deserve a special mention, as without their untiring support and patience these editions would certainly not have come to publication.

We thank them all.

Contents

User Guide

Organization

This book begins with a Section on basic anatomical concepts, which is followed by seven Sections, each dealing with one of the anatomical regions. Following the introduction to each Section, information is often presented in dissection order suitable for teaching, progressing from the surface to deeper structures. The limbs are described from proximal to distal with the joints considered at the ends of the appropriate Section.

Texts and Photographs

Where possible, topics are presented on self-contained spreads, the photographs accompanying the relevant text. Within the text, cross-references are given to other relevant text and illustrations.

Accompanying Diagrams

Each photograph is augmented by a line diagram in which colour is used to focus attention on particular structures in the dissection. Most of the colours are used consistently and conform to the following code:

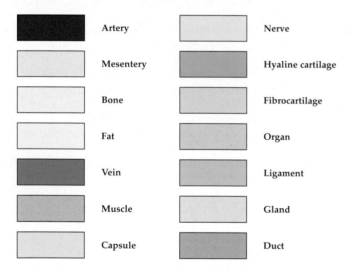

Labels and Leader Lines

The structures of particular interest in each diagram are labelled. If a single structure is named in a label with a branched leader line, the leader line and its branch(es) terminate on different parts of that structure. However, if two or more structures are named, the first has the main leader line terminating on it while the subsequent structures are indicated by branches given off at progressively shorter distances from the label. A leader line ending in an arrow head indicates a space or cavity.

Orientation Guides

Each diagram is accompanied by an orientation guide whose axes employ the following abbreviations:

L left   **P** posterior   **pr** proximal
R right   **A** anterior   **d** distal
S superior   **la** lateral
I inferior   **m** medial

Orientation guides in oblique views employ large and small arrow heads and long and short arrow shafts. The following examples illustrate orientation guides to specimens seen:

from in front;

from behind;

from the left side and slightly in front;

from the left side, slightly above and in front.

Terminology

The book conforms to *Terminologia Anatomica*, using the English terms.

Self-assessment

The photographs are unfettered by labels, leader lines and other superimposed markings; thus, the reader can readily use this book to test knowledge by either masking the whole of the accompanying diagram and studying the photograph alone or covering only the labels around the diagram.

TERMS OF POSITION AND MOVEMENT

To avoid ambiguity and confusion, anatomical terms of position and movement are defined according to an internationally accepted convention. This convention defines the 'anatomical position' as one in which the human body stands erect with the feet together and the face, eyes and palms of the hands directed forwards (Fig. 1.1).

With the subject in the anatomical position, three sets of planes, mutually at right angles, can be defined.

Fig. 1.2 Coronal section through the head.

Fig. 1.3 Sagittal section through the trunk. This section lies to the left of the median sagittal plane.

Fig. 1.1 Anatomical position and the terms used in anatomical description.

Vertical (or longitudinal) planes are termed either **coronal** or **sagittal**. **Coronal (or frontal) planes** (Fig. 1.2) pass from one side to the other while **sagittal planes** (Fig. 1.3) pass from front to back. One particular sagittal plane, the **median sagittal plane**, lies in the midline and divides the body into right and left halves (Fig. 1.4).

Horizontal (or **transverse**) **planes** (Fig. 1.5) transect the body from side to side and front to back.

Sections cut at right angles to the long axis of an organ or part of the body are also known as transverse. Similarly, longitudinal sections are cut parallel to the long axis.

The terms **medial** and **lateral** are used to indicate the position of structures relative to the median sagittal plane. For example, the ring finger lies lateral to the little finger but medial to the thumb. The front and back of the body are usually termed the **anterior** (or ventral) and **posterior** (or dorsal) surfaces respectively (Fig. 1.1). Thus one structure is described as anterior to another because it is placed further forwards.

Superior and **inferior** are terms used to indicate the relative head/foot positions of structures (Fig. 1.1). Those lying towards the head (or **cranial**) end of the body are described as superior to others which are inferior (or **caudal**). Thus the heart lies superior to the diaphragm; the diaphragm is inferior to the heart. In the limbs the terms **proximal** and **distal** have comparable meanings. For example, the elbow joint is proximal to the wrist but distal to the shoulder.

The terms **superficial** and **deep** indicate the location of structures in relation to the body surface. Thus the ribs lie superficial to the lungs but deep to the skin of the chest wall (Fig. 1.5).

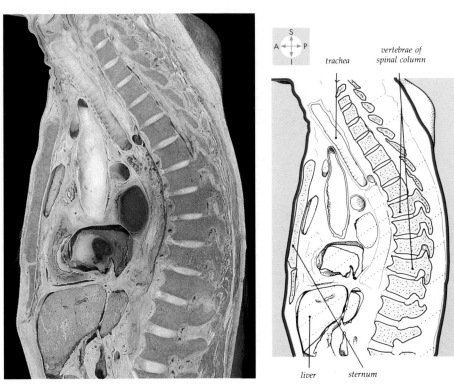

Fig. 1.4 Median sagittal section through the trunk.

Fig. 1.5 Transverse section through the thorax at the level of the intervertebral disc between the sixth and seventh thoracic vertebrae. Inferior aspect. Compare Fig. 2.69.

Movements at joints are also described by specific terms. From the anatomical position, forward movement of one part in relation to the rest of the body is called **flexion**. **Extension** carries the same part posteriorly (Fig. 1.6). However, because in the fetus the developing upper and lower limbs rotate in different directions, the movements of flexion and extension in all joints from the knee downwards occur in opposite directions to the equivalent joints in the upper limb. In **abduction** the structure moves away from the median sagittal plane in a lateral direction, whereas **adduction** moves it towards the midline (Fig. 1.7). For the fingers and toes the terms abduction and adduction are used in reference to a longitudinal plane passing along the middle finger or the second toe respectively. Movement around the longitudinal axis of part of the body is called rotation. In **medial** (or internal) **rotation** the anterior surface of a limb rotates medially whilst **lateral** (or external) **rotation** turns the anterior surface laterally (Fig. 1.8). Movements that combine flexion, extension, abduction, adduction and medial and lateral rotation (for instance, the 'windmilling' action seen at the shoulder joint) are known as **circumduction**.

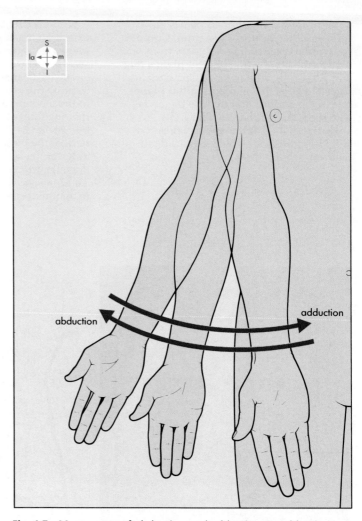

Fig. 1.7 Movements of abduction and adduction. In adduction, flexion of the shoulder joint allows the limb to be carried anterior to the trunk.

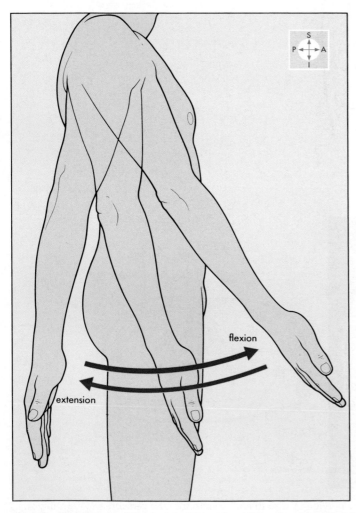

Fig. 1.6 Movements of flexion and extension of the shoulder joint.

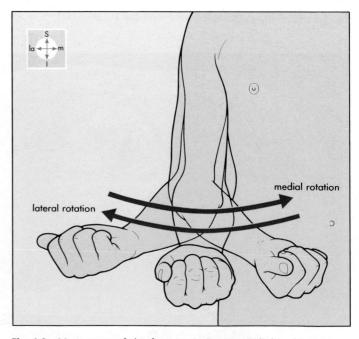

Fig. 1.8 Movement of the forearm indicates medial and lateral rotation at the shoulder joint. The elbow is flexed.

BASIC TISSUES AND STRUCTURES

Skin

Skin (Fig. 1.9) is a protective covering for the surface of the body and comprises a superficial layer, called the epidermis, and a deeper layer, the dermis. The epidermis is an epithelium consisting of a surface layer of dead cells which are continually shed and replaced by cells from its deeper germinal layer. The dermis is a layer of connective tissue containing blood vessels, lymphatics and nerves. In most areas of the body the skin is thin and mobile over the underlying structures. Specializations of the skin include fingernails and toenails, hair follicles and sweat glands. On the palms of the hands and soles of the feet (and corresponding surfaces of the digits), hair follicles are absent and the epidermis is relatively thick. The skin in these regions is also firmly anchored to the underlying structures, reducing its mobility during gripping and standing. Lines of tension occur within skin and are of importance to surgeons. Scars following surgical incisions made along these lines tend to be narrower than those made across the lines of tension.

Skin is usually well vascularized and receives blood from numerous subcutaneous vessels. Knowledge of this vascular supply is important when operations that involve the use of skin flaps are undertaken. Skin has a rich nerve supply, responding to touch, pressure, heat, cold, vibration and pain. In certain areas, such as the fingertips, the skin is especially sensitive to touch and pressure. Skin is innervated by superficial (cutaneous) branches of spinal or cranial nerves. The area of skin supplied by each cranial or spinal nerve is known as a dermatome (see Figs 1.35 & 1.36).

Subcutaneous tissue (superficial fascia)

Immediately deep to the skin is a layer of loose connective tissue, the subcutaneous tissue (Fig. 1.9), which contains networks of superficial veins and lymphatics and is traversed by cutaneous nerves and arteries. It also contains fat, which varies considerably in thickness from region to region and between individuals. For example, over the buttock the fat is particularly thick whilst on the back of the hand it is relatively thin.

Deep fascia

The deep fascia (Fig. 1.9) consists of a layer of dense connective tissue immediately beneath the subcutaneous tissue. Although thin over the thorax and abdomen, it forms a substantial layer in the limbs (for example, fascia lata; see page 231) and neck (for example, investing fascia; see page 286). Near the wrist and ankle joints the deep fascia is thickened to form retinacula, which maintain the tendons in position as they cross the joints. Deep fascia also provides attachment for muscles and gives anchorage to intermuscular septa, which separate the muscles into compartments.

Fig. 1.9 Multilevel 'step' dissection through the right midcalf to show layers of skin, fascia and intermuscular septa.

external
oblique

apo-
neurosis

external
oblique
(cut)

costal
cartilages

Fig. 1.10   External oblique is a flat muscle with an extensive aponeurosis.

Fig. 1.11   External oblique cut to show its thickness.

Fig. 1.12 Subscapularis is a multipennate muscle.

Fig. 1.13 Flexor pollicis longus is a unipennate muscle.

Muscle

Muscle is a tissue in which active contraction either shortens its component cells or generates tension along their length. There are three basic types: smooth muscle; cardiac striated muscle; voluntary striated muscle. 'Striated' and 'smooth' describe the microscopic appearance of the muscle.

Smooth muscle is present in the organs of the alimentary, genitourinary and respiratory systems and in the walls of blood vessels. Capable of slow sustained contraction, smooth muscle is usually controlled by the autonomic nervous system (see page 22), and, in some organs, by endocrine secretions (hormones).

Cardiac striated muscle (myocardium) is confined to the wall of the heart and is able to contract spontaneously and rhythmically. Its cyclical activity is coordinated by the specialized conducting tissue of the heart and can be modified by the autonomic nervous system.

Voluntary striated muscle (often called skeletal muscle) is the basic component of those muscles that produce movements at joints. These actions are controlled by the somatic nervous system (see page 21) and may be voluntary or reflex. Each muscle cell (fibre) has its own motor nerve ending, which initiates contraction of the fibre. Muscles may be attached to the periosteum of bones either directly or by fibrous connective tissue in the form of deep fascia, intermuscular septa or tendons. Direct fleshy attachment can be extensive but tendons are usually attached to small areas of bone. Muscles with similar actions tend to be grouped together, and in limbs these groups occur in compartments (for instance, extensor compartment of forearm).

Usually each end of a muscle has an attachment to bone. The attachment that remains relatively fixed when the muscle performs its prime action is known as the origin whereas the insertion is the more mobile attachment. However, in some movements the origin moves more than the insertion; therefore these terms are of only limited significance.

The muscle fibres within voluntary muscle are arranged in differing patterns which reflect the function of the muscle (Figs 1.10–1.15). Sometimes they are found as thin flat sheets (as in external oblique). Strap muscles (such as sartorius) have long fibres that reach without interruption from one end of the muscle to the other. Pennate muscles are characterized by fibres that run obliquely. Unipennate muscles (for example flexor pollicis longus) have fibres running from their origin to attach along only one side of the tendon of insertion. In bipennate muscles (such as dorsal interossei) the fibres are anchored to both sides of the tendon of insertion.

Multipennate muscles (for example subscapularis) have several tendons of origin and insertion with muscle fibres passing obliquely between them. Some muscles, for instance digastric, have two fleshy parts (bellies) connected by an intermediate tendon.

Most tendons are thick and round or flattened in cross-section, although some form thin sheets called aponeuroses (see Fig. 1.10). When tendons cross projections or traverse confined spaces they are often enveloped in a double layer of synovial membrane to minimize friction. Where they cross joints, tendons are often held in place by bands of thick fibrous tissue, which prevent 'bowstringing' when the joints are moved. Examples include the retinacula at the wrist and ankle joints, and tendon sheaths in the fingers and toes (Figs 1.16 & 1.17).

The nerve supply to a skeletal muscle contains both motor and sensory fibres, which usually enter the fleshy part of the muscle. Groups of muscles with similar actions tend to be supplied by nerve fibres derived from the same spinal cord segments.

As very metabolically active tissue, muscle has a rich arterial blood supply, usually carried by several separate vessels. The contraction and relaxation of muscles in the limbs compresses the veins in each compartment. As the veins contain unidirectional valves, this 'muscle pump' action assists the return of venous blood from the limbs to the trunk.

Cartilage

Cartilage is a variety of hard connective tissue which gains its nutrition by diffusion from blood vessels in the surrounding tissues. It is classified by its histological structure into hyaline cartilage, fibrocartilage and elastic cartilage.

sartorius

Fig. 1.14 Sartorius is a strap muscle.

dorsal interossei

Fig. 1.15 Dorsal interossei are bipennate muscles.

Hyaline cartilage occurs in costal cartilages (see Fig. 1.11), the cartilages of the larynx and trachea, and in developing bones. In synovial joints (see Fig. 1.23) it forms the glassy smooth articular surfaces which reduce friction during movement. Articular cartilage is partly nourished by diffusion from the synovial fluid in the joint cavity.

The inclusion of tough inelastic collagen fibres in the matrix constitutes fibrocartilage, which is stronger and more flexible than the hyaline type. Fibrocartilage is found in intervertebral discs (see Fig. 1.22), the pubic symphysis, the manubriosternal joint, and as articular discs in some synovial joints (for example, knee and temporomandibular).

Elastic cartilage, which occurs in the external ear and epiglottis, is the most flexible form of cartilage. It contains predominantly elastic fibres and has a yellowish appearance.

Cartilage may become calcified in old age, becoming harder and more rigid.

Fig. 1.16 Anterior view of the left hand, dissected to reveal its fibrous sheaths and tendons.

tendons

fibrous sheaths

tendons

extensor retinaculum

Fig. 1.17 Posterior view of the left hand, dissected to show the extensor retinaculum at the wrist.

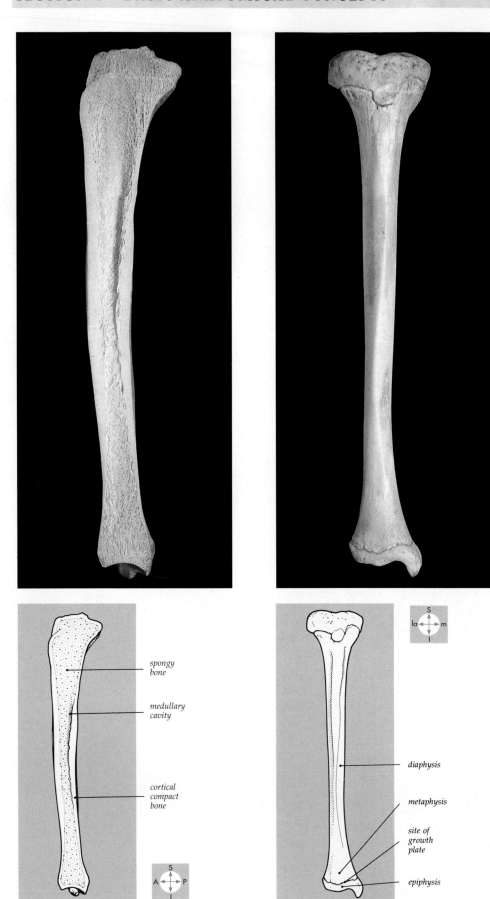

spongy
bone

medullary
cavity

cortical
compact
bone

diaphysis

metaphysis

site of
growth
plate

epiphysis

Fig. 1.18 Longitudinal section of an adult tibia.

Fig. 1.19 Anterior view of a child's tibia.

Bone

Bone forms the basis of the skeleton and is characterized by a hard calcified matrix which gives rigidity. In most bones two zones are visible. Near the surface the outer cortical layer of bone appears solid and is called compact bone whereas centrally the bone appears spongy and is known as spongy (cancellous) bone. Many bones contain a cavity (medulla) occupied by the bone marrow, a potential site of blood cell production (Fig. 1.18).

The numerous bones comprising the human skeleton vary considerably in shape and size and are classified into long bones (for example, femur), short bones (bones of the carpus), flat bones (parietal bone of skull), irregular bones (maxilla of skull) and sesamoid bones (patella). Sesamoid bones develop in tendons, generally where the tendon passes over a joint or bony projection. Some bones are described as pneumatized because of their air-filled cavities (for instance, ethmoid).

Bone is enveloped by a thin layer of fibrous tissue called periosteum (see Fig. 1.9) which provides anchorage for muscles, tendons and ligaments. Periosteum is a source of cells for bone growth and repair and is richly innervated and exquisitely sensitive to pain.

Bone has a profuse blood supply which is provided partly via the periosteal vessels and partly by nutrient arteries, which enter bones via nutrient foramina and also supply the marrow. Fractured bones often bleed profusely from damaged medullary and periosteal vessels.

Several names are given to the different parts of a long bone in relation to its development (Fig. 1.19). The shaft (or diaphysis) ossifies first and is separated by growth plates from the secondary centres of ossification (or epiphyses) which usually lie at the extremities of the bone. The part of a diaphysis next to a growth plate is called a metaphysis and has a particularly rich blood supply. When increase in bone length ceases, the growth plates disappear and the epiphyses fuse with the diaphysis.

Skeleton

The skeleton (Fig. 1.20) is composed of bones and cartilages held together by joints, and gives rigidity and support to the body. It has axial and appendicular components. The axial component includes the skull, vertebral column, ribs, costal cartilages and sternum. The appendicular skeleton comprises the bones of the upper and lower limbs and their associated girdles. In this book individual bones are described in the appropriate regions.

Fig. 1.20 Anterior and posterior views of the skeleton.

Joints

Joints are classified according to their structure into fibrous, cartilaginous and synovial types. In fibrous joints (Fig. 1.21) which are relatively immobile, the two bones are joined by fibrous tissue (for example, sutures seen between the bones of the skull).

Cartilage is interposed between bone ends in cartilaginous joints. Primary cartilaginous joints contain hyaline cartilage, are usually capable of only limited movement, and are described between the ribs and sternum. In secondary cartilaginous joints (Fig. 1.22), fibrocartilage unites the bone ends. These joints, which generally allow more movement than those of the primary type, all lie in the midline. Examples include the intervertebral discs, the manubriosternal joint and the pubic symphysis.

Fig. 1.21 The inferior tibiofibular joint is an example of a fibrous joint.

Fig. 1.22 Sagittal section to show an intervertebral disc, a secondary cartilaginous joint.

Synovial joints

The most common type of joint is the synovial joint, which is complex and usually highly mobile. They are classified according to the shape of the joint surfaces (such as plane, saddle, ball-and-socket) or by the type of movement they permit (such as sliding, pivot, hinge). In a typical synovial joint (Fig. 1.23) the articulating surfaces are coated with hyaline cartilage and the bones are joined by a fibrous capsule, a tubular sleeve which is attached around the periphery of the areas of articular cartilage. In every synovial joint all of the interior (except for intra-articular cartilage) is lined with synovial membrane. This thin vascular membrane secretes synovial fluid into the joint space, providing nutrition for the cartilage and lubrication for the joint.

The capsule is usually thickened to form strengthening bands known as capsular ligaments (for example, the pubofemoral ligament). In addition, fibrous bands, discrete from the capsule, may form extracapsular ligaments (such as the costoclavicular ligament). In some joints there are intracapsular ligaments (for instance, the ligament of the head of the femur) which are covered by synovial membrane. Tendons sometimes fuse with the capsule (as in the rotator cuff) or they may run within the joint, covered by synovial membrane, before gaining their bony attachment (for example, biceps brachii at the shoulder joint; Fig. 1.24).

articular cartilage

synovial cavity

collateral ligaments

Fig. 1.23 Coronal section through a metacarpophalangeal joint, a synovial joint. The collateral ligaments are thickenings of the joint capsule.

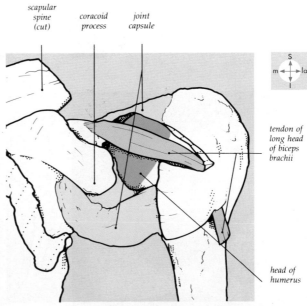

scapular spine (cut)

coracoid process

joint capsule

tendon of long head of biceps brachii

head of humerus

Fig. 1.24 Removal of part of the shoulder joint capsule reveals the intracapsular but extrasynovial tendon of the long head of biceps brachii.

Fluid containing sacs of synovial membrane called bursae (Fig. 1.25) separate some tendons and muscles from other structures. Bursae which lie close to joints may communicate with the cavity of the joint through a small opening in the capsule (as does the subscapularis bursa).

In some joints (for example, the knee) a disc of cartilage is interposed between the articular cartilage covering the bone ends (Fig. 1.26). This provides a matched shape for each bone end, thus allowing freer movement without compromising stability. In addition, different types of movement are permitted in each half of the joint.

Stability varies considerably from one synovial joint to another, as several factors limit excessive movement and contribute to the stability of the joint. These include the shape of the articulating surfaces, the strength of the capsule and associated ligaments, the tone of the surrounding muscles and, where present, intra-articular discs and ligaments. At the hip joint the ligaments and the shape of the bones provide the main stability whereas the tone of the surrounding muscles stabilizes the shoulder joint.

Fig. 1.25 Sagittal section through the elbow joint. The olecranon bursa does not communicate with the joint cavity.

Fig. 1.26 Disarticulated knee joint to show the menisci.

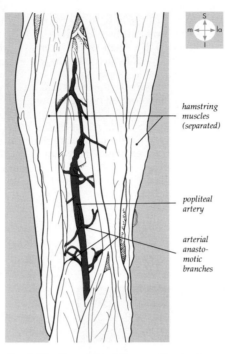

hamstring
muscles
(separated)

popliteal
artery

arterial
anasto-
motic
branches

Fig. 1.27 Branches of the popliteal artery anastomose around the knee joint.

Joints, particularly their capsules, receive a rich sensory innervation derived from the nerves supplying the muscles that act on the joint. For instance, the axillary nerve supplies the shoulder joint and deltoid.

Blood vessels around joints frequently take part in rich anastomoses, which allow alternative pathways for blood flow when the joint has moved to a different position and ensure an adequate supply to the synovial membrane (such as in the knee joint; Fig. 1.27).

Serous membranes and cavities

Pericardium, pleura and peritoneum comprise the serous membranes lining the cavities that separate the heart, lungs and abdominal viscera, respectively, from their surrounding structures. Where the membrane lines the outer wall of the cavity it is called parietal, and where it covers the appropriate organ it is called visceral. The parietal and visceral parts are in continuity around the root of the viscus and are separated from each other by a cavity, which normally contains only a thin film of serous fluid. The membranes are in close contact but are lubricated by the intervening fluid, which permits movement between the viscus and its surroundings (Fig. 1.28).

visceral
pleura

pleural
cavity

right lung

parietal
pleura

Fig. 1.28 Transverse section through the thorax at the level of T5 showing the right pleural cavity. Superior aspect.

Blood vessels

Blood vessels convey blood around the body and are classified into three main types, namely arteries, capillaries and veins.

Arteries are relatively thick-walled vessels which convey blood in a branching system of decreasing calibre away from the heart (Fig. 1.31). Some arteries are named after the region through which they pass (such as the femoral artery), while others are named according to the structures they supply (for instance, the renal artery). The largest vessels, such as the aorta, have elastic walls and therefore are called elastic arteries. They give rise to arteries whose walls are more muscular (muscular arteries), such as the radial artery in the forearm. A particularly thick smooth muscle coat is also a feature of the walls of the microscopic arterioles. The tone of arteriolar smooth muscle is under the control of the autonomic nervous system and hormones, and is an important factor in the maintenance of pressure in the arterial system. In general, there are few alternative pathways for arterial blood to reach its destination. However, in some regions (for example, joints and at the base of the brain), arterial supply is provided by more than one vessel (see Fig. 1.27). Such arteries may communicate directly with each other at sites known as arterial anastomoses.

Capillaries link the smallest arteries and the smallest veins and convey blood at low pressure through the tissues. Collectively these thin-walled microscopic vessels have a very extensive surface area, facilitating gaseous and metabolic exchange between the blood and tissues.

Veins carry blood at low pressure from the capillary bed back to the heart (see Fig. 1.32). They may be deep (accompanying arteries) or superficial (lying in the superficial fascia) (Fig. 1.29) and are usually linked by venous anastomoses. Veins accompanying arteries are often arranged as several interconnecting vessels called venae comitantes. In the limbs the deep veins can be compressed by local muscular action, thus assisting venous return. Many veins (excluding the venae cavae, those draining viscera and those within the cranium) contain unidirectional valves which direct the flow of blood towards the heart (Fig. 1.30). The venous pattern is often variable, and numerous anastomotic connections provide alternative pathways for venous return. In some regions numerous intercommunicating veins form meshworks called plexuses (such as the pelvic venous plexus). In the cranial cavity, venous blood is carried in special vessels formed by the dura mater lining the interior of the skull. These dural sinuses receive blood from the brain.

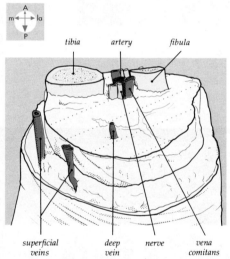

Fig. 1.29   Multilevel 'step' dissection through the right midcalf showing the vascular supply.

Fig. 1.30   Portion of saphenous vein seen opened longitudinally and in cross-section.

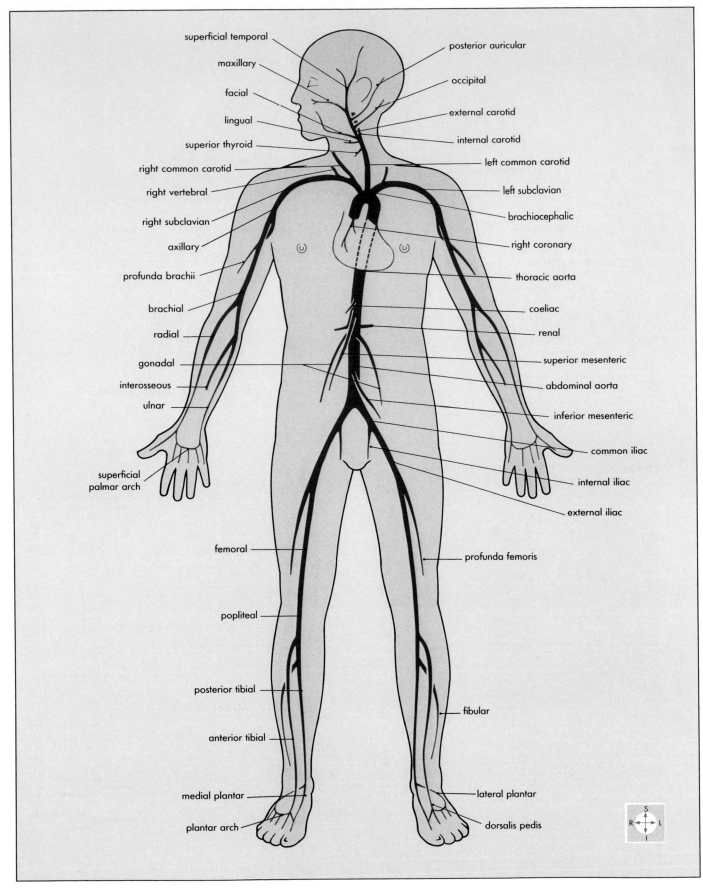

Fig. 1.31 Principal systemic arteries.

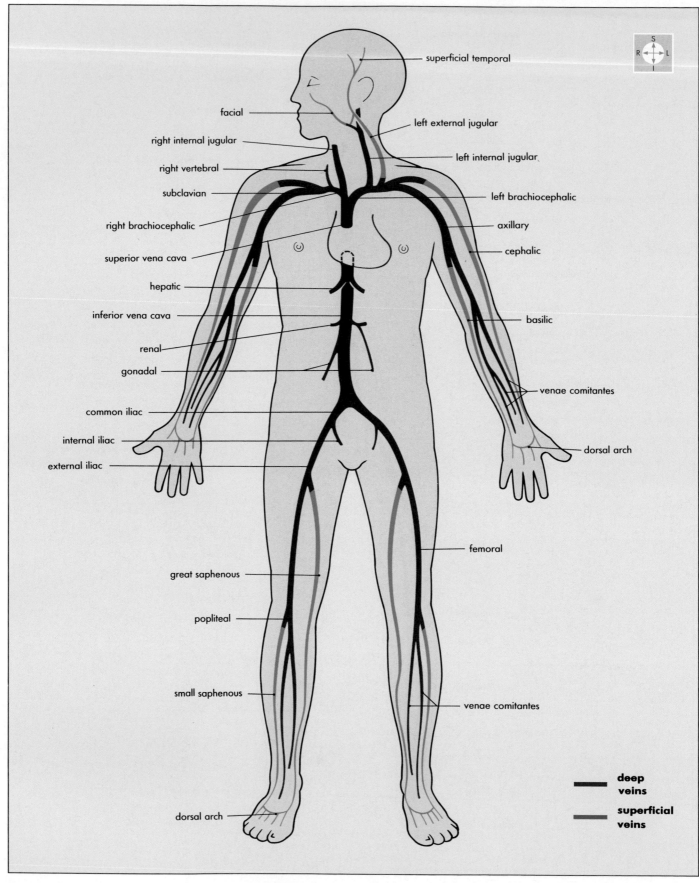

Fig. 1.32 Principal systemic veins.

Lymphatic vessels and nodes

Tissue fluid is collected by microscopic open-ended channels called lymphatics. From a particular region or organ these valved lymphatic vessels drain into aggregations of lymphoid tissue (called lymph nodes), which filter lymph. Groups of lymph nodes are often found close to an organ (for example, hilar nodes) or at the root of a limb (for example, axillary lymph nodes). Ultimately lymph drains into the venous system in the root of the neck through larger lymph channels called the thoracic duct and the right lymphatic trunk (Fig. 1.33).

Because they filter the fluid passing through them, lymph nodes may become involved in the spread of infection or malignancy (for example, cancer). Thus, the surgeon removing a cancerous organ may also excise the lymph nodes draining that organ.

Fig. 1.33   The main lymphatic nodes and vessels of the body.

The regular pattern of innervation in the trunk is modified in the limbs, each being supplied by several spinal nerves through a complex network, a plexus (such as the brachial plexus of the upper limb; Fig. 1.37). Plexus formation modifies the pattern of myotomes so that spinal cord segments innervate muscles according to their prime actions. For example, flexors of the elbow joint are supplied by the spinal cord segments C5 and C6. Sensory cell bodies are located in ganglia on peripheral nerves near the central nervous system (for instance, trigeminal ganglion, posterior root ganglia). However, the cell bodies of somatic motor nerves are located in the central nervous system.

Autonomic nerves

The autonomic nervous system innervates smooth and cardiac muscle, and glands. It is divided into two parts, sympathetic and parasympathetic, whose effects for the most part are antagonistic (for example, sympathetic stimulation increases while parasympathetic stimulation reduces heart rate). In both sympathetic and parasympathetic components, preganglionic myelinated axons leave the central nervous system and synapse on neurones in peripheral ganglia distributed throughout the body. The postganglionic

axons that pass to the effector organs are non-myelinated. Autonomic sensory fibres accompany autonomic efferent fibres in peripheral nerves but their cell bodies are located in the posterior root ganglia in company with somatic sensory neurones.

The parts of the central nervous system from which the autonomic nerves emerge differ for the sympathetic and parasympathetic components (Fig. 1.38).

Sympathetic nerves

Preganglionic sympathetic fibres leave the central nervous system in the spinal nerves of all the thoracic and the upper two lumbar segments (thoracolumbar outflow) and enter the ganglionated sympathetic trunks via white rami communicantes. The two sympathetic trunks lie on either side of the vertebral column and extend throughout most of its length. Each trunk consists of sympathetic ganglia and interconnecting nerve trunks.

Unmyelinated postganglionic axons destined for the blood vessels and sweat glands of the body wall, including the limbs, leave the ganglia by grey rami communicantes and are distributed by the spinal nerves. Special visceral branches pass directly from the trunks to reach the appropriate organ.

Postganglionic sympathetic nerve fibres are often conveyed to their destinations as

plexuses intimately related to the walls of arteries.

Parasympathetic nerves

In the parasympathetic system, myelinated preganglionic fibres leave the central nervous system as part of cranial nerves III, VII, IX and X and as part of sacral spinal nerves S2, S3 and S4 to form the craniosacral autonomic outflow. These preganglionic fibres synapse in ganglia lying close to or in the wall of the target organ. Relatively short non-myelinated postganglionic axons emerge from these ganglia to innervate the appropriate tissue. In the head there are four paired ganglia (ciliary, pterygopalatine, submandibular and otic) that receive preganglionic parasympathetic fibres from cranial nerves III, VII and IX. The postganglionic fibres from these ganglia supply the eye, and lacrimal, nasal and salivary glands. Preganglionic fibres from the vagus (X) nerve synapse with postganglionic neurones that innervate cervical, thoracic and abdominal viscera. Preganglionic fibres from the sacral nerves (pelvic splanchnic nerves or nervi erigentes) supply the pelvic organs. The parasympathetic ganglia associated with the vagus and sacral nerves usually comprise small clusters of cells in the walls of the innervated organs (Fig. 1.38).

brachial
plexus

Fig. 1.37   The axilla has been dissected to show the brachial plexus.

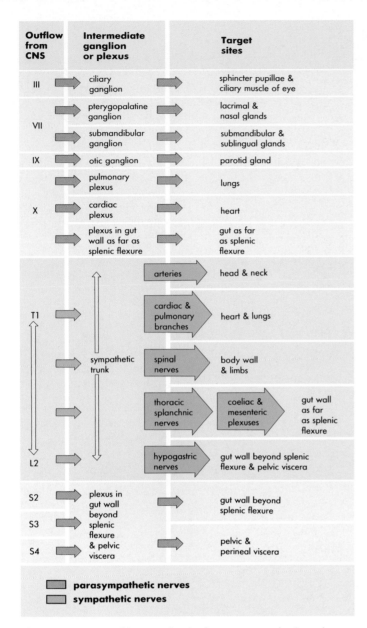

Outflow from CNS	Intermediate ganglion or plexus	Target sites
III	ciliary ganglion	sphincter pupillae & ciliary muscle of eye
VII	pterygopalatine ganglion	lacrimal & nasal glands
	submandibular ganglion	submandibular & sublingual glands
IX	otic ganglion	parotid gland
X	pulmonary plexus	lungs
	cardiac plexus	heart
	plexus in gut wall as far as splenic flexure	gut as far as splenic flexure
T1	arteries	head & neck
	cardiac & pulmonary branches	heart & lungs
	sympathetic trunk · spinal nerves	body wall & limbs
	thoracic splanchnic nerves · coeliac & mesenteric plexuses	gut wall as far as splenic flexure
L2	hypogastric nerves	gut wall beyond splenic flexure & pelvic viscera
S2	plexus in gut wall beyond splenic flexure & pelvic viscera	gut wall beyond splenic flexure
S3		
S4		pelvic & perineal viscera

parasympathetic nerves
sympathetic nerves

Fig. 1.38 Pattern of innervation in the parasympathetic and sympathetic autonomic nervous systems.

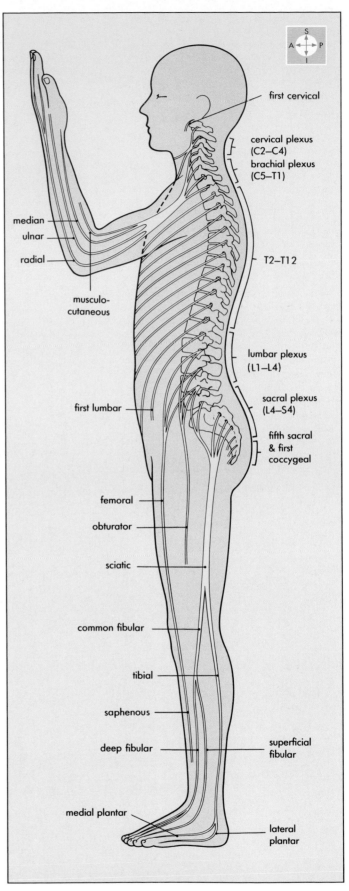

first cervical

cervical plexus (C2–C4)

brachial plexus (C5–T1)

median

ulnar

radial

musculo-cutaneous

T2–T12

lumbar plexus (L1–L4)

sacral plexus (L4–S4)

fifth sacral & first coccygeal

first lumbar

femoral

obturator

sciatic

common fibular

tibial

saphenous

deep fibular

superficial fibular

medial plantar

lateral plantar

Fig. 1.39 Lateral view of the distribution of the anterior rami of the spinal nerves.

2 THORAX

INTRODUCTION

The thorax is the region of the trunk that includes the sternum, costal cartilages, ribs and thoracic vertebrae, together with the structures they enclose. Superiorly the thorax is limited by the upper surfaces of the first ribs and their costal cartilages, the manubrium of the sternum and the first thoracic vertebra. The space bounded by these structures is the superior thoracic aperture (thoracic inlet) (Fig. 2.1), which allows structures to pass between the root of the neck and the thorax. Inferiorly, the cavity of the thorax is separated from the abdominal contents by a fibromuscular sheet called the diaphragm. The oesophagus and other intrathoracic structures pass through the diaphragm to gain or leave the abdomen. Since the diaphragm is convex superiorly, some of the organs within the abdomen are covered by the lower ribs and costal cartilages.

The ribs, costal cartilages and sternum form a semi-rigid framework that provides attachment for several muscles; some connect adjacent ribs and costal cartilages, others attach to the pectoral girdle or humerus or descend from the thorax to contribute to the musculature of the abdominal wall. The medial ends of the clavicles articulate with the upper border of the manubrium and flank the suprasternal notch. The manubrium articulates with the body of the sternum at the manubriosternal joint, which usually forms a horizontal ridge. This is a useful landmark during clinical examination because the second costal cartilages meet the sternum at this level. It is normal practice to count ribs starting at the second costal cartilages as the first ribs are obscured by the clavicles. Inferiorly the thoracic wall is limited by the costal margin, which is formed by the costal

Fig. 2.1   The boundaries of the superior thoracic aperture.

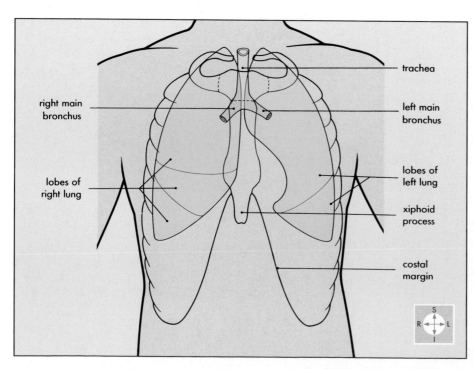

Fig. 2.2   The trachea, bronchi and lungs.

cartilages of the lower ribs. The costal margin extends upwards and medially as far as the lower end of the sternum and forms the upper boundary of the abdominal wall. The inferior portion of the sternum, the xiphoid process, can usually be identified in the midline between the costal margins. The space between adjacent ribs and costal cartilages is occupied by intercostal muscles, which are active during respiratory movements of the thoracic wall. Intercostal vessels and nerves run between these muscles in each space and give branches to adjacent tissues and the overlying skin. In both sexes, the nipples are surface features, the anatomical locations of which vary depending upon the build of the individual. The glandular components of the breast lie deep to the nipple, embedded in the fat of the subcutaneous tissues that cover the muscles of the chest wall. Posteriorly the upper ribs are covered by the scapulae and their muscles.

The space contained within the thoracic wall is occupied by several important organs. Some of these are confined to the thorax (e.g. heart) whilst others traverse the region passing from the neck into the abdomen (e.g. oesophagus). On each side the lung occupies a large proportion of the thoracic cavity (Fig. 2.2) and is surrounded by a serous sac called the pleura. Each membrane forms a closed cavity that usually contains a thin film of serous fluid enabling the lungs and thoracic wall to move freely over one another. Each pleural cavity is separated from its neighbour by a midline partition called the mediastinum. The mediastinum is the term used to describe all the structures that occupy this central portion, including the heart and its great vessels (Figs 2.3 & 2.4) and the intrathoracic parts of the trachea and oesophagus.

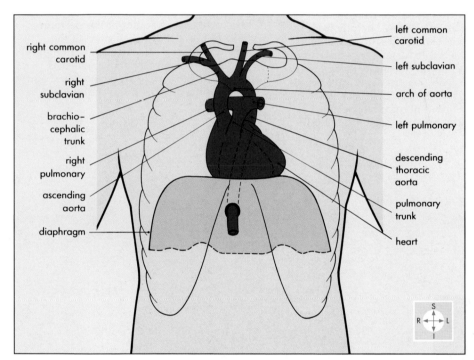

Fig. 2.3 The heart and great arteries.

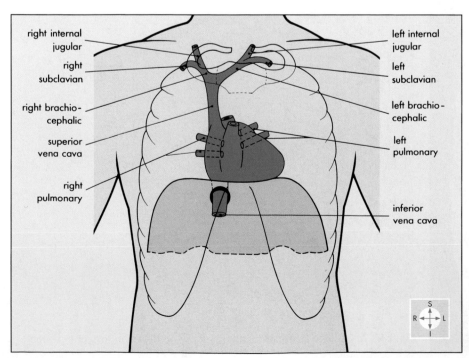

Fig. 2.4 The heart and great veins.

SKELETON OF THORAX

The skeleton of the thorax consists of twelve thoracic vertebrae, the twelve pairs of ribs and their costal cartilages, and the sternum (Fig. 2.5). Structures in continuity between the root of the neck and the upper part of the thoracic cavity pass through the superior thoracic aperture (thoracic inlet), which is bounded by the first thoracic vertebral body, the first pair of ribs and costal cartilages and the upper border of the sternum. The inferior thoracic aperture (thoracic outlet) through which structures pass between the thoracic and abdominal cavities is formed by the twelfth thoracic vertebral body, the twelfth and eleventh ribs and the costal margin (the fused costal cartilages of the seventh to the tenth ribs inclusive).

Ribs

Although the ribs differ in size and shape most (3–9 inclusive) have features in common and are described as 'typical ribs' (Fig. 2.6). Each typical rib consists of a head, neck, tubercle, shaft, upper and lower borders and inner and outer surfaces. The heads of the ribs are those parts which articulate with the thoracic vertebral bodies. The lower part of the head forms a synovial joint with its own vertebral body whilst the upper part articulates with the vertebra above. The intermediate part of the head lies against the intervertebral disc. The neck of the rib connects the head and the tubercle and lies in front of the transverse process. The tubercle of the rib faces posteriorly and the medial part of its surface forms a synovial joint with the articular facet on the transverse process of the corresponding vertebra. The shaft forms the remainder of the rib and ends anteriorly at a shallow depression, which receives the costal cartilage. Passing laterally from the tubercle, the shaft slopes downwards and backwards before turning forwards and outwards to form the angle. Lateral to the angle the shaft possesses a sharp lower border, which bounds the costal groove.

The first rib is atypical. Its head possesses an articular facet solely for its own vertebral body. The shaft is short and broad and has superior and inferior surfaces. In addition, its superior surface carries a ridge that forms a projection on the inner border of the rib, the scalene tubercle, to which is attached scalenus anterior. Two grooves lie across the shaft, one in front of the ridge (for the subclavian vein) and the other behind (for the subclavian artery and lowest trunk of the brachial plexus). The tenth, eleventh and twelfth ribs are also atypical, in that each head possesses a single facet and the rib is usually devoid of a tubercle and an angle.

Costal cartilages

All ribs possess costal cartilages and those of the upper seven pairs (true ribs) articulate with the sides of the sternum. Pairs 8–12 (false ribs) fall short of the sternum. Pairs 8–10 articulate with the cartilage immediately above whilst 11 and 12 (floating ribs) are pointed and end freely in the muscle of the abdominal wall.

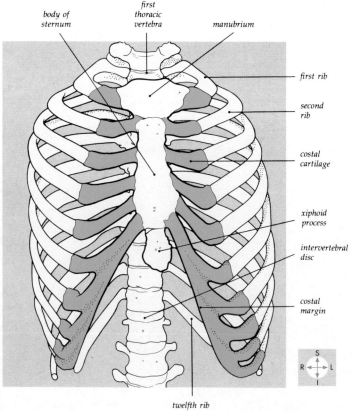

Fig. 2.5 Articulated bones of the thorax showing the relationships between the vertebral column, ribs, costal cartilages and sternum.

Sternum

The sternum is a flat bone and consists of the manubrium, the body (Fig. 2.7) and the xiphoid process. The manubrium articulates with the medial end of each clavicle at the sternoclavicular joint and with the first costal cartilage. Its upper margin is broad and forms part of the superior thoracic aperture. A palpable secondary cartilaginous joint (the manubriosternal joint) unites the manubrium and body and forms a useful guide to the second costal cartilage, which abuts the sternum at the lateral margin of the joint. The lateral margins of the body of the sternum are indented by the medial ends of the second to the seventh costal cartilages. The xiphoid process lies in the subcostal angle and projects downwards and backwards from the body of the sternum.

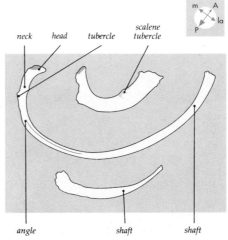

Fig. 2.6 The first, seventh and twelfth ribs showing their surface features and relative sizes.

Fig. 2.7 The manubrium and the body of the sternum. The xiphoid process is absent.

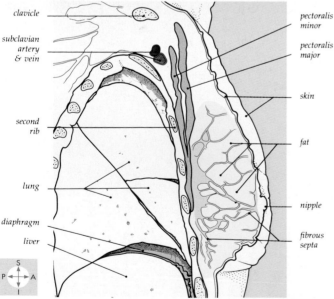

Fig. 2.8 Sagittal section through the right breast and underlying chest wall. In this dissection, the glandular structure of the breast cannot be distinguished.

THORACIC WALL

Breast

The breast (Fig. 2.8) consists of glandular tissue and a quantity of fat embedded in the subcutaneous tissue of the anterior chest wall. In the male and immature female the gland is rudimentary. Although the size and shape of the breast in the adult female are variable, the base (the part lying on the deep fascia covering pectoralis major, serratus anterior and rectus abdominis) is constant in position. In the adult female the base is roughly circular and extends between the second and sixth ribs. Medially the gland overlies the lateral border of the sternum. Part of the breast extends upwards and laterally and reaches the anterior fold of the axilla. This is the axillary tail (process) and is the only part of the breast to penetrate beneath the deep fascia.

The glandular elements consist of 15–20 lobes arranged radially, each draining into a lactiferous duct. These ducts open independently onto the surface of the nipple. The nipple is surrounded by an area of pink skin, the areola, which may develop brown pigmentation during pregnancy.

The gland is traversed by fibrous septa (Fig. 2.8), which subdivide the lobes and loosely attach the skin of the breast to the deep fascia covering the chest wall. Normally the breast is freely mobile over the underlying muscles.

Blood supply

The fat and glandular elements of the breast receive blood from arteries that also supply the deeper structures of the chest wall. These vessels include perforating branches from the internal thoracic artery and the second, third and fourth intercostal arteries. The lateral thoracic and thoracoacromial arteries arising from the axillary artery also supply the breast. The gland is drained by veins which accompany the arteries.

Lymph drainage

Within the substance of the breast the lymphatic vessels form a system of interconnecting channels that collect lymph from all parts of the organ. The superior and lateral aspects of the breast usually drain into central and apical axillary nodes via infraclavicular and pectoral nodes. The medial and inferior parts of the breast drain deeply into glands along the internal thoracic vessels and thence via the bronchomediastinal lymph trunk into the confluence of lymphatic vessels in the root of the neck (see page 292). Lymphatics may also cross the midline to communicate with vessels in the opposite breast.

Muscles

The outer surfaces of the ribs, costal cartilages and sternum give attachment to muscles involved in movements of the upper limb and the scapula, namely pectoralis major, pectoralis minor and serratus anterior. In addition, the external surfaces of the lower ribs provide attachment for rectus abdominis and the external oblique muscles of the anterior abdominal wall (see pages 128 & 130).

Pectoralis major

This large fan-shaped muscle (Fig. 2.9) attaches to the clavicle, sternum and upper costal cartilages and forms the bulk of the anterior wall of the axilla. The clavicular head is attached to the anterior surface of the medial half of the clavicle. The sternocostal head is anchored to the manubrium and body of the sternum, and to the upper six costal cartilages (see page 112). Laterally both parts of the muscle attach to the humerus along the lateral lip of the intertubercular sulcus (see page 112).

Pectoralis major is supplied by the medial and lateral pectoral nerves from the brachial plexus. Functionally it is a powerful adductor and flexor of the arm at the shoulder joint and also produces medial rotation of the humerus. When the upper limb is fixed the sternocostal part may act as an accessory muscle of inspiration by elevating the ribs.

Pectoralis minor

This small muscle (Fig. 2.10) lies deep to pectoralis major and is usually attached to the third, fourth and fifth ribs. The muscle converges on the medial border of the coracoid process of the scapula. Pectoralis minor is supplied by the medial and lateral pectoral nerves and assists in movements of protraction and rotation of the scapula.

Fig. 2.9 Pectoralis major, revealed by removal of the skin, the subcutaneous tissue and deep fascia.

Fig. 2.10 Pectoralis minor, exposed by removal of pectoralis major.

Serratus anterior

This large muscle lies between the scapula and chest wall and attaches to the lateral aspects of the upper eight ribs (Fig. 2.11), forming part of the medial wall of the axilla. The muscle fibres from the upper four ribs attach to the superior angle and to the costal surface of the medial border of the scapula. The fibres from ribs 5–8 converge on the costal surface of the inferior angle of the scapula.

Innervation is provided by the long thoracic nerve arising in the neck from the upper three roots (C5, C6 & C7) of the brachial plexus. The muscle is a powerful protractor of the scapula and assists trapezius in producing scapular rotation during abduction of the upper limb. In addition, the muscle helps to stabilize the scapula during movements of the upper limb.

Intercostal spaces

The interval between two adjacent ribs is called an intercostal space. On each side of the thorax there are 11 such spaces, numbered from above and occupied by muscles, membranes, nerves and vessels. The number given to each intercostal space and its neurovascular structures corresponds to that of the rib which limits the space superiorly. The nerves and vessels immediately inferior to the twelfth ribs are termed the subcostal nerves and vessels. The intercostal nerves and vessels supply the intercostal muscles and the parietal pleura deep to each space. Branches from these vessels also supply the overlying muscles of the body wall, the superficial fascia and skin. Most intercostal nerves have cutaneous branches that supply the skin covering the chest and abdominal walls.

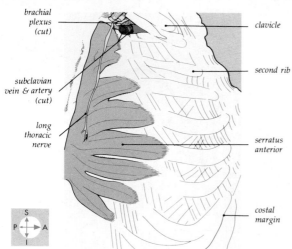

Fig. 2.11   Serratus anterior seen after removal of the pectoral muscles and displacement of the scapula backwards.

Fig. 2.12   External intercostal muscles, exposed by removal of the upper limb and serratus anterior.

Intercostal muscles

There are three layers of intercostal muscles which lie superficial, intermediate and deep. These are named the external, the internal and the innermost intercostal muscles.

External intercostal muscles

The fibres of the external intercostal muscles slope downwards and forwards from the lower border of one rib to the upper border of the subjacent rib (Fig. 2.12). The muscle extends from the tubercle of the rib posteriorly to the junction of the rib and its costal cartilage anteriorly. Between costal cartilages the muscle fibres are replaced by a thin fascial sheet, the external intercostal membrane, which reaches the lateral border of the sternum (Fig. 2.13).

Internal intercostal muscles

The internal intercostal muscles (Fig. 2.14) lie immediately deep to the external intercostal muscles. The fibres of the two muscles are mutually at right angles, those of the internal intercostal muscles running downwards and backwards from the lower border of one rib to the upper border of the subjacent rib. Anteriorly each muscle continues between the costal cartilages to reach the lateral border of the sternum (Fig. 2.13). Posteriorly each muscle extends only to the angles of the ribs, where it is replaced by the internal intercostal membrane, which continues as far as the tubercles of the ribs.

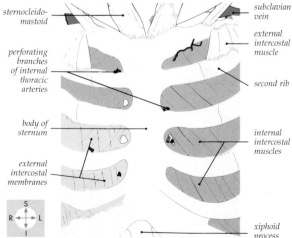

Fig. 2.13 External intercostal membranes and the anterior fibres of the internal intercostal muscles.

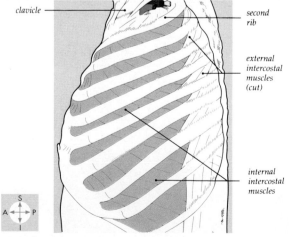

Fig. 2.14 Internal intercostal muscles, exposed by removal of the anterior parts of the external intercostal muscles.

Innermost intercostal muscles

These muscles lie on a plane deep to that of the internal intercostal muscles (Fig. 2.15). They form the lateral part of an incomplete layer of muscle which includes the transversus thoracis (sternocostalis) anteriorly (Fig. 2.16) and subcostalis posteriorly. Each innermost intercostal muscle connects the inner surface of one rib to that of its neighbours.

Nerve supply

All the intercostal muscles in a particular intercostal space are supplied by the corresponding intercostal nerve.

Actions

Although the main role of the intercostal muscles is in ventilation of the lungs, it must be emphasized that during normal quiet breathing the muscles of the thoracic wall make only a small contribution. Inspiration is usually brought about mainly by the diaphragm, whose descent increases the vertical diameter of the thorax. The transverse and anteroposterior diameters of

the thorax are increased, especially in deep inspiration, by the external intercostal muscles, which incline the ribs outwards, upwards and forwards so that the intercostal spaces are widened. During quiet breathing, expiration is largely due to the 'elastic' recoil of the lungs and thoracic wall and involves minimal activity by the intercostal muscles. Even when expiration is 'forced', for example during vigorous physical exertion or when coughing, the main muscular effort is provided by the muscles of the abdominal wall rather than the chest wall. However, the internal intercostal muscles contribute to forced expiration by drawing the ribs downwards and inwards, thereby narrowing the intercostal spaces.

Intercostal vessels and nerves

Each intercostal space has a principal artery, vein and nerve, which collectively form the neurovascular bundle (Fig. 2.15). This bundle lies in the neurovascular plane between the internal and innermost

intercostal muscles and runs along the upper part of the intercostal space occupying the costal groove of the rib. Usually the vein lies superiorly and the nerve inferiorly in the bundle. A collateral nerve and collateral vessels arise posteriorly from the neurovascular bundle and run forwards along the lower border of the intercostal space to supply the intercostal muscles.

Intercostal arteries

Intercostal arteries enter from both anterior and posterior ends of the intercostal space. Anteriorly the internal thoracic arteries (Fig. 2.16) arising from the subclavian arteries in the root of the neck (see page 292) provide branches that run laterally to supply the upper six pairs of intercostal spaces. On each side the lower five spaces receive anterior intercostal arteries from the musculophrenic artery, one of the terminal branches of the internal thoracic artery. These anterior arteries anastomose end-to-end with the posterior intercostal arteries.

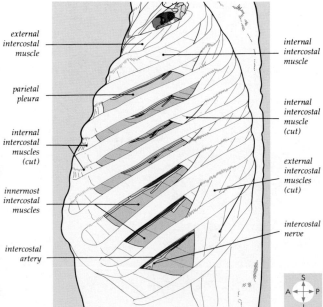

Fig. 2.15 Innermost intercostal muscles and intercostal nerves exposed after removing parts of the internal intercostal muscles. In the third intercostal space the innermost intercostal muscle has been removed to expose the parietal pleura.

Posterior intercostal arteries to the lower nine intercostal spaces arise as direct branches from the descending thoracic aorta (see Fig. 2.63). For the first and second spaces the posterior intercostal arteries are derived from the intercostal branch of the costocervical trunk. This trunk arises from the subclavian artery (see page 293) and its intercostal branch enters the thorax by crossing the neck of the first rib. The anastomoses between anterior and posterior intercostal arteries and between the scapular arteries and posterior intercostals are important because they enable blood to reach the descending aorta when the aortic arch is abnormally narrowed (coarctation of the aorta).

Intercostal veins

Anteriorly the intercostal veins from the lower five intercostal spaces drain into the musculophrenic veins. The upper six intercostal veins and the musculophrenic veins drain into the internal thoracic veins, which themselves are tributaries of the brachiocephalic veins in the root of the neck. Posteriorly the intercostal veins drain into the azygos venous system. On the right, those in the lower eight spaces terminate directly in the azygos vein (see Fig. 2.63). The veins from the second and third spaces combine into a single vessel, the right superior intercostal vein, which drains into the arch of the azygos vein. The first posterior intercostal vein (supreme intercostal vein) leaves the thorax to terminate in the root of the neck, usually in the right vertebral vein.

On the left, the lower eight posterior intercostal veins enter either the hemiazygos or accessory hemiazygos veins (see Fig. 2.64). The left superior intercostal vein drains the second and third spaces and crosses the left side of the arch of the aorta to terminate in the left brachiocephalic vein. As on the right, the first posterior intercostal vein (supreme intercostal vein) leaves the thorax to terminate usually in the vertebral, but occasionally in the brachiocephalic, vein.

Intercostal nerves

The intercostal nerves comprise the anterior rami of the upper eleven thoracic spinal nerves. Each intercostal nerve enters the neurovascular plane posteriorly (see Fig. 2.64) and gives a collateral branch that supplies the intercostal muscles of the space. Except for the first, each intercostal nerve gives off a lateral cutaneous branch near the midaxillary line which pierces the overlying muscle (see Fig. 1.34). This cutaneous nerve divides into anterior and posterior branches, which supply the adjacent skin. The intercostal nerves of the second to the sixth spaces enter the superficial fascia near the lateral border of the sternum and divide into medial and lateral cutaneous branches.

Most of the fibres of the anterior ramus of the first thoracic spinal nerve join the brachial plexus for distribution to the upper limb (see page 78). The small first intercostal nerve is the collateral branch and supplies only the muscles of the intercostal space, not the overlying skin.

The intercostal nerves of the lower five spaces continue in the neurovascular plane beyond the costal margin to supply the muscles and skin of the abdominal wall (see page 131).

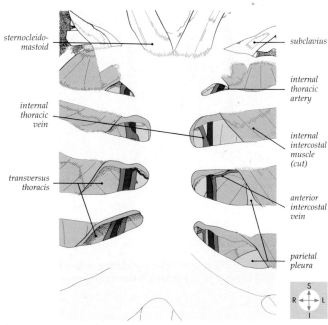

Fig. 2.16 Internal thoracic vessels, revealed by removal of the anterior parts of the intercostal muscles.

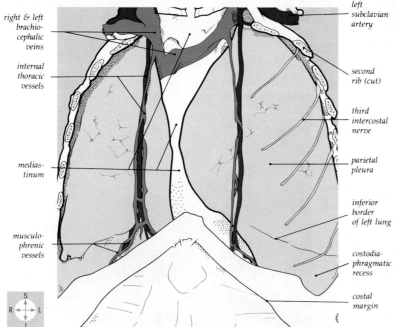

Fig. 2.17 Removal of the anterior chest wall has exposed the internal thoracic vessels and costal part of the parietal pleura, through which the lungs are visible.

PLEURA

The thoracic cavity lies within the walls of the thorax and is separated from the abdominal cavity by the diaphragm. The cavity contains the right and left lungs, each surrounded by a serous membrane called the pleura. Between the lungs is a central partition, the mediastinum, which includes the heart and great vessels, the trachea and the oesophagus. Superiorly, numerous mediastinal structures enter or leave the root of the neck through the superior thoracic aperture (see pages 292–293). Inferiorly, important structures including the aorta, inferior vena cava and oesophagus pass between the mediastinum and the abdomen through openings in the diaphragm (see page 183).

The pleura surrounds the lungs and lines the walls of the thoracic cavity and is subdivided into visceral and parietal parts. The visceral layer covers the surface of the lung and is continuous with the parietal layer around the mediastinal attachment of the lung at the lung root. The parietal layer covers the lateral aspect of the mediastinum, the upper surface of the diaphragm and the inner aspect of the chest wall (Fig. 2.17). Although the parietal and visceral layers are normally in contact, a space, the pleural cavity (Fig. 2.18), exists between them and contains a thin film of serous fluid. The fluid ensures close apposition of the two pleural surfaces and reduces friction during respiratory movements. Injury or disease may produce an accumulation of air (pneumothorax) or fluid (pleural effusion) within the pleural cavity, causing the lung to collapse.

Parietal pleura

The parietal pleura is named according to the surfaces it covers. Thus, the mediastinal pleura conforms to the contours of the structures forming the lateral surface of the mediastinum and is innervated by sensory branches of the phrenic nerve. Inferiorly the diaphragmatic pleura clothes the upper surface of the diaphragm. The central portion receives sensory branches from each phrenic nerve whilst the periphery is innervated by lower intercostal nerves. The pleura covering the inner surface of the thoracic wall is called the costal pleura and is innervated segmentally by the intercostal nerves (Fig. 2.17).

The periphery of the diaphragm slopes steeply downwards towards its attachment to the thoracic wall, creating a narrow gutter, the costodiaphragmatic recess. Within this recess, which is particularly deep laterally and posteriorly, the costal and diaphragmatic parts of the parietal pleura lie in mutual contact (see Fig. 4.104).

The parietal pleura extending into the root of the neck is called the cervical pleura and is innervated by the first intercostal nerve. It is applied to the undersurface of a firm fascial layer, the suprapleural membrane, which prevents upward movement of the apex of the lung and pleura during ventilation (see Fig. 7.15).

Surface markings of the parietal pleura

Because the parietal pleura is reflected from the thoracic wall onto both the mediastinum and the diaphragm, a line of pleural reflection can be mapped out on the body surface. Traced from its upper limit, approximately 2.5 cm above the medial third of the clavicle, this line descends behind the sternoclavicular joint and approaches the midline at the level of the manubriosternal joint. On the right the pleural reflection descends vertically to the level of the sixth costal cartilage while on the left the heart displaces the pleura laterally (Fig. 2.17) so that from the fourth to the sixth costal cartilages the line of reflection lies just lateral to the edge of the sternum. This displacement exposes part of the pericardium underlying the medial ends of the fourth and fifth intercostal spaces. Traced laterally from the sixth costal cartilage the surface marking is the same on each side, crossing the eighth rib in the midclavicular line and the tenth rib in the midaxillary line.

Posteriorly the parietal pleura continues horizontally, crosses the twelfth rib 5 cm from the midline and continues medially for a further 2.5 cm. Thus, a small area of parietal pleura lies below the level of the twelfth rib.

Visceral pleura

The visceral pleura (Fig. 2.18) is continuous with the mediastinal parietal pleura around the root of the lung. Structures entering or leaving the lung occupy the upper part of this pleural sleeve, the lower part consisting of an empty fold of pleura, the pulmonary ligament (see Fig. 2.25). The visceral pleura firmly adheres to the surface of the lung and extends into the depths of the fissures. Unlike the parietal layer, visceral pleura does not have a somatic innervation.

Surface markings of the visceral pleura

Since the visceral pleura covers the surface of the lung, its surface markings coincide with those of the lung (see page 41).

Fig. 2.18 Transverse section at the level of the fourth thoracic vertebra showing the arch of the aorta and the bifurcation of the trachea. Inferior aspect. Compare Fig. 2.67.

LUNGS

The two lungs lie in the thoracic cavity and are separated by the structures in the mediastinum (Fig. 2.19). Although the lungs of infants are pink, those of older individuals may have a mottled appearance due to deposits of inhaled carbon. Living lungs are elastic, enabling their volumes to change during ventilation, in contrast to embalmed lungs, which are rigid and often bear the imprints of adjacent structures. Each lung is covered in visceral pleura and is cone-shaped with the base or diaphragmatic surface directed downwards and the apex upwards. The costal surface is smoothly convex while the mediastinal surface is irregular and bears the hilum of the organ.

Fissures are usually present, and divide each lung into lobes (usually three lobes on the right and two on the left). Most of the lung consists of the peripheral part of the respiratory tract and the associated pulmonary vascular system. Having entered the lung, the bronchi and pulmonary vessels subdivide extensively (see Fig. 2.26).

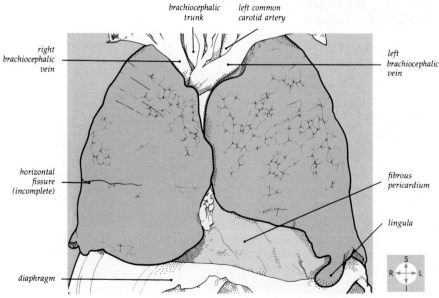

Fig. 2.19 Lungs, after removal of the anterolateral thoracic wall and parietal pleura. In this specimen the lungs overlie more of the mediastinum than is usual.

Fig. 2.20 Costal surface of the right lung, showing oblique and horizontal fissures and the upper, middle and lower lobes.

Fissures

Although variations occur, each lung is usually divided into upper and lower lobes by an oblique fissure. On the right the upper lobe is further subdivided by the horizontal fissure (Fig. 2.20), which runs from the anterior border of the lung into the oblique fissure and demarcates the middle lobe. On the left the horizontal fissure is usually absent and the middle lobe is represented by the lingula (Fig. 2.21).

Surfaces, borders and relations

The costal surface is convex and extends upwards into the cervical part of the pleura to form the apex of the lung, which is closely related to the corresponding subclavian artery and vein. The inferior surface (base) is markedly concave (Figs 2.22 & 2.23), conforming to the upward convexity of the dome of the diaphragm. The costal and diaphragmatic surfaces meet at the sharp inferior border. The anterior border is also sharp and is formed where the costal and mediastinal surfaces are in continuity. In contrast, the posterior border is rounded and rather indistinct.

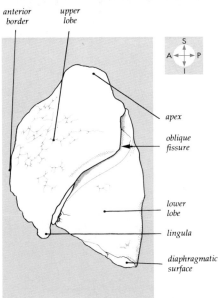

Fig. 2.21 Costal surface of the left lung showing the oblique fissure and upper and lower lobes.

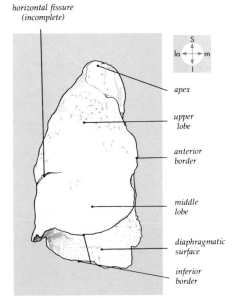

Fig. 2.22 Right lung showing its concave inferior surface and sharp anterior and inferior borders.

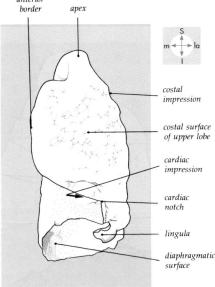

Fig. 2.23 Left lung showing the cardiac notch and lingula, both of which are particularly obvious in this specimen.

Surfaces

Most of the anterior surface of the heart consists of the right atrium and right ventricle (Fig. 2.33). The left ventricle contributes a narrow strip adjacent to the left border of the heart. The anterior surface is completed by the right and left auricles. The coronary sulcus descends more or less vertically across the anterior

surface and contains the right coronary artery surrounded by fat. The anterior surfaces of the right and left ventricles are separated by the anterior interventricular artery.

Most of the inferior (diaphragmatic) surface of the heart (Fig. 2.34) consists of the two ventricles, the left usually contributing the greater area. The posterior

interventricular vessels mark the boundary between these two chambers. The surface is completed by a small portion of the right atrium adjacent to the termination of the inferior vena cava.

The posterior surface or base of the heart (Fig. 2.35) consists mostly of the left atrium together with a small part of the right atrium.

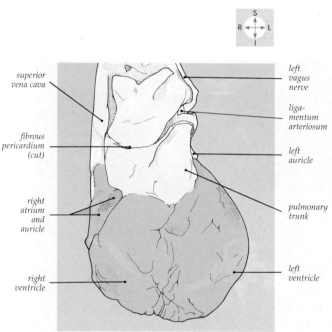

Fig. 2.33   Anterior surface of the heart.

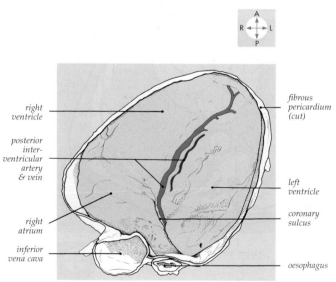

Fig. 2.34   Inferior surface of the heart. The inferior part of the fibrous pericardium has been removed with the diaphragm.

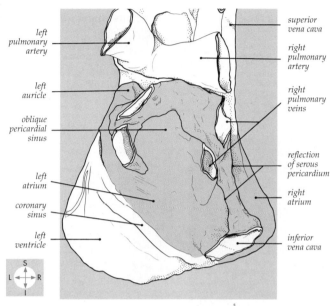

Fig. 2.35 The posterior surface of the heart showing the reflection of the serous pericardium and the site of the oblique pericardial sinus.

Chambers and valves

The cavities of the right and left atria are continuous with those of their respective ventricles through the atrioventricular orifices. Each orifice possesses an atrioventricular valve, which prevents backflow of blood from the ventricle into the atrium. The myocardium of the atria is separated from that of the ventricles by connective tissue, which forms a complete fibrous ring around each atrioventricular orifice. Interatrial and interventricular septa separate the cavities of the atria and ventricles. Valves, each with three semilunar cusps, guard the orifices between the right ventricle and pulmonary trunk (pulmonary valve) and the left ventricle and ascending aorta (aortic valve). All these valves close passively in response to differential pressure gradients.

Right atrium

The right atrium receives blood from the superior and inferior venae cavae and from the coronary sinus and cardiac veins which drain the myocardium. The superior vena cava enters the upper part of the chamber. Adjacent to its termination is a broad triangular prolongation of the atrium, the auricle (atrial appendage), which overlaps the ascending aorta (Fig. 2.36).

Internally the anterior wall of the right atrium possesses a vertical ridge, the crista terminalis (Fig. 2.36). From the crista muscular ridges (musculi pectinati) run to

the left and extend into the auricle. The posterior (septal) wall is relatively smooth but possesses a well defined ridge surrounding a shallow depression named the fossa ovalis. This fossa is the site of the foramen ovale, which, in the fetus, allows blood to pass directly from the right to the left atrium. The coronary sinus empties into the chamber close to the atrioventricular

orifice. Inferiorly the right atrium receives the inferior vena cava immediately after the vessel has pierced the central tendon of the diaphragm. A fold called the valve of the inferior vena cava (Fig. 2.36) projects into the chamber and is the remnant of a fetal structure that directed the flow of blood across the right atrium towards the foramen ovale.

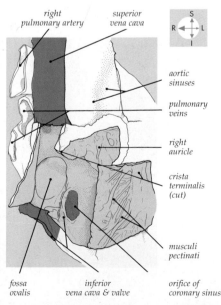

Fig. 2.36 Interior of the right atrium and auricle, exposed by reflection and excision of part of the anterior atrial wall.

Tricuspid valve

From the right atrium blood flows into the right ventricle through the right atrioventricular orifice, which is guarded by the tricuspid valve (Fig. 2.37). The valve possesses three cusps, the bases of which attach to the margins of the atrioventricular orifice while their free borders project into the cavity of the right ventricle (Fig. 2.38), where they are anchored by fibrous strands (chordae tendineae) to the papillary muscles of the ventricle. During ventricular contraction (systole) the papillary muscles pull on the chordae, preventing eversion of the valve cusps and reflux of blood into the atrium. The valve lies in the midline behind the lower part of the body of the sternum (see Fig. 2.32) and its sounds are heard best by auscultation over the xiphisternum.

Right ventricle

The right ventricle has the right atrium on its right and the left ventricle both behind and to its left. The chamber forms parts of the anterior and inferior surfaces of the heart and narrows superiorly at the infundibulum, which leads into the pulmonary trunk (Fig. 2.38). The walls of the right ventricle are thicker than those of the right atrium and internally possess

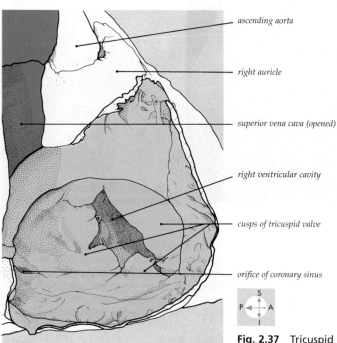

ascending aorta

right auricle

superior vena cava (opened)

right ventricular cavity

cusps of tricuspid valve

orifice of coronary sinus

Fig. 2.37   Tricuspid valve, revealed after removal of the lateral wall of the right atrium.

ascending aorta

pulmonary trunk & valve

right auricle

infundibulum of right ventricle

right coronary artery

cusps of tricuspid valve

chordae tendineae

papillary muscle

ventricular wall (cut)

Fig. 2.38   Interior of the right ventricle seen after removal of its anterior wall.

numerous muscular ridges called trabeculae carneae (see Fig. 2.43). One of these, the moderator band (see Fig. 2.54), often bridges the cavity of the chamber, connecting the interventricular septum to the anterior ventricular wall. When present, it carries the right branch of the atrioventricular bundle of conducting tissue (see page 56). Projecting from the ventricular walls into the interior of the

chamber are processes of myocardium, the papillary muscles, each attached at its apex to several chordae tendineae.

Pulmonary valve

The pulmonary orifice lies between the infundibulum and the pulmonary trunk and is guarded by the pulmonary valve (Figs 2.39 & 2.40), which consists of three

semilunar cusps. The valve closes during ventricular relaxation (diastole), preventing backflow of blood from the pulmonary trunk into the right ventricle. The valve lies behind the left border of the sternum at the level of the third costal cartilage (see Fig. 2.32). Sounds generated by this valve are loudest over the anterior end of the second left intercostal space.

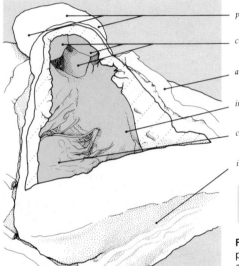

pulmonary trunk (cut) & sinuses

cusps of pulmonary valve

anterior interventricular artery

interventricular septum

cusp of tricuspid valve

inferior surface

Fig. 2.39 Ventricular surfaces of the cusps of the pulmonary valve seen after removal of part of the anterior wall of the right ventricle.

anterior interventricular artery

pulmonary sinus & valve

right coronary artery

right ventricle

left coronary artery

pulmonary vein

left atrium

aortic valve

superior vena cava

position of transverse pericardial sinus

Fig. 2.40 Pulmonary and aortic valves seen from above.

Left atrium

The left atrium lies behind the right atrium and forms the base of the heart. It possesses a hook-like auricle (left atrial appendage), which projects forwards to the left of the pulmonary trunk and infundibulum. The chamber receives superior and inferior pulmonary veins from each lung (see Fig. 2.35). The four pulmonary veins, together with the two venae cavae, are all enclosed in a sleeve of serous pericardium, forming the superior limit of the oblique pericardial sinus. The left atrium forms the anterior wall of this sinus, which separates the chamber from the fibrous pericardium and oesophagus. Most of the inner surface of the left atrium is smooth (Fig. 2.41), although musculi pectinati are present in the auricle.

Mitral (bicuspid) valve

The left atrium communicates anteroinferiorly with the left ventricle through the left atrioventricular orifice, which is guarded by the mitral valve. This valve possesses two cusps, whose bases attach to the margins of the atrioventricular orifice (Fig. 2.41) while their free borders and cusps are anchored by chordae tendineae to the papillary muscles within the left ventricle (Fig. 2.42). The valve prevents reflux during ventricular contraction. Although it lies in the midline at the level of the fourth costal cartilages (see Fig. 2.32), the sounds of the mitral valve are best heard over the apex of the heart.

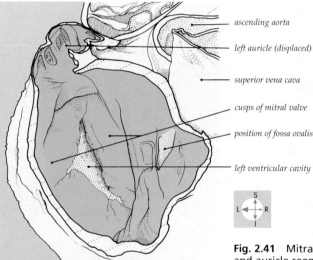

ascending aorta

left auricle (displaced)

superior vena cava

cusps of mitral valve

position of fossa ovalis

left ventricular cavity

Fig. 2.41   Mitral valve and interior of the left atrium and auricle seen after removal of the posterior wall of the chamber.

anterior interventricular artery

pulmonary sinus

ascending aorta

trabeculae carneae

papillary muscle (cut)

mitral valve & chordae tendinea

circumflex artery

coronary sinus (cut)

Fig. 2.42   Interior of the left ventricle seen after removal of part of its wall.

Left ventricle

From the left atrioventricular orifice the left ventricle extends forwards and to the left as far as the apex. The thickness of the wall of the chamber is normally three times that of the right ventricle (Fig. 2.43). Internally there are prominent trabeculae carneae and papillary muscles (see Fig. 2.46). The chamber narrows as it passes upwards and to the right behind the infundibulum to form the aortic vestibule (Fig. 2.44), the part of the ventricle that communicates with the ascending aorta through the aortic orifice.

Aortic valve

The aortic valve consists of three semilunar cusps (see Fig. 2.45), which prevent backflow of blood from the ascending aorta during ventricular diastole. The valve lies behind the sternum to the left of the midline at the level of the anterior end of the third left intercostal space (see Fig. 2.32). However, its sounds are best heard over the medial ends of the first and second right intercostal spaces.

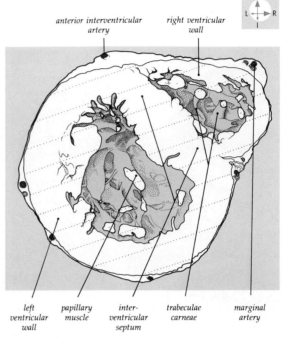

Fig. 2.43 Section through the heart showing the apical portions of the left and right ventricles.

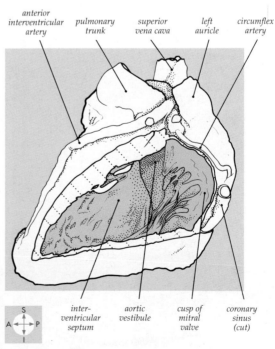

Fig. 2.44 Mitral valve and aortic vestibule, exposed by removal of part of the left ventricular wall.

Pulmonary trunk and ascending aorta

The pulmonary trunk and the ascending aorta lie within the fibrous pericardium, enclosed together in a sleeve of serous pericardium anterior to the transverse pericardial sinus (see Fig. 2.40). The pulmonary trunk extends upwards and backwards while the ascending aorta initially lies behind it and passes upwards and forwards, overlapped by the right auricle. At the origin of each vessel are three dilatations or sinuses (Fig. 2.45), one immediately above each of the cusps of the pulmonary and aortic valves. When ventricular contraction ceases, blood flows into the sinuses, thus pushing against the cusps and closing the valves. Two of the aortic sinuses give rise to the right and left coronary arteries.

The pulmonary trunk emerges from the pericardium and divides into right and left pulmonary arteries in the concavity of the aortic arch, anterior to the bifurcation of the trachea at the level of the fourth thoracic vertebra. As the ascending aorta pierces the fibrous pericardium it turns backwards and to the left, becoming the arch of the aorta.

Connecting the aortic arch to the pulmonary trunk (or to the commencement of the left pulmonary artery) is the ligamentum arteriosum (Fig. 2.46), the remnant of the fetal ductus arteriosus which conveyed blood from the pulmonary trunk to the aorta, bypassing the pulmonary circulation. Occasionally the ductus remains patent after birth, giving rise to serious circulatory abnormalities.

Fig. 2.45 Aortic and pulmonary valves viewed obliquely from above.

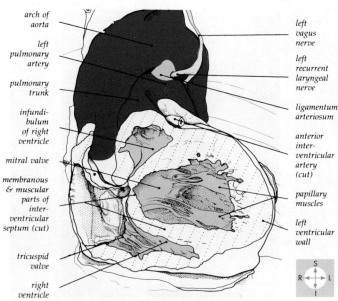

Fig. 2.46 Anterior view of the aorta, pulmonary trunk and ligamentum arteriosum. Most of the muscular part of the interventricular septum has been removed to show the interior of the left ventricle.

Blood vessels

The arterial supply to the heart is provided by the right and left coronary arteries, which arise from the ascending aorta just above the aortic valve (Fig. 2.47). They supply the myocardium, including the papillary muscles and conducting tissue. The principal venous return is via the coronary sinus and the cardiac veins.

Right coronary artery

This vessel arises from the anterior aspect of the root of the aorta and descends in the anterior coronary sulcus (Figs 2.47 & 2.48). At the inferior border it gives off a marginal branch, which runs to the left towards the apex of the heart. The right coronary artery continues on the inferior surface in the coronary sulcus (see Fig. 2.49) and terminates by anastomosing with the left coronary artery. On the inferior surface, the posterior (inferior) interventricular artery arises from the right coronary artery (occasionally the left coronary artery) and runs in the posterior interventricular groove towards the apex. The right coronary artery and its branches supply the anterior surface of the right atrium, the lower part of the left atrium, most of the right ventricle and parts of the left ventricle and interventricular septum. In addition, branches from this artery usually supply most of the conducting tissue of the heart (see page 56).

Fig. 2.47 Origins of the right and left coronary arteries from the root of the ascending aorta seen from above.

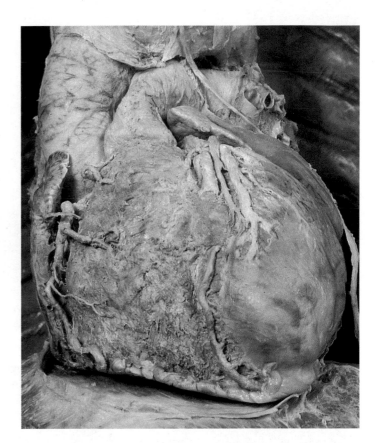

Fig. 2.48 Right and left coronary arteries and their branches on the anterior surface of the heart.

Left coronary artery

This artery takes origin from the posterior aspect of the root of the ascending aorta and runs to the left behind the pulmonary trunk where its major branch, the anterior interventricular artery, arises (Figs 2.47 & 2.50). The latter vessel descends in the anterior interventricular groove towards the apex of the heart. The left coronary artery continues as the circumflex artery in the posterior part of the coronary sulcus and terminates by anastomosing with the right coronary artery. The vessel supplies the posterior wall of the left atrium and auricle, most of the left ventricle and parts of the right ventricle and interventricular septum.

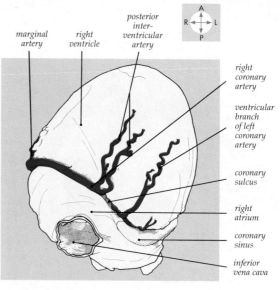

Fig. 2.49   Right and left coronary arteries and their branches on the inferior surface of the heart. The posterior interventricular artery is duplicated in this specimen.

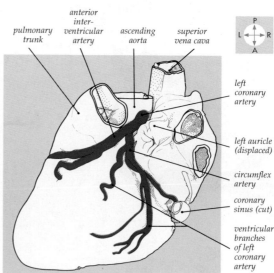

Fig. 2.50   Left coronary artery and its branches, viewed from the left.

Coronary sinus and cardiac veins

Most of the venous return from the heart is carried by the coronary sinus, which runs along the posterior part of the coronary sulcus and terminates in the right atrium.

The coronary sinus is formed near the left border of the heart by the union of the posterior vein of the left ventricle and the great cardiac vein (Fig. 2.51), which accompanies the anterior interventricular artery. Other veins enter the coronary sinus,

including the middle cardiac vein (Fig. 2.52), which accompanies the posterior interventricular artery. Some cardiac veins enter the right atrium independently (see Fig. 2.48).

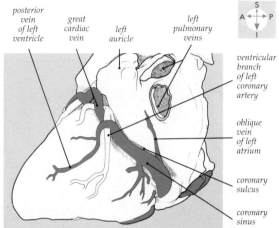

Fig. 2.51 Oblique view of the coronary sinus lying in the coronary sulcus.

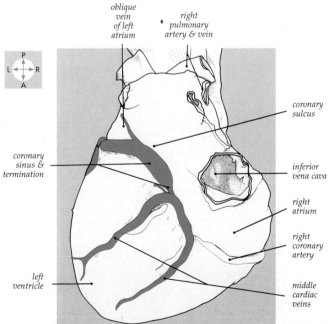

Fig. 2.52 Posteroinferior view of the termination of the coronary sinus in the right atrium.

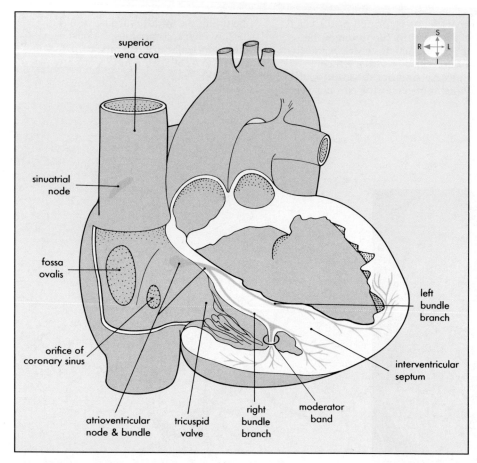

superior
vena cava

sinuatrial
node

fossa
ovalis

orifice of
coronary sinus

atrioventricular
node & bundle

tricuspid
valve

right
bundle
branch

moderator
band

interventricular
septum

left
bundle
branch

Fig. 2.53   Location of the conducting tissues.

Conducting system

Coordinated contraction of the myocardium is controlled by specialized conducting tissues, consisting of the sinuatrial (SA) node, the atrioventricular (AV) node, the atrioventricular bundle (of His) and its right and left branches (Fig. 2.53).

The sinuatrial node lies in the anterior wall of the right atrium close to the termination of the superior vena cava. It occupies part of the root of the auricle and the upper end of the sulcus terminalis. Numerous autonomic nerves supply the node and modify its rate of discharge. The SA node usually receives blood from an atrial branch of either the right or left coronary artery. From the SA node the cardiac excitation wave passes through the atrial myocardium to reach the AV node.

The AV node lies in the interatrial septum anterosuperior to the termination of the coronary sinus. It is continuous with the atrioventricular bundle, which passes through the fibrous ring separating the atria and ventricles. The bundle gains the upper part of the interventricular septum and promptly divides into right and left branches. The AV node and bundle are supplied by branches of the posterior interventricular artery.

Lying beneath the endocardium the right branch of the atrioventricular bundle descends in the interventricular septum and often passes in the moderator band (Fig. 2.54) to ramify within the anterior wall of the right ventricle. The left branch runs on the left side of the interventricular septum. Both branches divide repeatedly at the ventricular apices and spread out into the myocardium of the respective ventricles.

ascending
aorta
& right
coronary
artery

cusp of
tricuspid
valve

chordae
tendineae

infundi-
bulum

right
ventricular
wall (cut)

inter-
ventricular
septum

moderator
band

Fig. 2.54   Moderator band, seen through a window cut in the anterior wall of the right ventricle.

MEDIASTINAL STRUCTURES

Brachiocephalic veins

On each side the brachiocephalic vein is formed in the root of the neck by the union of the internal jugular and subclavian veins. At its origin the vein lies behind the sternoclavicular joint and in front of the first part of the subclavian artery.

The right brachiocephalic vein runs a short vertical course in the superior mediastinum to unite with the left brachiocephalic vein (Fig. 2.55) behind the medial end of the first right costal cartilage. It receives the right vertebral and internal thoracic veins, together with the right jugular and subclavian lymph trunks and the right lymph duct. The vessel is accompanied by the right phrenic nerve.

The left brachiocephalic vein enters the thorax and runs obliquely to the right, passing behind the manubrium. The vessel lies in front of the origin from the arch of the aorta of the left common carotid artery and the brachiocephalic trunk. At its commencement the vein is joined by the termination of the thoracic duct and, along its course, receives the left vertebral,

internal thoracic and superior intercostal veins and, usually, the inferior thyroid veins.

Superior vena cava

Formed by the union of the two brachiocephalic veins, this large vessel descends vertically (Fig. 2.55) and terminates in the right atrium of the heart. It lies to the right of the ascending aorta and to the left of the right phrenic nerve and receives the azygos vein before piercing the fibrous pericardium.

Arch of aorta and branches

The arch of the aorta lies within the superior mediastinum, in continuity with the ascending aorta. The vessel curves backwards and to the left to reach the left side of the fourth thoracic vertebral body, where it becomes the descending aorta. The arch possesses a concavity inferiorly, left and right sides, and a superior convexity.

The concavity is related to the bifurcation of the pulmonary trunk and the left main bronchus. The ligamentum arteriosum attaches the pulmonary trunk (or left pulmonary artery) to the concavity of the aortic arch and is closely related to

the left recurrent laryngeal nerve (see Figs 2.46 & 2.57).

The left side of the aortic arch is crossed by the left phrenic and vagus nerves (see Fig. 2.56) and covered by mediastinal pleura. The phrenic nerve lies in front of the vagus and passes onto the fibrous pericardium in front of the lung root. The vagus nerve inclines backwards to pass behind the lung root, having given off the left recurrent laryngeal nerve. The left superior intercostal vein passes forwards across the arch and usually terminates in the left brachiocephalic vein.

The right side of the arch is related, from in front backwards, to the superior vena cava, trachea, left recurrent laryngeal nerve, oesophagus and thoracic duct. These structures lie between the aorta and the right mediastinal pleura.

The convexity of the arch gives rise to the brachiocephalic trunk, left common carotid and left subclavian arteries (see Fig. 2.57), which ascend into the root of the neck. The brachiocephalic trunk is the first branch of the arch of the aorta and arises behind the left brachiocephalic vein. The trunk slopes upwards and to the right across the anterior surface of the trachea, leaving the thorax to the right of the trachea to divide in the root of the neck into the right subclavian and right common carotid arteries.

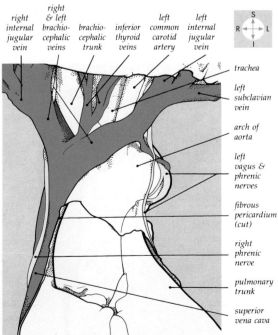

right internal jugular vein

right & left brachio-cephalic veins

brachio-cephalic trunk

inferior thyroid veins

left common carotid artery

left internal jugular vein

trachea

left subclavian vein

arch of aorta

left vagus & phrenic nerves

fibrous pericardium (cut)

right phrenic nerve

pulmonary trunk

superior vena cava

Fig. 2.55 Relationships of the brachiocephalic veins to the great arteries arising from the aortic arch.

The left common carotid artery arises behind the brachiocephalic trunk and ascends, in company with the left phrenic and vagus nerves, through the superior mediastinum on the left of the trachea into the root of the neck (Fig. 2.57).

The left subclavian artery is the most posterior artery arising from the aortic arch and lies immediately behind the left common carotid artery. It runs upwards and laterally, closely related to the pleura covering the apex of the left lung, entering the root of the neck behind the sternoclavicular joint.

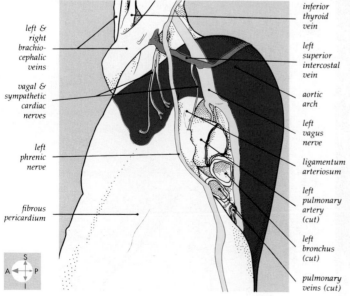

Fig. 2.56 Oblique view of the arch of the aorta showing the courses of the left vagus and phrenic nerves.

Fig. 2.57 Arch of the aorta and its branches viewed anteriorly.

Phrenic nerves

The right and left phrenic nerves (C3, C4 & C5) pass through the superior thoracic aperture behind the respective subclavian veins. Owing to the asymmetry of the mediastinal organs, the intrathoracic courses of the two nerves differ. The right phrenic nerve, covered by mediastinal pleura, accompanies the right brachiocephalic vein and the superior vena cava in front of the root of the right lung (Fig. 2.58). It descends vertically across the fibrous pericardium covering the right atrium and pierces the diaphragm alongside the inferior vena cava.

The left phrenic nerve, also covered by mediastinal pleura, lies lateral to the left common carotid artery and crosses the left side of the aortic arch to gain the fibrous pericardium in front of the left lung root (Fig. 2.56). The nerve then descends across the pericardium as far as the apex of the heart, where it pierces the diaphragm (see Fig. 2.59).

The phrenic nerves supply the muscle of the diaphragm, excluding the crura. They give sensory fibres to the fibrous and parietal serous pericardium and the mediastinal and diaphragmatic pleura, and sensory branches to the peritoneum covering the inferior surface of the diaphragm (see pages 38 & 185).

Trachea

The trachea descends through the neck, where normally it is palpable, and enters the thorax in the midline, immediately behind the upper border of the manubrium. It runs vertically through the superior mediastinum and, at the level of the aortic arch, divides into right and left main bronchi (see Fig. 2.60).

The right main bronchus is wider than the left and inclines steeply downwards to enter the right lung root. The right upper lobar bronchus often arises outside the hilum of the lung. The left main bronchus runs obliquely to the left within the concavity of the arch of the aorta, passing behind the left pulmonary artery to gain the left lung root.

The thoracic part of the trachea is crossed anteriorly by the brachiocephalic trunk and the left brachiocephalic vein (Fig. 2.58). In addition, the trachea is overlapped by the anterior margins of the pleura and lungs and the thymus (or its remnants). The trachea is related on the left to the arch of the aorta and left common carotid and subclavian arteries, on the right to the superior vena cava, the termination of the azygos vein, the right vagus nerve and the mediastinal pleura, and posteriorly to the oesophagus and the left recurrent laryngeal nerve. (The right recurrent laryngeal nerve does not enter the thorax but passes around the right subclavian artery in the root of the neck; see page 293.)

The vascular supply of the trachea is from the inferior thyroid arteries and veins. The recurrent laryngeal nerves supply sensory and parasympathetic secretomotor fibres to the mucous membrane and motor fibres to the smooth muscle (trachealis).

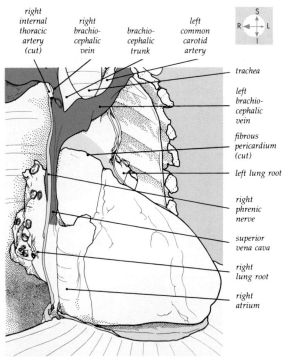

Fig. 2.58 Oblique view showing the course of the right phrenic nerve.

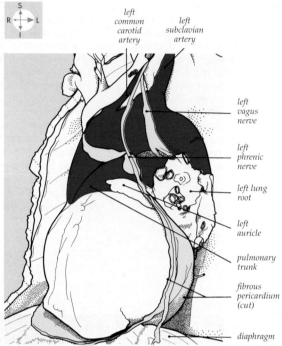

left common carotid artery

left subclavian artery

left vagus nerve

left phrenic nerve

left lung root

left auricle

pulmonary trunk

fibrous pericardium (cut)

diaphragm

Fig. 2.59   Oblique view of the intrathoracic course of the left phrenic nerve.

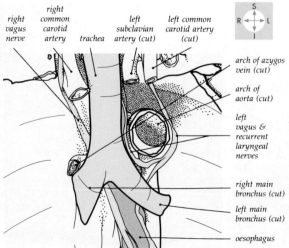

right vagus nerve

right common carotid artery

trachea

left subclavian artery (cut)

left common carotid artery (cut)

arch of azygos vein (cut)

arch of aorta (cut)

left vagus & recurrent laryngeal nerves

right main bronchus (cut)

left main bronchus (cut)

oesophagus

Fig. 2.60   Trachea and left and right main bronchi, exposed after removal of the anterior part of the aortic arch.

Oesophagus

The oesophagus descends through the root of the neck and
traverses the superior thoracic aperture behind the trachea. In the
superior mediastinum the oesophagus lies in front of the upper four
thoracic vertebral bodies and behind the trachea, the left main
bronchus and left recurrent laryngeal nerve. The aortic arch and the
thoracic duct are on its left while the azygos vein arches forwards
on its right (Fig. 2.61).

The oesophagus continues into the posterior mediastinum in front
of the fifth thoracic vertebra accompanied by the right and left
vagus nerves. It descends behind the fibrous pericardium and
inclines to the left to cross in front of the descending aorta. On its
right side the oesophagus is covered by mediastinal pleura. On the
left, once anterior to the descending aorta, it is related to pleura as
far as the diaphragm. Accompanied by branches of the vagus
nerves (see below), the oesophagus passes through the diaphragm
at the level of the tenth thoracic vertebra.

The oesophagus is supplied by branches from the inferior thyroid
arteries and from the descending thoracic aorta. Its lower part
receives branches from the left gastric artery that ascend through
the oesophageal opening in the diaphragm. Radicles of the left
gastric vein (a tributary of the portal vein) anastomose with veins
that drain venous blood from the oesophagus into the azygos
system. The upper part of the oesophagus is drained by the
brachiocephalic veins. Sensory and parasympathetic motor fibres to
the oesophagus are provided by the vagi and their recurrent
laryngeal branches.

Vagus (X) nerves

In the superior mediastinum the relationships of the right and left
vagi differ. The right vagus nerve (Fig. 2.61) enters the thorax
behind the bifurcation of the brachiocephalic artery and on the right
of the trachea. The nerve, covered by mediastinal pleura, inclines
backwards and passes behind the right lung root to gain the
oesophagus. The left vagus nerve descends behind the left common
carotid artery to cross the left side of the aortic arch, gives off the
left recurrent laryngeal nerve, and continues behind the left lung
root to reach the oesophagus.

The left recurrent laryngeal nerve (Fig. 2.61) passes around the
arch of the aorta adjacent to the ligamentum arteriosum and ascends
in the interval between the trachea and oesophagus. In the posterior
mediastinum the right and left vagus nerves divide on the surface of
the oesophagus to form a network, the oesophageal plexus. The
terminal branches of the plexus (the anterior and posterior vagal
trunks) enter the abdomen with the oesophagus (see page 178).

Descending thoracic aorta and branches

The descending aorta (Fig. 2.62) is continuous with the aortic arch
and initially lies to the left of the fifth thoracic vertebral body. As it
traverses the posterior mediastinum it inclines forwards and to the
right, gaining the midline anterior to the twelfth thoracic vertebra.
On the right, the upper part of the descending aorta is related to the
thoracic vertebral bodies and the oesophagus. The lower part and
all of its left side are covered by mediastinal pleura. The thoracic
duct and the azygos vein lie to the right of the aorta and anteriorly
it is crossed by the oesophagus sloping obliquely from the midline
to the left. The descending aorta leaves the thorax in front of the
twelfth thoracic vertebra and behind the median arcuate ligament of
the diaphragm with the thoracic duct and azygos vein (see Fig. 2.64).

Posterior intercostal arteries from the descending aorta supply the
third to the eleventh intercostal spaces on both sides. They
anastomose with the anterior intercostal arteries derived from either
the internal thoracic or the musculophrenic arteries. Other branches
from the aorta supply the right and left bronchi and the oesophagus.

Thoracic duct

Arising from the upper part of the cisterna chyli (see page 177), the
thoracic duct passes into the thorax, lying between the azygos vein

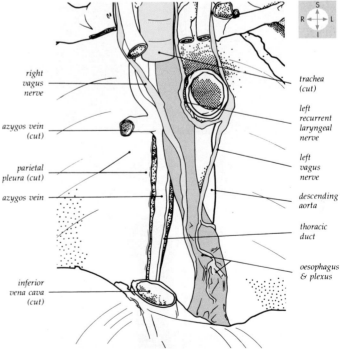

Fig. 2.61 Intrathoracic part of the oesophagus and accompanying
vagus nerves after removal of the main bronchi and the lower part
of the trachea.

and descending aorta, and with these structures (Figs 2.61 & 2.62) ascends through the posterior mediastinum to gain the superior mediastinum on the left of the oesophagus. The duct then curves forwards and to the left, crossing the apex of the left lung to enter the root of the neck where it terminates in the confluence of the left internal jugular and subclavian veins.

Azygos venous system

This system of veins drains blood from most of the posterior thoracic wall and from the bronchi, the pericardium and part of the intrathoracic oesophagus. The azygos vein enters the thorax through the aortic opening and receives posterior intercostal veins from the lower eight spaces on the right (Fig. 2.63). Veins from the second and third spaces drain into the right superior intercostal vein, which terminates in the azygos vein as it arches over the right lung root to join the superior vena cava. The venous return from the first space drains into the right brachiocephalic vein. The azygos vein also receives the hemiazygos veins.

Fig. 2.62 Descending aorta and thoracic duct, exposed after removal of the thoracic part of the oesophagus.

Fig. 2.63 Azygos vein, right intercostal nerves and posterior intercostal vessels, exposed after removal of the parietal pleura.

The hemiazygos and accessory hemiazygos veins drain the lower eight posterior intercostal spaces on the left side. The lowermost four spaces usually empty into the hemiazygos vein, which crosses the midline to terminate in the azygos vein (Fig. 2.64). Veins from the next four intercostal spaces usually join to form the accessory hemiazygos vein, which also crosses to end in the azygos. Sometimes the hemiazygos and accessory hemiazygos veins drain into the azygos vein by a single vessel. The second and third spaces on the left are drained by the left superior intercostal vein (see Fig. 2.56), which crosses the aortic arch to end in the left brachiocephalic vein. The first left intercostal space drains into the corresponding brachiocephalic vein.

Thoracic sympathetic trunk

The thoracic part of the sympathetic trunk (chain) runs along the lateral aspects of the thoracic vertebral bodies (Figs 2.64 & 2.65). In continuity with the cervical and abdominal parts, the thoracic sympathetic trunk consists of a series of interconnected enlargements (ganglia) occurring at intervals along its length. Usually each thoracic spinal nerve is connected to its own ganglion by two branches, a white (preganglionic) and a grey (postganglionic) ramus communicans. Not infrequently, adjacent ganglia fuse together and, most often, the inferior cervical and first thoracic ganglia fuse to form the stellate ganglion.

Branches

Fine nerve filaments running from the sympathetic trunk contribute to the autonomic prevertebral plexuses supplying the thoracic organs, including the heart (cardiac plexuses), lungs (pulmonary plexuses) and the oesophagus (oesophageal plexus). The lower thoracic ganglia give rise to a collection of autonomic fibres that form the greater (Fig. 2.65), lesser and least splanchnic nerves, destined to supply intra-abdominal structures which are gained by piercing the crura of the diaphragm. All thoracic spinal nerves receive from the grey rami communicantes sympathetic postganglionic fibres, which are distributed to various structures of the body wall (for example, blood vessels, hair follicles and sweat glands) by the segmental spinal nerves.

Fig. 2.64 Oblique view of left sympathetic trunk, hemiazygos vein, intercostal nerves and posterior intercostal vessels after removal of the descending aorta and parietal pleura on the left side of the midline.

Fig. 2.65 Oblique view of right sympathetic trunk and posterior intercostal vessels and intercostal nerves after removal of the parietal pleura.

Observation Skills

Identify the structures indicated. The answers are supplied at the foot of the page.

Fig. 2.66 Transverse CT image at the level of the second thoracic vertebra. Compare Fig. 2.70.

Fig. 2.67 Transverse CT image at the level of the fourth thoracic vertebra. Compare Fig. 2.18.

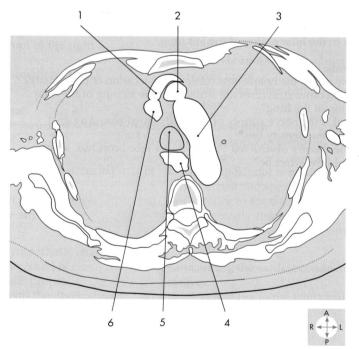

Answers

Fig. 2.66 1 = right internal jugular vein, 2 = infrahyoid strap muscle, 3 = trachea, 4 = medial end of left clavicle, 5 = left internal jugular vein, 6 = left common carotid artery, 7 = left subclavian vein, 8 = left subclavian artery, 9 = oesophagus, 10 = right common carotid artery, 11 = right subclavian artery.

Fig. 2.67 1 = left brachiocephalic vein, 2 = brachiocephalic trunk arising from arch of aorta, 3 = aortic arch, 4 = oesophagus, 5 = trachea, 6 = termination of right brachiocephalic vein.

Identify the structures indicated. The answers are supplied at the foot of the page.

Fig. 2.68 Transverse CT image at the level of the fifth thoracic vertebra. Compare Fig. 2.27.

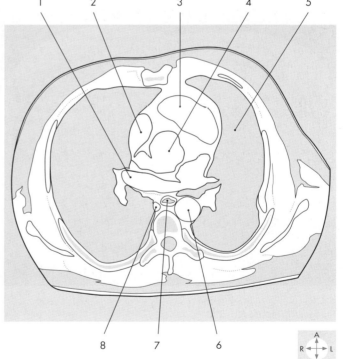

Fig. 2.69 Transverse CT image at the level of the seventh thoracic vertebra. Compare Fig. 1.5.

Answers

Fig. 2.68 1 = superior vena cava, 2 = ascending aorta, 3 = bifurcation of pulmonary trunk into right and left pulmonary arteries, 4 = descending aorta, 5 = pulmonary veins.

Fig. 2.69 1 = right pulmonary vein entering left atrium, 2 = right atrium, 3 = right ventricle, 4 = infundibulum of left ventricle, 5 = left lung, 6 = descending aorta, 7 = oesophagus, 8 = azygos vein.

Identify the structures indicated. The answers are supplied at the foot of the page.

Fig. 2.70   Transverse section at the level of the third thoracic vertebra. Inferior aspect. Compare Fig. 2.66.

Fig. 2.71   Transverse section at the level of the sixth thoracic vertebra. Inferior aspect. Compare Fig. 2.31.

Answers

Fig. 2.70   1 = pectoralis major, 2 = pectoralis minor, 3 = right brachiocephalic vein, 4 = left brachiocephalic vein, 5 = brachiocephalic trunk, 6 = left common carotid artery, 7 = left lung, 8 = left axillary vein, 9 = left subclavian artery, 10 = oesophagus, 11 = thoracic spinal cord, 12 = trachea, 13 = lymph nodes.

Fig. 2.71   1 = right atrium, 2 = fibrous pericardium, 3 = internal thoracic vessels, 4 = sternum, 5 = right ventricle, 6 = aortic valve, 7 = anterior interventricular artery, 8 = left ventricle, 9 = descending aorta, 10 = azygos vein, 11 = oesophagus, 12 = pericardial cavity, 13 = pleural cavity, 14 = oblique fissure, 15 = lower lobe of right lung.

3 UPPER LIMB

INTRODUCTION

The upper limb (extremity) comprises several bones and their joints (Fig. 3.1), clothed by soft tissues. For descriptive purposes the limb is divided into regions (Fig. 3.2), each enveloped by fascia and containing muscles with nerve and vascular supplies. The scapula with its associated muscles and soft tissues comprise the scapular region, the muscles attaching between the front of the chest wall and the upper limb (together with the overlying fascia, breast and skin) constitute the pectoral region. The scapula and the clavicle, which together form the pectoral girdle, articulate at the acromioclavicular joint. The clavicle articulates with the trunk at the sternoclavicular joint and the scapula with the humerus at the glenohumeral (shoulder) joint.

Between the proximal part of the limb and the chest wall is the axilla, a region traversed by the principal nerves and vessels passing between the upper limb and the root of the neck.

The arm is that part of the upper limb between the shoulder and the elbow. The muscles of the arm are disposed in anterior (flexor) and posterior (extensor) compartments, separated by the humerus and the medial and lateral intermuscular septa (Fig. 3.3). In front of the elbow joint (at which the humerus, radius and ulna articulate) lies the cubital fossa, a region traversed by vessels and nerves passing between the arm and the forearm.

The forearm lies between the elbow and the wrist, and its muscles are arranged in anterior (flexor) and posterior (extensor) compartments, separated by the radius, ulna, and interosseous membrane (Fig. 3.4). Rotation at the proximal and distal radioulnar joints permits the hand to function in any position between the extremes of supination (palm facing up), and pronation (palm facing down).

The forearm articulates with the carpus at the wrist (radiocarpal) joint. Together with the flexor retinaculum, the bones of the carpus form the carpal tunnel, which links the anterior compartment of the forearm and the palm of the hand. The structures of the palm lie anterior to the metacarpals while posteriorly is the dorsum of the hand. The digits are named, from lateral to medial, the thumb and the index, middle, ring and little fingers.

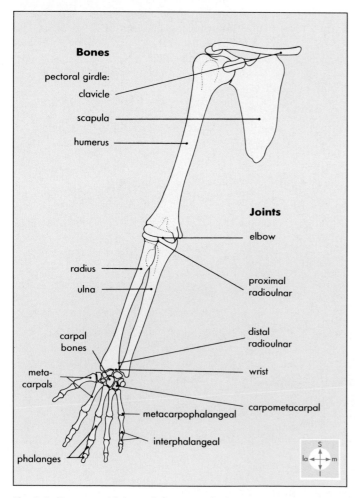

Bones

pectoral girdle:
clavicle
scapula
humerus

Joints

elbow

radius
ulna

proximal radioulnar

carpal bones

distal radioulnar

meta-carpals

wrist

carpometacarpal

metacarpophalangeal

interphalangeal

phalanges

Fig. 3.1 Bones and joints of the upper limb.

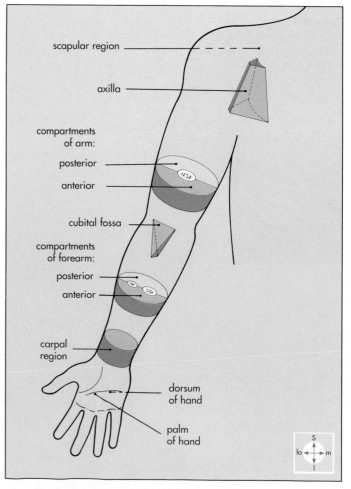

scapular region

axilla

compartments of arm:
posterior
anterior

cubital fossa

compartments of forearm:
posterior
anterior

carpal region

dorsum of hand

palm of hand

Fig. 3.2 Parts of the upper limb.

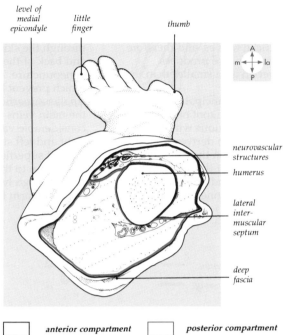

level of medial epicondyle *little finger* *thumb*

neurovascular structures

humerus

lateral inter-muscular septum

deep fascia

☐ *anterior compartment* ☐ *posterior compartment*

Fig. 3.3 Transverse section midway between glenohumeral and elbow joints to show the compartments of the arm.

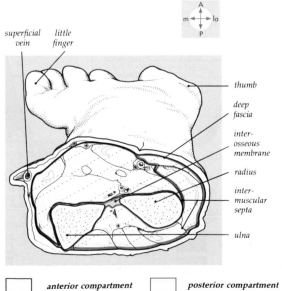

superficial vein *little finger*

thumb

deep fascia

inter-osseous membrane

radius

inter-muscular septa

ulna

☐ *anterior compartment* ☐ *posterior compartment*

Fig. 3.4 Transverse section midway between elbow and wrist joints to show the compartments of the forearm.

DELTOID

Deltoid is a large multipennate muscle responsible for the rounded contour of the shoulder region (Fig. 3.10). The muscle overlies the shoulder joint and the attachments of the short scapular muscles to the upper end of the humerus (Fig. 3.11). Proximally it has a continuous attachment to the lateral third of the clavicle and to the acromion and spine of the scapula. The distal attachment is to a roughened area, the deltoid tuberosity, midway down the lateral surface of the shaft of the humerus (see Fig. 3.23). Deltoid acts only on the shoulder joint, where it is the main abductor. During this movement, produced by the acromial fibres, the joint is stabilized by the clavicular fibres and those from the scapular spine. Acting alone the anterior fibres produce flexion whereas the posterior fibres extend the shoulder joint. Deltoid is supplied by the axillary nerve, a terminal branch of the posterior cord of the brachial plexus.

Axillary nerve

The axillary nerve leaves the axilla through the quadrangular space (see Fig. 3.64) accompanied by the posterior circumflex humeral artery. In its course the nerve is closely related to the surgical neck of the humerus and to the capsule of the shoulder joint. It supplies deltoid and teres minor, the shoulder joint and skin overlying the lower part of deltoid. Damage to the nerve may occur during dislocation of the shoulder joint, resulting in weakness of abduction, impaired sensation and, subsequently, in loss of the normal contour of the shoulder as the deltoid muscle becomes wasted.

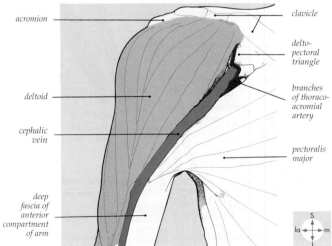

Fig. 3.10   Anterior view of deltoid. The cephalic vein lies in the deltopectoral groove. Deformity of the clavicle is due to a healed fracture.

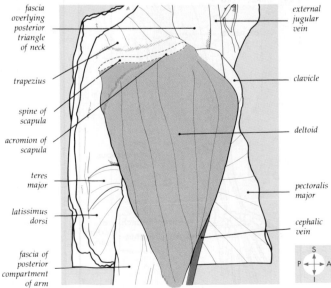

Fig. 3.11   Lateral view. Deltoid has a continuous proximal attachment to the spine and acromion of the scapula and the lateral part of the clavicle.

AXILLA

The axilla is the space between the root of the upper limb and the chest wall. It is traversed by the principal vessels and nerves that pass between the upper limb and the root of the neck. The shape and size of the axilla vary according to the position of the shoulder joint but when the limb is in the anatomical position the axilla is shaped like a truncated pyramid with a narrow apex (inlet) superiorly, a broad base and three walls (Fig. 3.12).

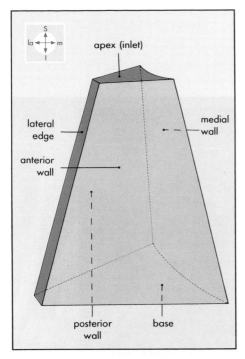

Fig. 3.12 Shape of the axilla.

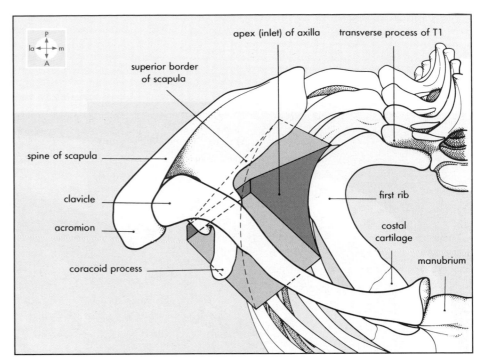

Fig. 3.13 Axilla from above showing the boundaries of its apex.

Walls

The upper ribs and intercostal spaces, covered by serratus anterior, form the medial wall (see Fig. 3.15), which is convex laterally. The anterior wall consists of pectoralis major overlying pectoralis minor and subclavius (Fig. 3.14; see Fig. 3.16) while the posterior wall is formed by subscapularis, teres major and latissimus dorsi. The muscles of the anterior and posterior walls converge on the humerus (see Fig. 3.15) so that the axilla is limited laterally by the narrow intertubercular sulcus of the humerus. The base of the axilla, convex upwards, is formed by fascia passing between the inferior margins of the anterior and posterior walls. The triangular apex of the axilla provides continuity between the root of the neck and the upper limb and is bounded by the clavicle, the superior border of the scapula and the first rib (Fig. 3.13).

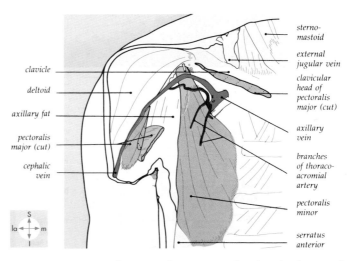

Fig. 3.14 Structures that pass above pectoralis minor in the anterior wall of the axilla. Pectoralis major and fascia around pectoralis minor have been removed.

heads, which are terminal branches of the lateral and medial cords. In the upper part of the arm the nerve lies lateral to the brachial artery but at midarm level it crosses anterior to the vessels and finally lies medial to the artery (see Fig. 3.24), a position retained in the cubital fossa. The ulnar nerve is a terminal branch of the

medial cord and, together with the medial cutaneous nerve of forearm, initially lies medial to the brachial artery but leaves the artery at midarm level (see Fig. 3.24). It then pierces the medial intermuscular septum and enters the posterior compartment to lie between the septum and the medial head of triceps.

CUBITAL FOSSA

The cubital fossa is a triangular space in front of the elbow joint, bounded laterally by brachioradialis and medially by pronator teres (Fig. 3.28). By convention, the fossa is limited proximally by an

basilic vein

medial cutaneous nerve of arm

cephalic vein

medial cutaneous nerve of forearm

biceps brachii

subcutaneous tissue

median cubital vein

lateral cutaneous nerve of forearm

perforating vein

Fig. 3.25 Cutaneous nerves and superficial veins overlying the right cubital fossa. Subcutaneous tissue has been retained medial to the basilic vein.

biceps brachii

basilic vein

branch of posterior cutaneous nerve of forearm

tendon & aponeurosis of biceps brachii

perforating vein

deep fascia of forearm

brachio-radialis

lateral cutaneous nerve of forearm

Fig. 3.26 Roof of the cubital fossa after removal of subcutaneous tissue, veins and nerves. A perforating vein communicates with deep veins by passing through the deep fascia.

medial head of triceps

brachial artery & venae comitantes

aponeurosis of biceps brachii (cut)

tendon of biceps brachii

median nerve

pronator teres

radial artery & vena comitans

Fig. 3.27 Contents of the cubital fossa. The aponeurosis of biceps brachii and deep fascia have been removed.

imaginary line drawn between the two humeral epicondyles. The roof is formed by deep fascia, reinforced by the aponeurosis of biceps (Fig. 3.26). The subcutaneous tissue overlying the roof contains branches of the lateral and medial cutaneous nerves of forearm and superficial veins such as the median cubital vein, which links the cephalic and basilic veins (Fig. 3.25). The arrangement of these superficial veins may vary considerably between individuals.

The fossa is traversed by nerves and vessels passing between the arm and the forearm. Its contents (Figs 3.27 & 3.29), embedded in fatty connective tissue, are, from medial to lateral, the median nerve, the brachial artery and its venae comitantes, the tendon of biceps and the radial nerve.

Distally the terminal branches of the radial nerve, the superficial and deep radial (posterior interosseous) nerves, and the terminal branches of the brachial artery (namely the radial and ulnar arteries) also lie within the fossa. The floor of the cubital fossa (Fig. 3.29) is formed by supinator and brachialis overlying the capsule of the elbow joint.

Fig. 3.28 Boundaries of the cubital fossa after removal of the roof and contents.

Fig. 3.29 Brachioradialis and pronator teres have been retracted to reveal the floor of the cubital fossa and expose the radial nerve.

ANTERIOR COMPARTMENT OF FOREARM

The anterior compartment of the forearm contains a superficial and a deep group of muscles, which include flexors of the wrist, fingers and thumb, and two muscles that act as pronators. The compartment is traversed by the median and ulnar nerves and by the radial and ulnar arteries with their venae comitantes. A layer of deep fascia continuous with a similar layer on the posterior aspect of the limb encloses the compartment and provides additional attachment for the superficial muscles. In front of the carpus, deep fascia forms the flexor retinaculum (Fig. 3.30), which lies anterior to tendons in the carpal tunnel (see page 119). Subcutaneous tissue overlying the compartment contains cutaneous nerves and tributaries of the cephalic and basilic veins.

Superficial muscles

The superficial muscles are, from lateral to medial, pronator teres, flexor carpi radialis, palmaris longus and flexor carpi ulnaris (Fig. 3.31). Flexor digitorum superficialis is also included in this group but is partly covered by the other muscles.

All the superficial muscles attach proximally to the common flexor origin on the front of the medial epicondyle of the humerus (see Fig. 3.34). In addition, pronator teres attaches to the medial side of the coronoid process of the ulna and flexor carpi ulnaris attaches to the medial border of the olecranon and the adjacent part of the subcutaneous border of the ulna. Flexor digitorum superficialis has an additional attachment to the ulnar collateral ligament of the elbow, the coronoid process and the anterior oblique line of the radius.

Distally pronator teres attaches half-way along the lateral aspect of the shaft of the radius and forms the medial border of the cubital fossa. The muscle pronates the forearm. Flexor carpi radialis attaches to the bases of the second and third metacarpal bones (see Fig. 3.37). It is a flexor and abductor of the wrist joint. Palmaris longus, a vestigial muscle that may be absent, has a long thin tendon, which attaches to the palmar aponeurosis. The muscle is a weak flexor of the wrist joint. Flexor carpi ulnaris attaches distally to the pisiform and, via ligaments from the pisiform, to the hook of the hamate and the base of the fifth metacarpal. It is the most medial of the superficial muscles and is a flexor and adductor of the wrist.

Flexor digitorum superficialis (Fig. 3.32) is relatively large and is the deepest of this group of muscles. Distally it gives rise to four tendons, one for each finger, which pass into the hand deep to the flexor retinaculum. In the carpal tunnel the

radial artery

flexor digitorum superficialis

median nerve

ulnar nerve

flexor retinaculum

flexor digitorum superficialis tendons

fibrous flexor sheath

Fig. 3.30 Flexor retinaculum revealed by removal of subcutaneous tissue and most of the deep fascia. The retinaculum is partly obscured by some of the intrinsic muscles of the hand.

pronator teres

flexor carpi radialis

brachioradialis

flexor carpi ulnaris

extensor carpi radialis longus

radial artery

flexor digitorum superficialis

abductor pollicis longus (cut)

ulnar nerve

median nerve

Fig. 3.31 Flexor carpi radialis and flexor carpi ulnaris seen after removal of deep fascia and the flexor retinaculum. This specimen lacks palmaris longus.

tendons have a characteristic grouping (Fig. 3.32). Within each finger the tendon forms two slips, which pass around the

profundus tendon and then partly reunite before attaching to the sides of the middle phalanx (see Fig. 3.37). The muscle flexes

PALM AND DIGITS

The hand comprises the wrist (carpus), the palm (metacarpus) and the digits (Figs 3.37 & 3.38). The palm of the hand (Fig. 3.39) contains the palmar aponeurosis,

intrinsic muscles, tendons originating from muscles in the anterior compartment of the forearm, and palmar vessels and nerves. The intrinsic muscles comprise the thenar and hypothenar groups, the lumbricals and interossei, and adductor pollicis. The tendons enter the palm

through the carpal tunnel (see Fig. 3.98) deep to the flexor retinaculum. The skin of the anterior surface of the hand is thick, devoid of hair and contains many sweat glands. It is firmly bound to the underlying deep fascia, producing characteristic creases.

the wrist and the metacarpophalangeal and proximal interphalangeal joints of the fingers.

The superficial muscles all pass anterior to the elbow and therefore act as weak flexors of that joint in addition to their roles in the movements of the wrist and hand. Collectively the carpal flexors and extensors stabilize the wrist joint during movements of the fingers and thumb.

All the superficial muscles are innervated by the median nerve, except flexor carpi ulnaris, which is supplied by the ulnar nerve.

Deep muscles

The deep muscles are flexor pollicis longus, flexor digitorum profundus and pronator quadratus. Their attachments to

the radius and ulna are illustrated in Fig. 3.34. Distally the flexor pollicis longus tendon (see Fig. 3.35) passes through the carpal tunnel and attaches to the base of the distal phalanx of the thumb. The muscle flexes the interphalangeal and metacarpophalangeal joints of the thumb. Flexor digitorum profundus (see Fig. 3.35) gives rise to four tendons, which traverse the carpal tunnel deep to the tendons of flexor digitorum superficialis (see Fig. 3.40). In the palm the tendons diverge, one entering each finger. Each tendon passes between the slips of the corresponding superficialis tendon, continuing distally to attach to the base of the terminal phalanx. The muscle is a flexor of the fingers and of the wrist joint. Pronator quadratus, a small rectangular muscle lying transversely between the anterior surfaces of the shafts of the radius and ulna (Fig. 3.33), pronates the forearm.

The deep muscles are innervated by the anterior interosseous nerve, except for the medial part of flexor digitorum profundus, which is supplied by the ulnar nerve.

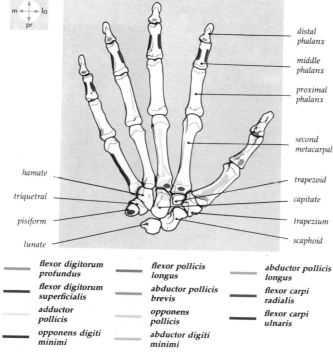

Fig. 3.37 Bones of the hand. The distal attachments of the forearm flexor muscles and of the thenar and hypothenar muscles and the attachments of adductor pollicis are indicated.

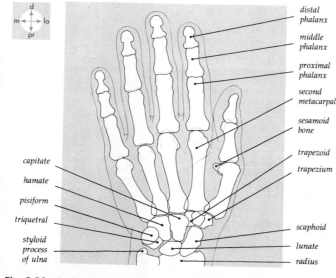

Fig. 3.38 Radiograph of an adult hand.

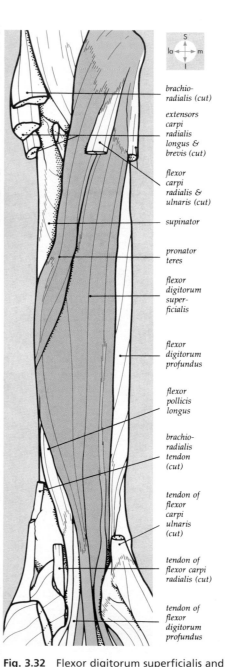

Fig. 3.32 Flexor digitorum superficialis and pronator teres revealed by division of flexors carpi ulnaris and radialis, and of brachioradialis. The vessels and nerves in the forearm have been removed.

Fig. 3.33 Pronator quadratus exposed by division of flexor pollicis longus and flexor digitorum profundus.

Vessels

The brachial artery usually divides into the radial and ulnar arteries in the cubital fossa

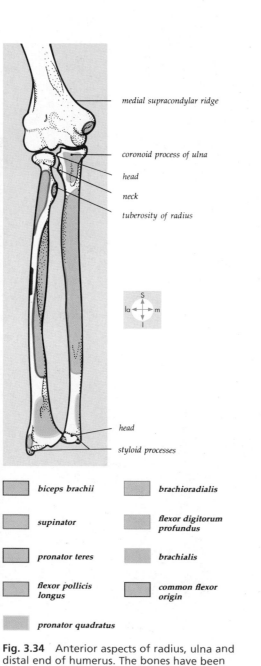

(Fig. 3.36). The radial artery passes distally, under brachioradialis, lying on the flexor muscles. In the lower forearm the vessel is accompanied by the superficial branch of the radial nerve and, near the wrist, is subcutaneous and palpable against the anterior surface of the radius. The artery winds round the lateral aspect of the wrist, traverses the 'anatomical snuff box' and subsequently enters the palm to form the deep palmar arch (see Fig. 3.54). In the forearm the artery gives branches to muscles and contributes to anastomoses around the elbow and wrist joints.

The ulnar artery passes deep to the arch formed by the radial and ulnar attachments of flexor digitorum superficialis and continues between the superficial and deep flexor muscles. In the distal part of the forearm the artery is joined on its medial side by the ulnar nerve. It lies beneath flexor carpi ulnaris but at the wrist emerges

to lie lateral to the tendon of this muscle. The ulnar artery crosses superficial to the flexor retinaculum and, as it enters the hand, divides into superficial and deep palmar branches. The ulnar artery gives branches to the muscles of the anterior compartment and to the anastomoses around the elbow and wrist joints. Its largest branch, the common interosseous

medial supracondylar ridge

coronoid process of ulna

head

neck

tuberosity of radius

head

styloid processes

biceps brachii		*brachioradialis*
supinator		*flexor digitorum profundus*
pronator teres		*brachialis*
flexor pollicis longus		*common flexor origin*
pronator quadratus		

Fig. 3.34 Anterior aspects of radius, ulna and distal end of humerus. The bones have been separated slightly.

artery (Fig. 3.36), arises near the origin of the ulnar artery and promptly divides into posterior and anterior interosseous branches. The posterior interosseous artery enters the posterior compartment of the forearm (see Fig. 3.77). The larger anterior interosseous artery passes distally in the anterior compartment, lying on the interosseous membrane, accompanied by the anterior interosseous nerve. The vessel supplies the deep flexor muscles and gives nutrient branches to the radius and ulna. Distally it penetrates the interosseous membrane to assist in the anastomoses around the wrist.

Venae comitantes accompany the arteries of the anterior compartment and drain proximally into veins around the brachial artery.

Nerves

The median nerve enters the forearm from the cubital fossa between the two heads of pronator teres. It crosses anterior to the ulnar artery (Fig. 3.36) and descends between the superficial and deep flexors. At the wrist the median nerve is remarkably superficial, lying medial to the tendon of flexor carpi radialis and just deep to the palmaris longus tendon. The median nerve

fused tendons of superficial flexors (cut)

brachioradialis (cut)

tendon of biceps brachii (cut)

supinator

flexor pollicis longus

flexor digitorum profundus

tendon of brachioradialis (cut)

tendon of flexor carpi ulnaris (cut)

tendon of flexor carpi radialis (cut)

lumbricals

tendons of flexor digitorum superficialis (cut)

Fig. 3.35 Flexor digitorum profundus and flexor pollicis longus exposed by removal of the superficial flexors. As in this specimen, the index component of flexor digitorum profundus is often separate from the rest of the muscle.

passes through the carpal tunnel into the hand, where it divides into terminal branches (see Fig. 3.52). The nerve supplies all the superficial muscles of the anterior compartment except flexor carpi ulnaris. The anterior interosseous branch of the median nerve (Fig. 3.36) supplies all the deep muscles of the compartment except the medial part of flexor digitorum

profundus. This branch lies between flexor digitorum profundus and flexor pollicis longus and passes behind pronator quadratus to supply the wrist. In the forearm the median nerve also gives a palmar cutaneous branch, which crosses superficial to the flexor retinaculum and supplies skin of the lateral part of the palm.

The ulnar nerve passes behind the medial epicondyle and enters the forearm between the two heads of flexor carpi ulnaris. Lying on flexor digitorum profundus and covered by flexor carpi ulnaris, it traverses the medial side of the anterior compartment, accompanied in the lower part of the forearm by the ulnar artery. Near the wrist the ulnar nerve emerges lateral to the flexor carpi ulnaris tendon and crosses superficial to the flexor retinaculum with the ulnar artery on its lateral side. The nerve terminates in the hand by dividing into superficial and deep branches (see page 92). The ulnar nerve supplies the elbow joint and gives branches to flexor carpi ulnaris and the medial part of flexor digitorum profundus. It also provides a palmar cutaneous nerve supplying skin on the medial aspect of the palm, and dorsal cutaneous branches that innervate the medial part of the dorsum of the hand (see Fig. 3.78).

brachial artery & vena comitans

radial nerve

median nerve

deep head of pronator teres

common interosseous artery

posterior interosseous artery

anterior interosseous nerve

anterior interosseous artery

ulnar nerve

ulnar artery

radial artery

median ne

superfici

flexor super

flex r

Fig. 3.36 Vessels an compartment of the flexor muscles and divided and most have been remov the wrist and the metacarpophalangeal and proximal interphalangeal joints of the fingers.

The superficial muscles all pass anterior to the elbow and therefore act as weak flexors of that joint in addition to their roles in the movements of the wrist and hand. Collectively the carpal flexors and extensors stabilize the wrist joint during movements of the fingers and thumb.

All the superficial muscles are innervated by the median nerve, except flexor carpi ulnaris, which is supplied by the ulnar nerve.

Deep muscles

The deep muscles are flexor pollicis longus, flexor digitorum profundus and pronator quadratus. Their attachments to the radius and ulna are illustrated in Fig. 3.34. Distally the flexor pollicis longus tendon (see Fig. 3.35) passes through the carpal tunnel and attaches to the base of the distal phalanx of the thumb. The muscle flexes the interphalangeal and metacarpophalangeal joints of the thumb. Flexor digitorum profundus (see Fig. 3.35) gives rise to four tendons, which traverse the carpal tunnel deep to the tendons of flexor digitorum superficialis (see Fig. 3.40). In the palm the tendons diverge, one entering each finger. Each tendon passes between the slips of the corresponding superficialis tendon, continuing distally to attach to the base of the terminal phalanx. The muscle is a flexor of the fingers and of the wrist joint. Pronator quadratus, a small rectangular muscle lying transversely between the anterior surfaces of the shafts of the radius and ulna (Fig. 3.33), pronates the forearm.

The deep muscles are innervated by the anterior interosseous nerve, except for the medial part of flexor digitorum profundus, which is supplied by the ulnar nerve.

brachio-radialis (cut)

extensors carpi radialis longus & brevis (cut)

flexor carpi radialis & ulnaris (cut)

supinator

pronator teres

flexor digitorum super-ficialis

flexor digitorum profundus

flexor pollicis longus

brachio-radialis tendon (cut)

tendon of flexor carpi ulnaris (cut)

tendon of flexor carpi radialis (cut)

tendon of flexor digitorum profundus

Fig. 3.32 Flexor digitorum superficialis and pronator teres revealed by division of flexors carpi ulnaris and radialis, and of brachioradialis. The vessels and nerves in the forearm have been removed.

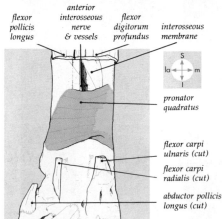

flexor pollicis longus

anterior interosseous nerve & vessels

flexor digitorum profundus

interosseous membrane

pronator quadratus

flexor carpi ulnaris (cut)

flexor carpi radialis (cut)

abductor pollicis longus (cut)

Fig. 3.33 Pronator quadratus exposed by division of flexor pollicis longus and flexor digitorum profundus.

Vessels

The brachial artery usually divides into the radial and ulnar arteries in the cubital fossa (Fig. 3.36). The radial artery passes distally, under brachioradialis, lying on the flexor muscles. In the lower forearm the vessel is accompanied by the superficial branch of the radial nerve and, near the wrist, is subcutaneous and palpable against the anterior surface of the radius. The artery winds round the lateral aspect of the wrist, traverses the 'anatomical snuff box' and subsequently enters the palm to form the deep palmar arch (see Fig. 3.54). In the forearm the artery gives branches to muscles and contributes to anastomoses around the elbow and wrist joints.

The ulnar artery passes deep to the arch formed by the radial and ulnar attachments of flexor digitorum superficialis and continues between the superficial and deep flexor muscles. In the distal part of the forearm the artery is joined on its medial side by the ulnar nerve. It lies beneath flexor carpi ulnaris but at the wrist emerges to lie lateral to the tendon of this muscle. The ulnar artery crosses superficial to the flexor retinaculum and, as it enters the hand, divides into superficial and deep palmar branches. The ulnar artery gives branches to the muscles of the anterior compartment and to the anastomoses around the elbow and wrist joints. Its largest branch, the common interosseous

medial supracondylar ridge

coronoid process of ulna

head

neck

tuberosity of radius

head

styloid processes

biceps brachii		**brachioradialis**
supinator		**flexor digitorum profundus**
pronator teres		**brachialis**
flexor pollicis longus		**common flexor origin**
pronator quadratus		

Fig. 3.34 Anterior aspects of radius, ulna and distal end of humerus. The bones have been separated slightly.

artery (Fig. 3.36), arises near the origin of the ulnar artery and promptly divides into posterior and anterior interosseous branches. The posterior interosseous artery enters the posterior compartment of the forearm (see Fig. 3.77). The larger anterior interosseous artery passes distally in the anterior compartment, lying on the interosseous membrane, accompanied by the anterior interosseous nerve. The vessel supplies the deep flexor muscles and gives nutrient branches to the radius and ulna. Distally it penetrates the interosseous membrane to assist in the anastomoses around the wrist.

Venae comitantes accompany the arteries of the anterior compartment and drain proximally into veins around the brachial artery.

Nerves

The median nerve enters the forearm from the cubital fossa between the two heads of pronator teres. It crosses anterior to the ulnar artery (Fig. 3.36) and descends between the superficial and deep flexors. At the wrist the median nerve is remarkably superficial, lying medial to the tendon of flexor carpi radialis and just deep to the palmaris longus tendon. The median nerve

passes through the carpal tunnel into the hand, where it divides into terminal branches (see Fig. 3.52). The nerve supplies all the superficial muscles of the anterior compartment except flexor carpi ulnaris. The anterior interosseous branch of the median nerve (Fig. 3.36) supplies all the deep muscles of the compartment except the medial part of flexor digitorum

profundus. This branch lies between flexor digitorum profundus and flexor pollicis longus and passes behind pronator quadratus to supply the wrist. In the forearm the median nerve also gives a palmar cutaneous branch, which crosses superficial to the flexor retinaculum and supplies skin of the lateral part of the palm.

The ulnar nerve passes behind the medial epicondyle and enters the forearm between the two heads of flexor carpi ulnaris. Lying on flexor digitorum profundus and covered by flexor carpi ulnaris, it traverses the medial side of the anterior compartment, accompanied in the lower part of the forearm by the ulnar artery. Near the wrist the ulnar nerve emerges lateral to the flexor carpi ulnaris tendon and crosses superficial to the flexor retinaculum with the ulnar artery on its lateral side. The nerve terminates in the hand by dividing into superficial and deep branches (see page 92). The ulnar nerve supplies the elbow joint and gives branches to flexor carpi ulnaris and the medial part of flexor digitorum profundus. It also provides a palmar cutaneous nerve supplying skin on the medial aspect of the palm, and dorsal cutaneous branches that innervate the medial part of the dorsum of the hand (see Fig. 3.78).

fused tendons
of superficial
flexors (cut)

brachioradialis
(cut)

tendon of
biceps brachii (cut)

supinator

flexor pollicis
longus

flexor digitorum
profundus

tendon of
brachioradialis
(cut)

tendon of flexor
carpi ulnaris (cut)

tendon of
flexor carpi
radialis (cut)

lumbricals

tendons of flexor
digitorum
superficialis
(cut)

Fig. 3.35   Flexor digitorum profundus and flexor pollicis longus exposed by removal of the superficial flexors. As in this specimen, the index component of flexor digitorum profundus is often separate from the rest of the muscle.

brachial artery
& vena comitans

radial nerve

median nerve

deep head of
pronator teres

common
interosseous artery

posterior
interosseous artery

anterior
interosseous nerve

anterior
interosseous artery

ulnar nerve

ulnar artery

radial artery

median nerve

superficial radial nerve

flexor digitorum
superficialis tendons (cut)

flexor carpi
radialis tendon (cut)

flexor retinaculum

Fig. 3.36   Vessels and nerves of the anterior compartment of the forearm. The superficial flexor muscles and brachioradialis have been divided and most of the venae comitantes have been removed.

PALM AND DIGITS

The hand comprises the wrist (carpus), the palm (metacarpus) and the digits (Figs 3.37 & 3.38). The palm of the hand (Fig. 3.39) contains the palmar aponeurosis, intrinsic muscles, tendons originating from muscles in the anterior compartment of the forearm, and palmar vessels and nerves. The intrinsic muscles comprise the thenar and hypothenar groups, the lumbricals and interossei, and adductor pollicis. The tendons enter the palm through the carpal tunnel (see Fig. 3.98) deep to the flexor retinaculum. The skin of the anterior surface of the hand is thick, devoid of hair and contains many sweat glands. It is firmly bound to the underlying deep fascia, producing characteristic creases.

flexor digitorum profundus	flexor pollicis longus	abductor pollicis longus
flexor digitorum superficialis	abductor pollicis brevis	flexor carpi radialis
adductor pollicis	opponens pollicis	flexor carpi ulnaris
opponens digiti minimi	abductor digiti minimi	

Fig. 3.37 Bones of the hand. The distal attachments of the forearm flexor muscles and of the thenar and hypothenar muscles and the attachments of adductor pollicis are indicated.

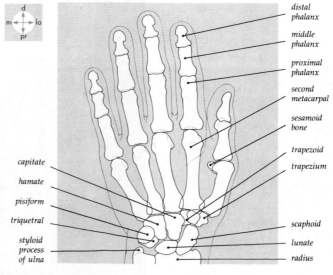

Fig. 3.38 Radiograph of an adult hand.

Deep fascia of palm

The deep fascia of the palm is thickened centrally to form the triangular palmar aponeurosis (Fig. 3.39) and is thinner at each side where it covers the thenar and hypothenar muscles. Proximally the palmar aponeurosis attaches to the flexor retinaculum and is continuous with the tendon of palmaris longus. Distally the aponeurosis gives rise to four pairs of digital slips, which cross the metacarpophalangeal joints and attach to the proximal phalanges of the fingers via the fibrous flexor sheaths. The aponeurosis covers the superficial palmar arch, the median nerve and the tendons of the long flexors of the digits.

Lateral and medial septa pass from the edges of the palmar aponeurosis to the first and fifth metacarpal bones respectively. These septa separate the thenar and hypothenar muscles from a 'central palmar space', which is traversed by the palmar digital vessels and nerves and by the tendons of the long flexor muscles of the fingers.

Fig. 3.39 Palmar aponeurosis exposed by removal of skin and subcutaneous tissue.

Fig. 3.40 Tendons of flexor digitorum superficialis in the palm. The palmar aponeurosis, flexor retinaculum and palmar vessels and nerves have been removed.

The subcutaneous tissue of the medial side of the palm usually contains palmaris brevis (see Fig. 3.39), a small muscle attaching to the overlying skin and to the palmar aponeurosis.

Flexor tendons in the hand

The tendons of flexor pollicis longus, flexor digitorum profundus and flexor digitorum superficialis enter the hand deep to the flexor retinaculum (see Fig. 3.99). On reaching the appropriate digit each tendon traverses a tunnel formed by the fibrous flexor sheath and the phalanges (see Fig. 3.40). The fibrous sheath is attached to the edges of the anterior surfaces of the phalanges (Fig. 3.41) and continues as far as the distal phalanx (Fig. 3.42). The sheath is thinner and more flexible in front of the interphalangeal joints, allowing flexion of the digit without 'bowstringing' of the tendons and thus facilitating gripping. Within the flexor sheaths the tendons are invested by synovial membrane and receive vincula tendinum, small folds of synovium that convey blood vessels to the tendons.

Fig. 3.41   Transverse section through the index finger at the level of the proximal phalanx.

Fig. 3.42   Digital fibrous flexor sheaths. The partially cut away sheath of the middle finger exposes the tendons of flexor digitorum superficialis and profundus, whose phalangeal attachments are revealed on the ring and little fingers.

Thenar muscles

Abductor pollicis brevis, flexor pollicis brevis and opponens pollicis form the thenar eminence on the lateral side of the palm. They attach proximally to the trapezium and scaphoid and to the lateral part of the flexor retinaculum (see Fig. 3.37).

Abductor pollicis brevis (Fig. 3.43) lies superficial to the other thenar muscles and passes from the scaphoid to the base of the proximal phalanx of the thumb. The muscle abducts the thumb, moving the digit anteriorly at right angles to the plane of the palm.

Flexor pollicis brevis, lying deep and medial to the abductor, passes from the trapezium to the proximal phalanx of the thumb. The muscle flexes the carpometacarpal and metacarpophalangeal joints, drawing the thumb across the palm (maintaining the thumbnail at right angles to the palmar plane).

Opponens pollicis (Fig. 3.44), the deepest of the thenar muscles, attaches proximally to the trapezium and distally to the shaft of the first metacarpal. The muscle produces opposition of the thumb, allowing pulp-to-pulp contact with the fingers. This movement combines flexion, adduction and rotation of the first metacarpal at its carpometacarpal joint.

The thenar muscles are supplied by the recurrent branch of the median nerve (Figs 3.43 & 3.44).

Fig. 3.43 Muscles of the thenar eminence exposed by removal of deep fascia. Abductor pollicis brevis is superficial to flexor pollicis brevis and opponens pollicis.

Fig. 3.44 Opponens pollicis and flexor pollicis brevis exposed by removal of abductor pollicis brevis.

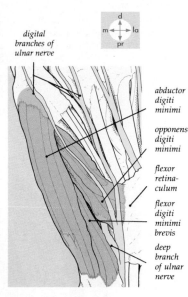

Fig. 3.45 Hypothenar muscles exposed by removal of the deep fascia.

Hypothenar muscles

Abductor digiti minimi, flexor digiti minimi brevis and opponens digiti minimi (Fig. 3.45) form the hypothenar eminence and attach proximally to the pisiform, the hook of the hamate and the adjacent part of the flexor retinaculum. Abductor digiti minimi passes from the pisiform to the base of the proximal phalanx of the little finger and abducts the digit, moving it medially in the plane of the palm. Flexor digiti minimi brevis attaches between the hamate and base of the proximal phalanx of the little finger and flexes the metacarpal and proximal phalanx of the little finger. Opponens digiti minimi passes from the hamate to the shaft of the fifth metacarpal and on contraction deepens the hollow of the palm.

The hypothenar muscles are supplied by the deep branch of the ulnar nerve (Fig. 3.45).

Deep muscles

The deep muscles of the hand consist of adductor pollicis, the palmar and dorsal interossei, and the lumbricals.

Adductor pollicis (Fig. 3.46) has transverse and oblique heads. The transverse head attaches to the shaft of the third metacarpal bone, and the oblique head to the trapezoid, capitate and bases of the second and third metacarpals. Both heads pass laterally to attach to the base of the proximal phalanx of the thumb by a common tendon which usually contains a sesamoid bone. The muscle adducts and flexes the thumb at its carpometacarpal and metacarpophalangeal joints and is supplied by the deep branch of the ulnar nerve (see Fig. 3.54).

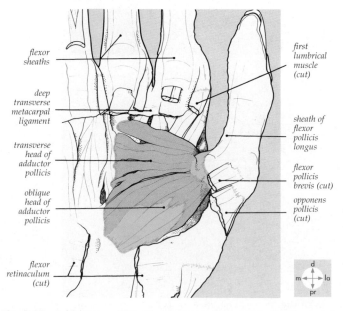

Fig. 3.46 Adductor pollicis. The muscles of the thenar eminence, long flexor tendons, and palmar and digital vessels and nerves have been removed.

The interossei consist of three palmar and four dorsal muscles (Fig. 3.47). Each palmar interosseous muscle (Fig. 3.48) arises by a single head from the anterior border of the shaft of the second, fourth or fifth metacarpal. Each dorsal interosseous muscle (see Fig. 3.49) arises by two heads from the contiguous sides of the shafts of the adjacent metacarpals. Distally the tendon of each interosseous muscle attaches to the base of the proximal phalanx and to the extensor expansion of

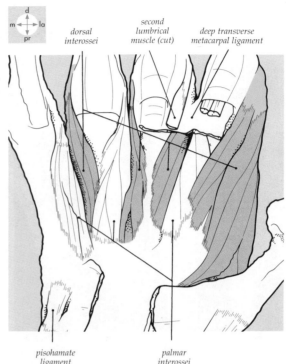

Fig. 3.47 Palmar and dorsal interossei exposed by removal of the long flexor tendons and adductor pollicis. The dorsal interossei have much more bulk than the palmar interossei.

Fig. 3.48 Palmar interossei. The dorsal interossei and deep transverse metacarpal ligaments have been excised.

the appropriate digit (Fig. 3.51). The interossei move the fingers in the plane of the palm (coronal plane); movement of a finger away from the long axis of the middle finger is called abduction while movement towards the middle finger is adduction. The palmar interossei adduct and the dorsal interossei abduct the fingers. In addition, the interossei flex the metacarpophalangeal joints and extend the interphalangeal joints. All the interossei are supplied by the deep branch of the ulnar nerve (see Fig. 3.54).

The lumbricals are four small muscles attaching proximally to the tendons of flexor digitorum profundus (Fig. 3.50). Distally each lumbrical attaches to the radial side of the extensor expansion of the appropriate finger. The muscles extend the interphalangeal joints and flex the metacarpophalangeal joints. The first and second lumbricals usually have only one head each and are supplied by the median nerve whereas the third and fourth (medial) usually have two heads and are supplied by the ulnar nerve.

Digital extensor expansions

Each finger possesses an extensor expansion or hood (Fig. 3.51) which receives the tendons of the appropriate long extensor muscle(s), interossei and lumbricals. The broad proximal part of the expansion overlies the metacarpophalangeal joint. Distally the expansion tapers and attaches by a central slip to the base of the middle phalanx and by two marginal slips to the base of the distal phalanx.

Fig. 3.49 Dorsal interossei exposed by removal of deep fascia and tendons of extensor digitorum.

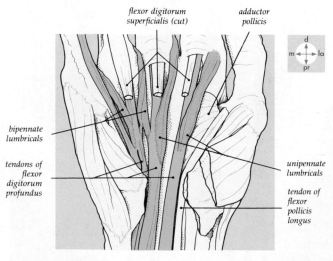

Fig. 3.50 Removal of the tendons of flexor digitorum superficialis has revealed the attachments of the lumbrical muscles to the tendons of flexor digitorum profundus.

Blood vessels

The arterial supply to the hand is derived from branches of the ulnar and radial arteries, which form superficial and deep palmar arches linking the two main arteries and ensuring a rich blood supply to the palm and fingers.

The ulnar artery enters the hand superficial to the flexor retinaculum and gives a deep branch that accompanies the deep branch of the ulnar nerve. The main artery continues as the superficial palmar arch (Fig. 3.52), which passes distally to the level of the thumb web, lying deep to the palmar aponeurosis but anterior to the digital nerves and flexor tendons. The superficial palmar arch gives four palmar digital branches, which supply the adjacent sides of the fingers (see Fig. 3.53) and medial side of the little finger, and is completed laterally by a branch of the radial artery.

The radial artery enters the palm from the dorsum of the hand between the two heads of the first dorsal interosseous muscle (Fig. 3.49). The artery gives branches to the thumb and index finger and continues as the deep palmar arch (see Fig. 3.54), which lies over the bases of the metacarpal bones, deep to the flexor tendons, and is about 1 cm proximal to the superficial arch. The deep arch provides perforating branches, which anastomose with dorsal metacarpal arteries, and three palmar metacarpal arteries, which anastomose with the palmar digital arteries of the superficial arch. The deep arch is completed medially by the deep branch of the ulnar artery. Other vessels such as dorsal metacarpal arteries from the dorsal carpal arch may provide an important supply of blood to the hand.

Most venous blood from the fingers and palm drains into superficial veins on the dorsum of the hand to enter the cephalic or basilic veins.

second lumbrical muscle (cut)

distal phalanx

attachment to distal phalanx

capsules of interphalan- geal joints

attachment to middle phalanx

second dorsal interosseous muscle (cut)

tendon of extensor digitorum

third dorsal interosseous muscle (cut)

Fig. 3.51 Dorsal view of the digital expansion of the middle finger. The expansion has been flattened proximally to show the attachments of lumbrical and interosseous muscles.

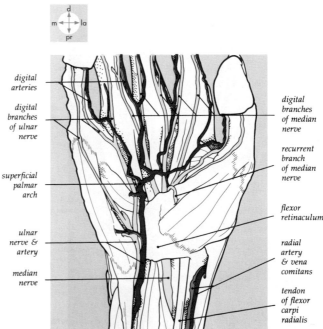

digital arteries

digital branches of ulnar nerve

superficial palmar arch

ulnar nerve & artery

median nerve

digital branches of median nerve

recurrent branch of median nerve

flexor retinaculum

radial artery & vena comitans

tendon of flexor carpi radialis

Fig. 3.52 Superficial vessels and nerves of the palm. Skin, subcutaneous tissue and the palmar aponeurosis have been removed.

the remainder of the medial border of the scapula and the spines of the second to fifth thoracic vertebrae.

All three muscles elevate the scapula and assist in scapular rotation during adduction of the upper limb. The dorsal scapular nerve from the brachial plexus, (C5), supplies the rhomboids and may innervate levator scapulae which is also supplied by branches from the cervical plexus (C3 & C4).

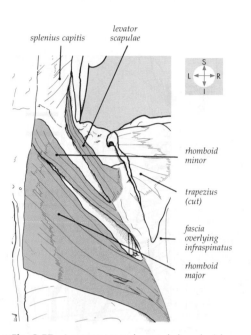

Fig. 3.57 Levator scapulae and rhomboids exposed by removal of trapezius.

Latissimus dorsi

Latissimus dorsi (Fig. 3.58) is a large triangular muscle overlying much of the dorsal aspect of the trunk. The muscle attaches to the spinous processes of the lower six thoracic vertebrae and through the lumbar fascia to the spines of the lumbar vertebrae and the sacrum. The most inferior fibres attach to the posterior part of the iliac crest. Fibres also attach to the lower four ribs and to the inferior angle of the scapula. All the fibres converge on a narrow tendon in the posterior fold of the axilla. The tendon winds round the lower border of teres major to attach to the intertubercular sulcus of the humerus.

The muscle is a powerful adductor and extensor of the humerus at the shoulder joint, particularly when the upper limb is abducted and flexed. Latissimus dorsi is also a medial rotator at the shoulder joint and assists with rotation and retraction of the scapula. In movements such as rising from an armchair, if the humerus is fixed, both muscles contract to raise the trunk. This action is particularly important in patients with paralysed lower limbs. Latissimus dorsi is supplied by a single neurovascular bundle which contains the thoracodorsal nerve (a branch of the posterior cord of the brachial plexus; see Fig. 3.18) and the thoracodorsal vessels, which are branches of the subscapular vessels. In reconstructive surgery, the muscle and its overlying skin may be mobilized on this neurovascular pedicle to provide a large myocutaneous flap.

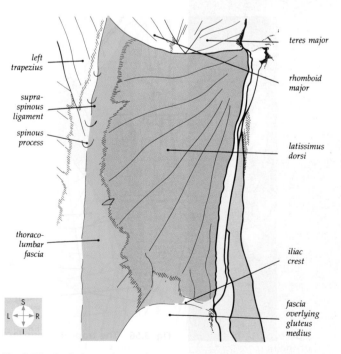

Fig. 3.58 Latissimus dorsi. The anterior border lies parallel to the cut skin edge and the thoracic attachment has been exposed by removal of trapezius.

SHORT SCAPULAR MUSCLES

These short muscles, the four rotator cuff muscles and teres major, span the shoulder (glenohumeral) joint, attaching to the scapula and to the proximal part of the humerus (Fig. 3.59 and see Fig. 3.62).

Rotator cuff muscles

This important group of muscles, namely subscapularis, supraspinatus, infraspinatus and teres minor, is intimately related to the shoulder joint. By attaching not only to the tubercles of the humerus but also to the capsule of the joint they hold the humeral head firmly in the glenoid fossa and help stabilize the joint.

Subscapularis

Subscapularis (Fig. 3.60) attaches proximally to the medial part of the costal surface of the scapula. Its tendon, separated from the neck of the scapula by the subscapular bursa, is attached to the lesser tubercle of the humerus. The muscle is supplied by the subscapular nerves from the posterior cord of the brachial plexus. Subscapularis produces medial rotation of the arm at the shoulder joint.

superior angle

acromion

suprascapular notch

coracoid process

medial border

inferior angle

subscapularis

serratus anterior

pectoralis minor

biceps brachii and coracobrachialis

latissimus dorsi

teres major

Fig. 3.59 Anterior aspects of scapula and proximal end of humerus. The head of the humerus is partly obscured by the overlying coracoid process of the scapula.

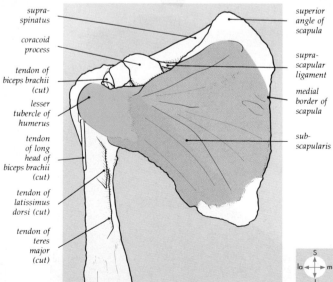

supra-spinatus

coracoid process

tendon of biceps brachii (cut)

lesser tubercle of humerus

tendon of long head of biceps brachii (cut)

tendon of latissimus dorsi (cut)

tendon of teres major (cut)

superior angle of scapula

supra-scapular ligament

medial border of scapula

sub-scapularis

Fig. 3.60 Anterior view of subscapularis. The attachment of serratus anterior to the medial border of the scapula has been excised.

POSTERIOR COMPARTMENT OF ARM

The posterior compartment of the arm contains triceps brachii, the radial nerve accompanied by the profunda brachii artery with its venae comitantes, and the ulnar nerve.

Triceps brachii

Proximally this muscle attaches to the scapula and the humerus by three heads. The tendon of the long head (Fig. 3.65) attaches to the infraglenoid tubercle of the scapula, and the lateral head attaches to the posterior aspect of the shaft of the humerus above the radial groove (spiral groove, sulcus of the radial nerve) (Fig. 3.67). Both the long and lateral heads lie superficial to the medial head (Fig. 3.66), which has an extensive origin from the lateral and medial intermuscular septa and from the shaft of the humerus below the radial groove. Distally the three heads fuse and triceps attaches by a single tendon to the olecranon process of the ulna. Frequently a bursa lies deep to the tendon, separating it from the capsule of the elbow joint. The three heads are supplied separately by branches of the radial nerve. Triceps is a powerful extensor of the elbow joint. The long head alone spans the shoulder joint and may assist in stabilizing that joint, particularly in full abduction.

Vessels and nerves

Radial nerve

The radial nerve, a terminal branch of the posterior cord, leaves the axilla by passing below teres major and between the humerus and the long head of triceps (see Fig. 3.64). In the posterior compartment the nerve passes between the medial and lateral heads of triceps and in the radial groove is intimately related to the shaft of the humerus (Fig. 3.68). It then leaves the posterior compartment by piercing the lateral intermuscular septum to reach the lateral part of the cubital fossa in front of the elbow joint (see Fig. 3.29). In the arm the radial nerve gives muscular branches to the medial and lateral heads of triceps and to brachioradialis and extensor carpi radialis longus, and cutaneous branches to the lateral aspect of the arm and the posterior aspect of the forearm. The branch to the long head of triceps usually arises in the axilla.

Profunda brachii artery

The profunda brachii artery, a proximal branch of the brachial artery (see Fig. 3.18), supplies the posterior compartment and accompanies the radial nerve in the radial groove of the humerus (Fig. 3.68). It gives muscular branches and contributes to the

anastomosis around the elbow joint. The venae comitantes of the profunda brachii artery drain into the axillary vein.

Ulnar nerve

The ulnar nerve passes from the anterior to the posterior compartment by piercing the

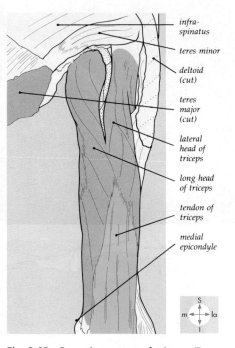

Fig. 3.65 Posterior aspect of triceps. Teres major and the posterior fibres of deltoid have been excised.

infra-spinatus
teres minor
deltoid (cut)
teres major (cut)
lateral head of triceps
long head of triceps
tendon of triceps
medial epicondyle

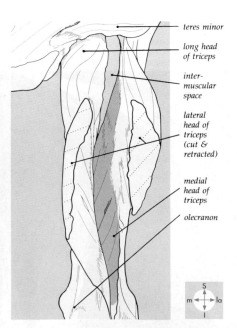

Fig. 3.66 The medial head of triceps has been exposed by removal of deltoid and division and retraction of the lateral head.

teres minor
long head of triceps
inter-muscular space
lateral head of triceps (cut & retracted)
medial head of triceps
olecranon

medial intermuscular septum at about midarm level (see Fig. 3.24), and descends between the septum and the medial head of triceps. At the elbow it passes posterior to the medial epicondyle of the humerus, medial to the joint, and enters the forearm between the humeral and ulnar heads of flexor carpi ulnaris. The nerve gives no branches in the arm.

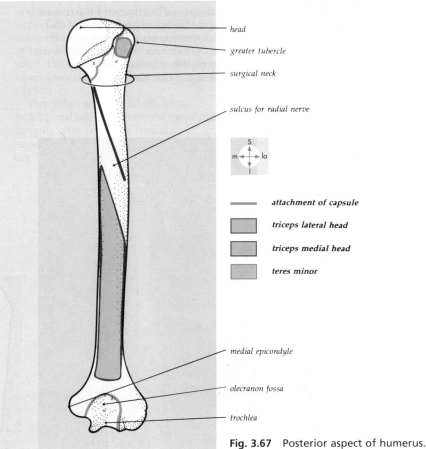

head

greater tubercle

surgical neck

sulcus for radial nerve

attachment of capsule

triceps lateral head

triceps medial head

teres minor

medial epicondyle

olecranon fossa

trochlea

Fig. 3.67 Posterior aspect of humerus.

teres major

tendon of latissimus dorsi

radial nerve

medial head of triceps

nerve to lateral head of triceps

profunda brachii artery

nerve to medial head of triceps

shaft of humerus

radial nerve

venae comitantes

Fig. 3.68 The radial nerve and profunda brachii artery in the radial groove, seen after retraction of the cut lateral head of triceps. The long head has been excised.

Deep muscles

The proximal attachments of four of the deep muscles are illustrated in Fig. 3.73. The tendon of extensor indicis (Fig. 3.74) passes distally, medial to that of extensor digitorum, and attaches to the extensor expansion of the index finger. The extensor pollicis longus tendon passes distally around the ulnar (medial) side of the dorsal tubercle of the radius (Fig. 3.74), then crosses the radial extensors of the carpus to attach to the base of the distal phalanx of the thumb (Fig. 3.75). The muscle extends the thumb and its carpometacarpal joint. The tendons of extensor pollicis brevis and abductor pollicis longus (Fig. 3.75) lie together as they cross the radial carpal extensors and brachioradialis. Extensor pollicis brevis attaches to the base of the proximal phalanx of the thumb, which it extends. Abductor pollicis longus attaches to the base of the first metacarpal bone, which it extends and abducts.

Although these four deep muscles act primarily on the joints of the hand, they also span the wrist joint; but their actions here are weak. They are all innervated by the posterior interosseous (deep branch of the radial) nerve.

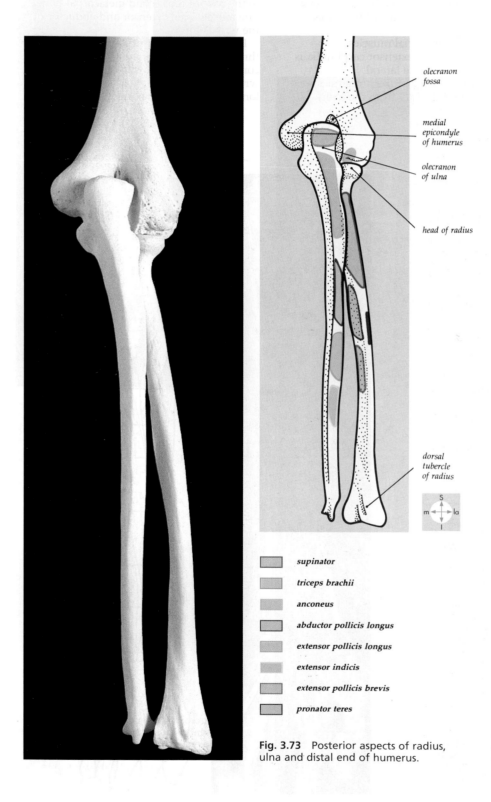

olecranon fossa

medial epicondyle of humerus

olecranon of ulna

head of radius

dorsal tubercle of radius

supinator

triceps brachii

anconeus

abductor pollicis longus

extensor pollicis longus

extensor indicis

extensor pollicis brevis

pronator teres

Fig. 3.73 Posterior aspects of radius, ulna and distal end of humerus.

Extension of the thumb creates a hollow on the posterolateral aspect of the wrist called the 'anatomical snuff box'. It is limited anteriorly by the tendons of abductor pollicis longus and extensor pollicis brevis and posteriorly by extensor pollicis longus. Superficial to the snuff box lie the origin of the cephalic vein and branches of the superficial radial nerve supplying the dorsum of the hand. The tendons of the two radial carpal extensors and the radial artery pass through the snuff box. The bony floor comprises the radial styloid process, scaphoid, trapezium and base of the first metacarpal bone. Fracture of the scaphoid bone often produces pain, swelling and tenderness in the snuff box.

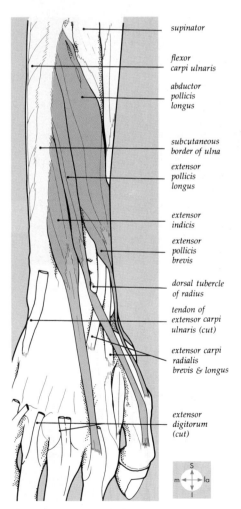

supinator

flexor carpi ulnaris

abductor pollicis longus

subcutaneous border of ulna

extensor pollicis longus

extensor indicis

extensor pollicis brevis

dorsal tubercle of radius

tendon of extensor carpi ulnaris (cut)

extensor carpi radialis brevis & longus

extensor digitorum (cut)

Fig. 3.74 Extensor indicis and extensors pollicis longus and brevis, after division of extensor digitorum. The tendon of extensor indicis lies on the ulnar (medial) side of the index tendon of extensor digitorum.

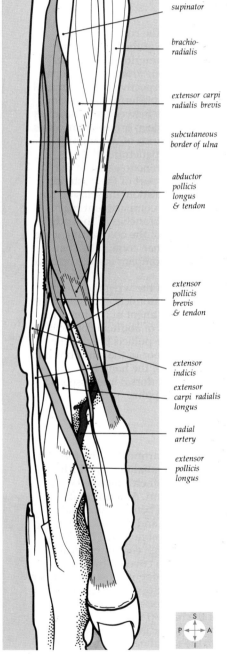

supinator

brachio-radialis

extensor carpi radialis brevis

subcutaneous border of ulna

abductor pollicis longus & tendon

extensor pollicis brevis & tendon

extensor indicis

extensor carpi radialis longus

radial artery

extensor pollicis longus

Fig. 3.75 Abductor pollicis longus and extensors pollicis longus and brevis. At the wrist the radial carpal extensors are crossed by the tendons of these three muscles passing to the thumb.

CLAVICULAR AND SHOULDER JOINTS

Three joints contribute to the considerable mobility of the arm; movement occurs between the humerus and the scapula at the shoulder (glenohumeral) joint, and the scapula moves on the chest wall through the joints at each end of the clavicle. Although few muscles attach to the clavicle, the numerous muscles attached to the scapula and upper humerus all contribute to movement at the clavicular joints. Indeed, movement at the shoulder joint is almost always associated with movement at the sternoclavicular and acromioclavicular joints.

Clavicular joints

The sternoclavicular and acromioclavicular joints are subcutaneous and easily palpable in the living subject. Each has a tubular capsule lined by synovial membrane.

At the sternoclavicular joint (Fig. 3.80), the medial end of the clavicle articulates with the notch on the upper border of the manubrium and with the first costal cartilage. The joint is partitioned by an intracapsular disc of fibrocartilage that attaches superiorly to the clavicle, inferiorly to the first costal cartilage and around its periphery to the capsule. There are two accessory ligaments. Above the capsule is the interclavicular ligament which joins the medial ends of the clavicles. Just lateral to the joint is the costoclavicular (rhomboid) ligament, which attaches the clavicle firmly to the first costal cartilage. Stability depends on the disc and accessory ligaments, which limit both medial displacement and elevation of the medial end of the clavicle. The sternoclavicular joints are separated from the origins of the brachiocephalic veins and other structures in the root of the neck by the sternohyoid and sternothyroid muscles.

At the acromioclavicular joint (Fig. 3.81) the lateral end of the clavicle articulates with the medial aspect of the acromion of the

Fig. 3.80 Sternoclavicular joints. On the left, the joint capsule and subclavius have been excised to reveal the cartilaginous disc and costoclavicular ligament. Pleura is exposed in the first left intercostal space.

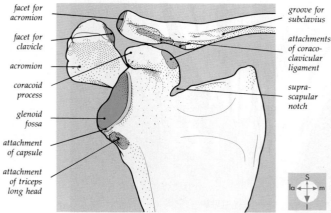

Fig. 3.81 Oblique anterior view of scapula and lateral part of clavicle. The bones have been separated to show the articular surfaces of the acromioclavicular joint and the sites of attachment of the coracoclavicular ligament.

scapula. The joint capsule attaches to the edges of the articular surfaces that lie obliquely, the clavicular facet facing laterally and inferiorly. Stability of the joint is provided mostly by the strong coracoclavicular ligament linking the coracoid process and the undersurface of the clavicle near its lateral end. This ligament consists of conoid and trapezoid parts.

Both the sternoclavicular and acromioclavicular joints are supplied by branches of the supraclavicular nerves (C3 & C4).

The lateral end of the clavicle may be elevated or depressed and drawn forwards or backwards. The axes of these movements occur at the costoclavicular and coracoclavicular ligaments rather than through the clavicular joints. Thus, the medial end of the clavicle is elevated during depression of the scapula and

moves posteriorly when the scapula is protracted. Full abduction of the upper limb requires rotation of the scapula so that the glenoid fossa tilts upwards. Rotation of the clavicle through 40° at the sternoclavicular joint supplements the 20° of movement available at the acromioclavicular joint, permitting the scapula to rotate through about 60°. The principal muscles of scapular rotation are trapezius and serratus anterior. Protraction is produced by pectoralis minor and serratus anterior and retraction by trapezius and the rhomboids.

The clavicle forms a strut that supports the scapula against the medial pull of muscles such as pectoralis major and latissimus dorsi. The clavicular joints are stabilized by their accessory ligaments which are so strong that trauma, such as falling onto the outstretched limb, is more

likely to fracture the clavicle than rupture the ligaments.

Shoulder joint

The shoulder (glenohumeral) joint is synovial, of the ball-and-socket type, and is capable of a wide range of movement. The hemispherical head of the humerus is directed medially and backwards and articulates with the much smaller glenoid fossa of the scapula (Fig. 3.82). The fossa faces anterolaterally and is slightly deepened by the glenoid labrum, a cartilaginous lip round its edge.

The joint capsule (Fig. 3.83) forms a loose sleeve attaching medially to the glenoid labrum. Its humeral attachment is around the anatomical neck except inferiorly on the medial side, where it descends to the level of the surgical neck.

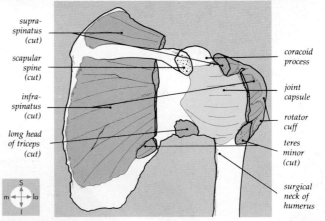

Fig. 3.82 Transverse section at the level of the humeral head showing the relations of the shoulder joint. Superior aspect.

Fig. 3.83 Posterior aspect of the shoulder joint. The acromion and parts of the rotator cuff muscles have been excised to reveal the joint capsule.

Synovial membrane lines the fibrous capsule and covers the intracapsular part of the humeral shaft (Fig. 3.84). The cavity of the joint usually communicates with the subscapular bursa through a deficiency in the anterior part of the capsule. Indistinct thickenings in the capsule form the glenohumeral ligaments. Between the greater and lesser tubercles (Fig. 3.85) the capsule forms the transverse humeral ligament beneath which the tendon of the long head of biceps enters the joint from the intertubercular groove. The tendon is surrounded by a tubular sheath of synovial membrane as it passes over the humeral head to attach to the supraglenoid tubercle (Fig. 3.86).

The joint is intimately related to subscapularis, supraspinatus, infraspinatus and teres minor (Figs 3.86 & 3.87) whose tendons fuse with the capsule to form the rotator cuff (see Fig. 3.83). Above the joint is the coracoacromial arch formed by the coracoid process, the acromion and the intervening coracoacromial ligament. The arch is separated from supraspinatus by the subacromial bursa.

Articular nerves are derived from the suprascapular and subscapular nerves and also from the axillary nerve which passes very close to the joint. As this nerve leaves the axilla through the quadrangular space (see Fig. 3.64), it lies immediately inferior to the capsule. The vascular supply is provided by branches of the circumflex humeral and suprascapular arteries.

Flexion of the shoulder joint (up to 180°) is produced mainly by the clavicular fibres of pectoralis major and the anterior fibres of deltoid. Extension (limited to about 45°) is produced by latissimus dorsi and the posterior fibres of deltoid. At the shoulder joint itself, about 120° of abduction is possible, produced by supraspinatus and deltoid; simultaneous rotation of the scapula through 60° permits full elevation of the arm above the head. Adduction, produced by teres major, latissimus dorsi and pectoralis major, is limited by the area of the articular surface of the humerus. Medial rotation is produced by pectoralis

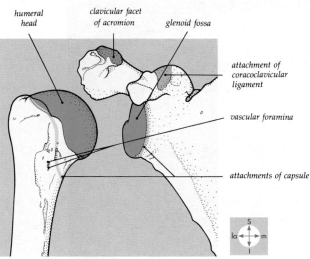

Fig. 3.84   The bones that form the shoulder joint have been separated to reveal their articular surfaces.

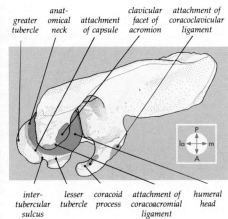

Fig. 3.85   Superior view of scapula and upper end of humerus. The acromion and coracoacromial ligament prevent upward displacement of the humeral head.

major, subscapularis, teres major and the anterior fibres of deltoid, and lateral rotation by infraspinatus, teres minor and the posterior fibres of deltoid.

Although the coracoacromial arch prevents upward displacement of the humerus, stability of the shoulder joint relies principally on the rotator cuff muscles that hold the humeral head firmly in the glenoid fossa. Despite the labrum, the glenoid fossa is a shallow socket. The capsular ligaments are lax in most positions and tighten only near the extremes of movement. Dislocation of the joint, either traumatic or associated with weakness of the short muscles, is therefore relatively common and may result in damage to the axillary nerve.

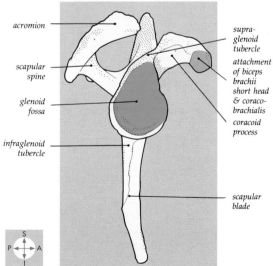

Fig. 3.86 Lateral aspect of scapula showing the pear-shaped glenoid fossa. The positions of supraspinous, infraspinous and subscapular fossae can be appreciated.

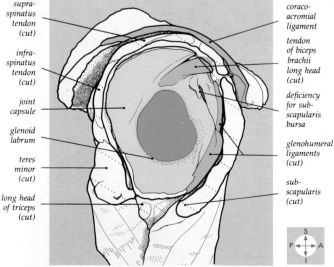

Fig. 3.87 The scapular component of a disarticulated shoulder joint showing the relations and internal features of the joint.

ELBOW JOINT

The elbow is a synovial hinge joint between the distal end of the humerus and the proximal ends of the radius and ulna (Fig. 3.88). Laterally the capitulum of the humerus articulates with the slightly concave upper surface of the head of the radius. Medially the trochlea of the humerus articulates with the deep trochlear notch of the ulna.

The joint capsule (Figs 3.89 & 3.90) attaches proximally to the shaft of the humerus above the radial and coronoid fossae anteriorly, and to the margins of the olecranon fossa posteriorly. Distally it attaches to the anular ligament of the proximal radioulnar joint and to the margins of the trochlear notch of the ulna. Synovial membrane lines the capsule and clothes the underlying pads of fat that project into the radial, coronoid and olecranon fossae of the humerus. The cavity of the elbow joint is continuous with that of the proximal radioulnar joint.

There are two collateral ligaments (Figs 3.89 & 3.90). The radial (lateral) collateral ligament passes between the lateral epicondyle and the anular ligament. The ulnar (medial) collateral ligament attaches proximally to the medial epicondyle whilst distally its fibres diverge and attach to the medial aspects of the coronoid and olecranon processes of the ulna. Stability of the joint depends on the integrity of these collateral ligaments, which hold the trochlea of the humerus firmly in the trochlear notch.

Rotation of the ulna is prevented by the shape of the articular surfaces of the trochlea. Dislocation of the joint is usually associated with ligamentous or bony injury.

Only flexion and extension occur at the elbow joint. Flexion (about 150°) is produced mainly by biceps and brachialis with a contribution from brachioradialis when the elbow is partially flexed. Extension is produced by triceps assisted by anconeus. The flexors and extensors of the wrist and hand arising from the humerus close to the joint do not contribute significantly to elbow movements.

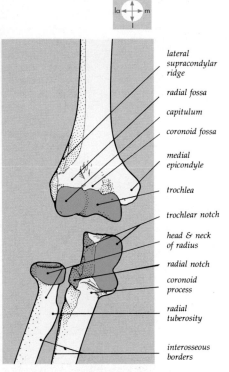

lateral supracondylar ridge
radial fossa
capitulum
coronoid fossa
medial epicondyle
trochlea
trochlear notch
head & neck of radius
radial notch
coronoid process
radial tuberosity
interosseous borders

Fig. 3.88 The bones that form the elbow and proximal radioulnar joints have been separated to reveal their articular surfaces.

capsule (opened)
radial fossa
radial collateral ligament
annular ligament
ulna
coronoid fossa
non-articular part of trochlea
articular cartilage
ulnar collateral ligament

Fig. 3.89 Anterior aspect of elbow joint. The capsule has been opened to expose the interior of the joint.

Behind the elbow joint lies the tendon of triceps (Fig. 3.91). Immediately anterior to the capsule are brachialis and the tendon of biceps in the cubital fossa (see Fig. 3.29). The brachial artery and median nerve are separated from the capsule by brachialis.

The ulnar nerve lies behind the medial epicondyle in contact with the ulnar collateral ligament.

The elbow receives blood from the anastomosis around the joint formed by branches of the brachial, radial and ulnar arteries. The vessels supplying the joint are accompanied by articular nerves derived from branches of the musculocutaneous, radial, ulnar (and sometimes the median) nerves.

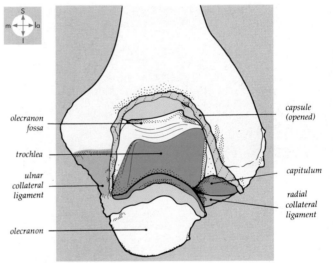

Fig. 3.90 Posterior aspect of flexed elbow joint. The capsule has been opened to reveal the olecranon fossa.

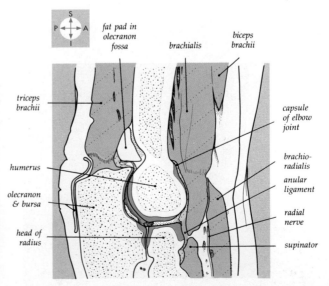

Fig. 3.91 Oblique longitudinal section of elbow (extended) and proximal radioulnar joints showing the articular surfaces and relations of the joints.

RADIOULNAR JOINTS

The radius and ulna articulate at the proximal and distal radioulnar joints which are synovial. At the proximal joint the head of the radius articulates with the radial notch of the ulna (see Fig. 3.88). The head and neck are encircled by the anular ligament, which attaches to the anterior and posterior margins of the notch on the ulna (Fig. 3.92) and blends with the capsule and radial collateral ligament of the elbow. Thus the cavity of the proximal joint is continuous with that of the elbow.

The distal radioulnar joint occurs between the head of the ulna and the ulnar notch of the radius (Fig. 3.93). An articular disc (a triangular cartilage) attaches the ulnar styloid process to the distal end of the radius and separates the cavity of the distal joint from that of the wrist.

The anular ligament of the proximal joint and the articular disc of the distal joint prevent separation of the radius and ulna, yet allow the radius to rotate freely. In addition, the shafts of the bones are joined by the interosseous membrane, whose fibres incline downwards and medially from the interosseous border of the radius to that of the ulna. The membrane may be regarded as a fibrous radioulnar joint.

The movements of supination and pronation occur through approximately 180° at the radioulnar joints. During pronation the radius rotates across the ulna and twists the forearm and hand so that the palm faces posteriorly. Supination returns the limb to the anatomical position. The axis of the movement passes through the head of the radius and the styloid process of the ulna. Supination is the more powerful movement and is produced by biceps and supinator, although biceps is ineffective when the elbow is fully extended. Pronation is produced by pronator teres and pronator quadratus. Also, when the elbow is flexed, brachioradialis rotates the forearm and returns the limb to the midposition from the extremes of supination or pronation.

In a fall onto the hand, the interosseous membrane may transmit force from the radius to the ulna, protecting the radial head from compression against the capitulum of the humerus. However, since the membrane does not oppose distraction, a sudden tug on the hand may dislocate the radial head downwards from within the anular ligament of the proximal radioulnar joint.

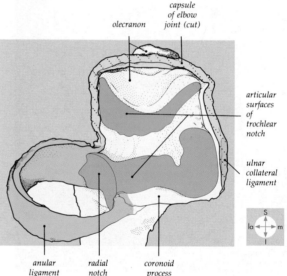

Fig. 3.92 Anterior view of proximal end of ulna with attached anular ligament, showing articular surfaces of trochlear and radial notches.

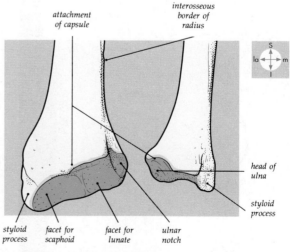

Fig. 3.93 Anterior view of distal ends of radius and ulna. The bones have been separated to reveal the ulnar notch.

WRIST JOINT

Mobility of the hand on the forearm is provided by a series of synovial joints. Most of the movement occurs at the radiocarpal (wrist) joint, supplemented by movement between the carpal bones themselves.

Radiocarpal joint

At the radiocarpal joint the distal end of the radius and the attached articular disc articulate with the proximal row of carpal bones including, from lateral to medial, the scaphoid, lunate and triquetral (Fig. 3.94). The articular disc attaches to the radius and the root of the ulnar styloid process and separates the cavity of the radiocarpal joint from that of the inferior radioulnar joint (Fig. 3.95). The capsule, lined by synovial membrane, attaches to the edges of the articular surfaces and is strengthened by collateral ligaments that pass from the styloid processes of the ulna and radius to the adjacent carpal bones. The movements of this joint are considered on page 118.

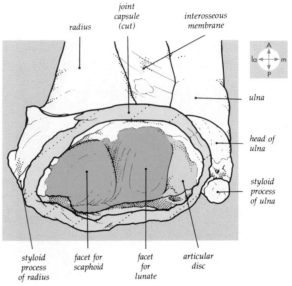

Fig. 3.94 Articular surface of the distal end of the radius and adjacent articular disc.

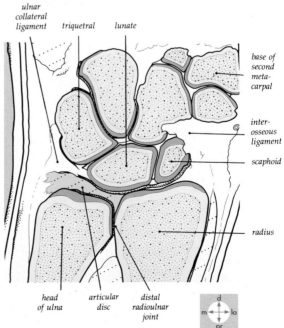

Fig. 3.95 Coronal section of the wrist joint showing articular surfaces and articular disc.

JOINTS OF CARPUS

The carpal bones are arranged in two rows: a proximal row, consisting of, from lateral to medial, scaphoid, lunate, triquetral and pisiform; and a distal row consisting of trapezium, trapezoid, capitate and hamate bones (Fig. 3.96).

Intercarpal joints

The joints between the carpal bones are supported by anterior, posterior and interosseous ligaments. The cavities of these joints usually communicate (Fig. 3.96) and function as a single unit called the 'midcarpal joint' (Fig. 3.97).

The pisiform, a sesamoid bone in the tendon of flexor carpi ulnaris, has a separate joint with the triquetral (Fig. 3.98), and is firmly anchored distally to the hook of the hamate and base of the fifth metacarpal bone by pisohamate and pisometacarpal ligaments (see Fig. 3.47). The relations of the intercarpal joints are illustrated in Fig. 3.98.

Movements

Movements at the radiocarpal and intercarpal joints are complementary, allowing flexion, extension, adduction and abduction of the hand on the forearm. Although the long flexors and extensors of the digits act on the radiocarpal and intercarpal joints, flexion is due principally to the two carpal flexors, and extension to the three carpal extensors. Adduction is produced mainly by the simultaneous contraction of the flexors and extensors on the ulnar side of the forearm and abduction by contraction of the muscles on the radial side.

The radiocarpal and intercarpal joints are stabilized by the extensors and flexors of the wrist during action of the long flexors and/or extensors of the digits. In

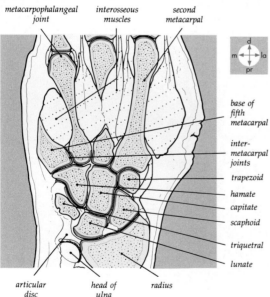

Fig. 3.96 Coronal section of the hand showing the joints of the carpal region. The thumb and little finger lay anterior to the plane of section.

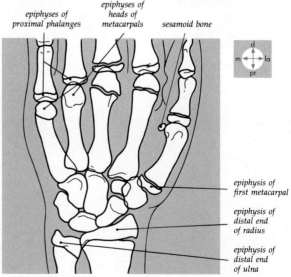

Fig. 3.97 Radiograph of the hand of an adolescent showing metacarpal and carpal bones. Epiphyseal plates are present.

many activities, movement between the hand and forearm combines extension and abduction, achieved by the two radial carpal extensors.

Carpal tunnel

The carpal tunnel (canal) is a fibro-osseous passage linking the anterior compartment of the forearm with the palm of the hand. The walls of the tunnel consist anteriorly of the flexor retinaculum and posteriorly of the two rows of carpal bones which form a deep groove on their flexor surfaces. The retinaculum (Fig. 3.99) lies transversely across the anterior aspect of the wrist, attaching to the trapezium and scaphoid laterally, and to the pisiform and hook of the hamate medially. The tendon of

palmaris longus gains partial attachment to the retinaculum and enters the hand in front of the carpal tunnel (see Fig. 3.39). The tendon is accompanied on its medial side by the ulnar artery and nerve which pass lateral to the pisiform but medial to the hook of the hamate. However, the median nerve and the other tendons entering the palm pass deep to the flexor retinaculum and traverse the carpal tunnel.

Within the tunnel (Fig. 3.98) the tendons of flexor digitorum superficialis lie anterior to those of flexor digitorum profundus. These tendons all possess a common synovial sheath, which is usually in continuity with the digital synovial sheath of the little finger but not with those of the other fingers. The tendon of flexor pollicis longus also traverses the

tunnel, invested by a separate synovial sheath which continues into the thumb. The tendon of flexor carpi radialis lies laterally in a groove on the trapezium, isolated from the main part of the carpal tunnel.

The median nerve traverses the tunnel immediately deep to the flexor retinaculum, lying approximately at the midpoint of the wrist close to the tendon of palmaris longus, anterior to the tendon of flexor pollicis longus and medial to the flexor carpi radialis tendon. Compression of the median nerve may occur within the carpal tunnel, giving rise to a condition called the 'carpal tunnel syndrome'. The syndrome may be treated operatively by dividing the flexor retinaculum to decompress the tunnel.

Fig. 3.98 Transverse section through the carpus showing the carpal tunnel and its contents.

Fig. 3.99 Flexor retinaculum and the superficial relations and structures entering the carpal tunnel.

INTRODUCTION

The abdomen is separated from the thorax above by the diaphragm, and below is continuous with the pelvis at the pelvic inlet. Passing through the diaphragm are the aorta, oesophagus and inferior vena cava. Because the diaphragm is strongly convex upwards, the upper abdominal organs lie deep to the lower ribs and costal cartilages. The pelvic inlet is an arbitrary plane sloping downwards and forwards through which run the small and large intestines, the ureters and several vessels and nerves.

The posterior abdominal wall includes muscles that attach to the last rib, the hip bone and the lumbar vertebrae. Laterally their fasciae merge with the anterolateral abdominal wall whose three layers of muscle broaden out and become aponeurotic before meeting in the midline anteriorly. Close to this median raphe is a vertical strap-like muscle, rectus abdominis, running from the pubis to the anterior chest wall.

The inguinal canal, an oblique passage through the anterolateral abdominal wall, conveys the spermatic cord in the male and the round ligament of the uterus in the female (Fig. 4.1).

The nerves and vessels of the abdominal wall run between the muscles and supply all layers from skin to parietal peritoneum. Most of the arteries, and their accompanying veins and lymphatics, arise from the thoracic wall or the inguinal region while the innervation is provided by spinal nerves. The cutaneous distribution of these nerves displays considerable overlap, as shown in Fig. 4.2.

The abdominal wall muscles accommodate to volume changes of the abdominal and pelvic hollow organs, increase intra-abdominal pressure during forced expiration and straining, and produce movements of the lumbar spine.

The shape of the abdominal cavity is shown in Figs 4.3 and 4.4. Projecting into the abdomen, the lumbar vertebrae form a substantial midline ridge anterior to which run the aorta and inferior vena cava. On each side of the lumbar vertebrae are deep paravertebral gutters. The liver lies predominantly to the right of the midline while the spleen and most of the stomach lie to the left (Fig. 4.5). The digestive organs, including the duodenum, jejunum, ileum and colon, lie anterior to the suprarenal glands, kidneys and ureters (Fig. 4.6). The abdominal organs vary considerably in their size, shape and relative position, the stomach and intestines expanding and contracting as they accommodate to their contents. The upper abdominal organs move with the diaphragm and in response to changes in body position, for example from upright to lying down.

The peritoneum is a serous sac with parietal and visceral layers that are normally in close apposition. The parietal peritoneum lines the abdominal wall and the undersurface of the diaphragm, whilst the visceral layer coats many of the abdominal organs. Some organs have an almost complete covering and are termed intraperitoneal, for example the stomach, jejunum, ileum and liver. They are relatively mobile and attached by double layers of peritoneum between which run

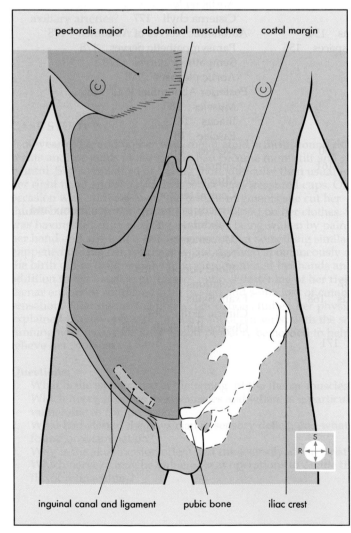

Fig. 4.1 Abdominal wall to show the position of the inguinal canal and the way some of the abdominal muscles overlap the rib cage.

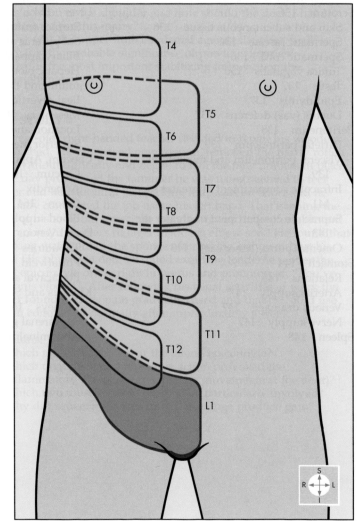

Fig. 4.2 Dermatomes of abdominal wall, showing how they overlap.

vessels and nerves. Such folds form mesenteries, for example the mesentery of the small intestine, or ligaments such as the falciform ligament of the liver, or omenta like the greater omentum that hangs like an apron from the stomach. Other organs, such as the pancreas and kidneys, have no mesenteries and only partial peritoneal covering, usually on the anterior surface.

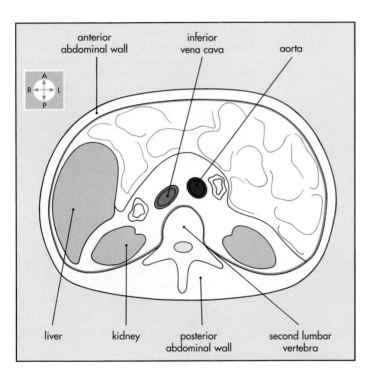

Fig. 4.3 Transverse section through the abdomen to demonstrate the shape of the cavity.

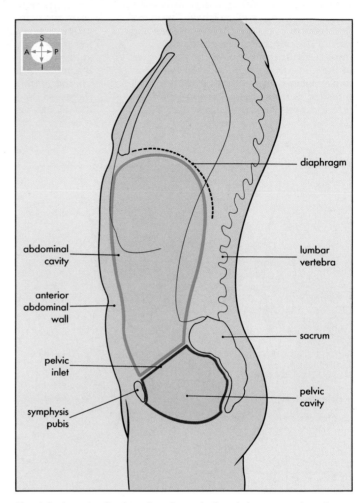

Fig. 4.4 Longitudinal section through the abdomen to show its shape and superior and inferior boundaries.

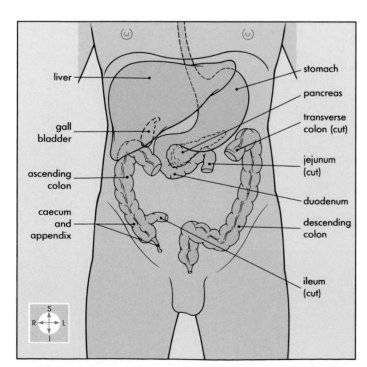

Fig. 4.5 The digestive organs within the abdomen.

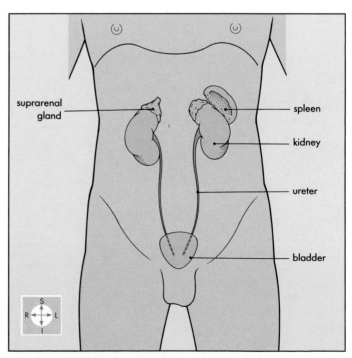

Fig. 4.6 The kidneys and related organs.

The aorta descends in the midline and bifurcates to form the common iliac arteries (Fig. 4.7). From its anterior surface spring three branches to the digestive organs. The coeliac trunk supplies the derivatives of the embryonic foregut: stomach and proximal duodenum, liver, gall bladder, spleen and part of the pancreas. The superior mesenteric artery supplies the derivatives of the midgut: the remainder of the pancreas and small intestine and the large intestine as far as the transverse colon. The inferior mesenteric artery supplies the hindgut: descending and sigmoid colon and rectum. Paired branches arise from the aorta to the suprarenal glands, kidneys, gonads and abdominal wall.

On the right the renal vein and the suprarenal and gonadal veins join the inferior vena cava directly (Fig. 4.8). On the left the renal vein is longer and receives the suprarenal and gonadal veins. Blood from the spleen, stomach and intestines drains via the portal venous system to the liver, thence to the inferior vena cava by way of the hepatic veins (Fig. 4.9).

Lymph from the abdominal organs drains by vessels and nodes that accompany the arterial supply. There are nodes within mesenteries and around the aorta, from which vessels drain upwards to enter the cysterna chyli. The latter gives rise to the thoracic duct carrying lymph upwards through the thorax.

Most viscera receive autonomic innervation via both sympathetic and parasympathetic plexuses around the blood vessels, particularly the aorta and its branches. The thoracic splanchnic nerves, branches of the thoracic portion of the sympathetic trunk, pierce the diaphragm close to its aortic opening. Parasympathetic fibres travel in the vagus nerve which supplies the stomach, liver and biliary system, the small intestine and the proximal part of the large intestine. The distal portion of the colon is supplied by parasympathetic nerves from sacral segments of the spinal cord.

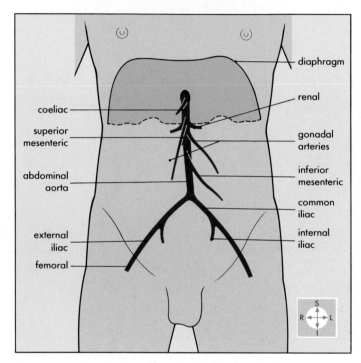

Fig. 4.7   Principal arteries of the abdomen.

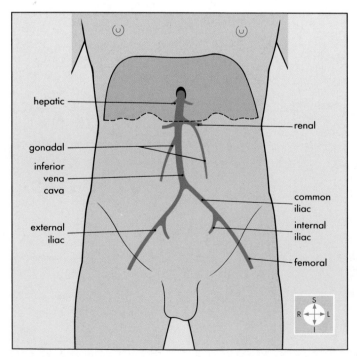

Fig. 4.8   Principal systematic veins of abdomen.

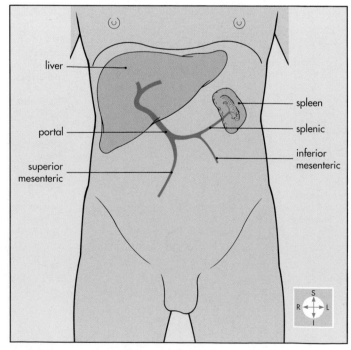

Fig. 4.9   The portal venous system.

ANTERIOR ABDOMINAL WALL

The skin and subcutaneous tissue of the anterior abdominal wall overlie four muscles that move the trunk, control intra-abdominal pressure and support the abdominal contents. The main nerves and blood vessels lie in the neurovascular plane, deep to all but one of the muscles. Deep to the muscles are the transversalis fascia, extraperitoneal fat and the parietal peritoneum.

Skin and subcutaneous tissue

The midline umbilicus marks the site of former attachment of the umbilical cord. In a lean person it usually lies midway between the xiphisternum and the symphysis pubis, at the level of the fourth lumbar vertebra, but its position is variable.

The subcutaneous tissue has an outer fatty layer, which is particularly thick in obese individuals, and a deeper membranous layer, which lies on the external oblique muscle (Fig. 4.10). Although thin over most of the abdominal wall, the membranous layer becomes substantial inferiorly. Laterally it descends into the thigh and attaches to the fascia lata while medially it continues around the external genitalia into the perineum (see page 218).

The subcutaneous tissue receives its blood from small branches of the arteries that supply the abdominal muscles. The superficial veins drain either upwards towards the axilla or downwards to the groin. The nerve supply to the skin is segmental and is provided by cutaneous branches of the lower thoracic spinal nerves and the first lumbar nerve (see Fig. 4.2).

Muscles

On each side of the midline there are four principal muscles. Three of these are flat muscles, arranged in layers in the lateral part of the abdominal wall. External oblique is the most superficial, internal oblique lies deep to it and the deepest layer is transversus abdominis. As each of these muscles is traced anteriorly and medially its fleshy part gives way to an aponeurosis (Fig. 4.10). The aponeuroses of the flat muscles form a sheath around the fourth muscle, rectus abdominis. In the midline the aponeuroses from both sides interdigitate to form the linea alba whilst inferiorly they attach to the pubic crest. These muscles are innervated by the lower six thoracic nerves and the first lumbar nerve (see page 131).

Immediately above the groin the inguinal canal traverses the lowest part of the abdominal wall and transmits the spermatic cord in the male and the round ligament of the uterus in the female (see page 133).

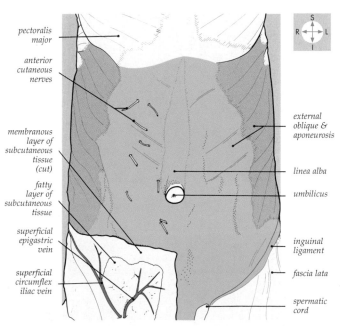

pectoralis major

anterior cutaneous nerves

membranous layer of subcutaneous tissue (cut)

fatty layer of subcutaneous tissue

superficial epigastric vein

superficial circumflex iliac vein

external oblique & aponeurosis

linea alba

umbilicus

inguinal ligament

fascia lata

spermatic cord

Fig. 4.10 External oblique muscles and aponeuroses. Some subcutaneous tissue, veins and cutaneous nerves have been preserved on one side.

External oblique

The muscle fibres of external oblique slope downwards and forwards (Fig. 4.11). Superiorly a series of fleshy slips attaches to the outer surfaces of the lower eight ribs, the upper slips interdigitating with serratus anterior, the lower ones with latissimus dorsi. The most posterior fibres attach inferiorly to the iliac crest; elsewhere the fibres give way to the aponeurosis which passes medially in front of rectus abdominis to reach the linea alba. The aponeurosis possesses a free lower border that extends from the anterior superior iliac spine to the pubic tubercle and forms the inguinal ligament (see Fig. 4.10), which marks the boundary between the abdominal wall and the anterior aspect of the thigh.

Immediately above the medial end of the inguinal ligament, the external oblique aponeurosis presents an aperture, the superficial inguinal ring, which is the medial opening of the inguinal canal (see page 130).

Internal oblique

Internal oblique attaches to the lateral two-thirds of the inguinal ligament, to the anterior part of the iliac crest and to the thoracolumbar fascia (Fig. 4.13), through which it is anchored to the lumbar vertebrae. Most of its fibres slope forwards and upwards. The uppermost fibres attach to the costal margin between the ninth and twelfth ribs while the remainder give way to the aponeurosis of the muscle (Fig. 4.12).

Some aponeurotic fibres reach the linea alba by passing anterior to rectus abdominis whilst others pass behind rectus (see below). The lowest fibres arch medially and downwards, contributing to the roof of the inguinal canal. They unite with the underlying fibres of transversus to form the inguinal falx (conjoint tendon), which descends to the pecten pubis (pectineal line) on the pubic bone.

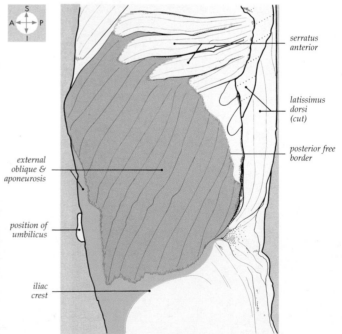

serratus anterior

latissimus dorsi (cut)

posterior free border

external oblique & aponeurosis

position of umbilicus

iliac crest

Fig. 4.11   The left external oblique showing its attachments to the lower ribs and the iliac crest.

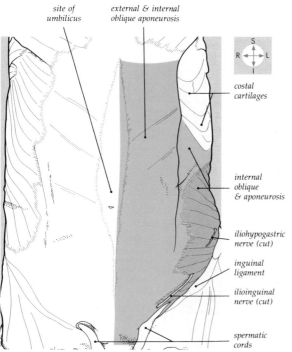

site of
umbilicus

external & internal
oblique aponeurosis

costal
cartilages

internal
oblique
& aponeurosis

iliohypogastric
nerve (cut)

inguinal
ligament

ilioinguinal
nerve (cut)

spermatic
cords

Fig. 4.12 Most of the left external oblique has been excised to reveal the underlying internal oblique muscle.

ribs
(numbered)

internal oblique
& aponeurosis

thoracolumbar fascia

iliohypogastric
nerve (cut)

iliac crest

ilioinguinal
nerve

Fig. 4.13 Left internal oblique and attachments, revealed by removal of the external oblique. In this specimen the costal attachments of serratus anterior include the ninth rib.

Transversus abdominis

The upper part of this muscle arises from the inner aspects of the lower six costal cartilages (Fig. 4.15) by fleshy slips which interdigitate with the costal attachments of the diaphragm. The middle part of the muscle fuses with the thoracolumbar fascia while the lowest fibres attach to the iliac crest and the lateral half of the inguinal ligament. Most of the fibres run horizontally forwards and are replaced, near the lateral border of rectus, by an aponeurosis (Figs 4.14 & 4.16). The upper part of the aponeurosis reaches the linea alba by passing posterior to rectus abdominis while the inferior part passes anterior to it (see below).

The lowest fibres of transversus abdominis attach to the lateral part of the inguinal ligament and arch over the inguinal canal and, fusing with those of the overlying internal oblique, contribute to the inguinal falx.

Rectus abdominis

Rectus abdominis runs vertically on each side of the linea alba, from the pubis to the front of the chest wall (Fig. 4.14). The inferior attachment is to the anterior aspect of the pubic symphysis and to the pubic crest. The muscle widens superiorly and attaches to the anterior surfaces of the fifth, sixth and seventh costal cartilages. Its gently convex lateral border forms a surface feature called the linea semilunaris. Rectus abdominis is characterized by transverse tendinous intersections, usually at the levels of the xiphisternum, the umbilicus and midway between the two.

Rectus sheath

Rectus abdominis is enclosed in a sheath formed by the aponeuroses of the flat abdominal muscles. The anterior wall of the sheath, which is anchored to the tendinous intersections, covers the entire length of the muscle (see Fig. 4.12). By contrast, the posterior wall is not attached to the muscle and falls short of its superior and inferior extremities. Superiorly the posterior wall of the sheath terminates at the costal margin, above which rectus is in direct contact with the costal cartilages. Inferiorly the posterior wall continues only a short distance below the umbilicus, where it thins out or ends abruptly. In the latter case the posterior wall has a recognizable inferior margin, the arcuate line (see Fig. 4.16), below which the posterior surface of rectus is in direct contact with the transversalis fascia.

The composition of the rectus sheath varies at different levels. The anterior wall above the costal margin consists solely of the external oblique aponeurosis, but from that level down to the level of the arcuate line it is supplemented by the anterior layer of the internal oblique aponeurosis. Above the arcuate line the posterior wall of the sheath consists of transversus abdominis and the posterior layer of the internal oblique aponeurosis. Below the level of the arcuate line all three aponeuroses pass anterior to rectus and form the anterior wall.

In addition to rectus abdominis, the rectus sheath contains the small triangular pyramidalis muscle, the superior and inferior epigastric vessels (Figs 4.14 & 4.16) and the terminal parts of the lower six intercostal nerves that supply rectus and the overlying skin.

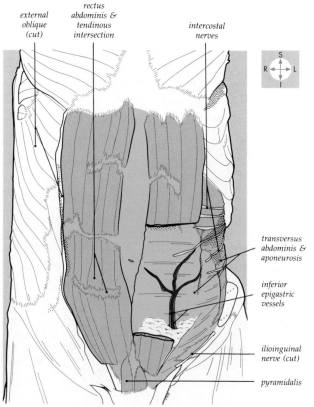

Fig. 4.14 Rectus abdominis muscles and neurovascular plane. The anterior walls of both rectus sheaths, the left oblique muscles and part of the left rectus abdominis have been removed.

Actions of abdominal muscles

The abdominal muscles flex the lumbar spine, rectus abdominis being particularly powerful in this action. Lateral flexion and rotation of the trunk are produced by coordinated contraction of the oblique muscles on both sides of the midline. Acting collectively, the abdominal muscles increase intra-abdominal pressure and, if the respiratory passages are open, the diaphragm is pushed upwards as in forced expiration, sneezing and coughing. Increased abdominal pressure with the airway closed (straining) occurs when lifting heavy objects and during defecation, childbirth and vomiting.

Structures deep to muscles

The deep surfaces of transversus and rectus abdominis are covered by the transversalis fascia, which forms part of a complete fascial sheet lying deep to the muscles surrounding the peritoneal cavity. Several names are given to this continuous fascial sheet and are derived from the muscles to which the fascia relates. For example, the diaphragmatic and iliac fasciae cover the diaphragm and iliacus respectively. Above the midpoint of the inguinal ligament an aperture in the transversalis fascia (the deep inguinal ring) forms the lateral opening of the inguinal canal.

Deep to the transversalis fascia is the extraperitoneal fat, which contains four vestigial structures converging on the umbilicus. Descending from the liver is the round ligament of the liver (ligamentum teres hepatis; see page 139), the remnant of the left umbilical vein. Ascending in the midline from the urinary bladder is the urachus or median umbilical ligament, the remnant of the embryonic allantois (see Fig. 4.16). Inclining upwards from each side of the pelvis is the obliterated umbilical artery.

The deepest layer of the abdominal wall is the parietal peritoneum (see Fig. 4.16). Although the peritoneum and the abdominal musculature are adherent in most areas, they are only loosely attached between the pubis and umbilicus. Therefore an enlarging bladder intervenes between them and the organ can be approached surgically through the abdominal wall without traversing the peritoneal cavity.

Nerves and vessels

The skin, muscles and parietal peritoneum of the anterior abdominal wall are innervated by the lower six thoracic nerves and the first lumbar nerve.

Lower thoracic nerves

At the costal margin, thoracic nerves seven to eleven leave their intercostal spaces and enter the neurovascular plane of the abdominal wall between transversus abdominis and internal oblique (Fig. 4.15). The seventh and eighth nerves slope upwards, the ninth runs horizontally and the tenth and eleventh incline downwards. The nerves pierce rectus abdominis and the anterior layer of the rectus sheath to emerge as anterior cutaneous branches that supply the overlying skin (see Fig. 4.10).

The subcostal nerve (T12) takes the line of the twelfth rib across the posterior abdominal wall. It continues around the flank in the neurovascular plane and terminates in a similar manner to the lower intercostal nerves.

Fig. 4.15 Removal of the external and internal oblique muscles has revealed the transversus abdominis muscle and aponeurosis. Running across its surface are the lower intercostal, subcostal and iliohypogastric nerves.

The roof is formed by the lowest fibres of internal oblique and transversus abdominis (Fig. 4.20). These fibres arch over the canal and pass medially and downwards to form the inguinal falx (conjoint tendon), which attaches to the crest and pectineal line of the pubis. The anterior wall of the canal is formed by the external oblique aponeurosis, supplemented laterally by fibres of internal oblique that attach to the lateral part of the inguinal ligament (Fig. 4.19). The posterior wall is formed by the transversalis fascia, reinforced medially by the conjoint tendon. Deep to the transversalis fascia are the inferior epigastric vessels, which lie just medial to the deep ring (Fig. 4.21).

The inguinal canal is a site of potential weakness in the abdominal wall through which intra-abdominal structures may pass, producing an inguinal hernia (see below). However, several features of the canal's anatomy minimize this weakness. The obliquity of the canal ensures that the superficial and deep inguinal rings do not overlie one another (see Fig. 4.17). Furthermore, the strongest part of the anterior wall lies in front of the deep ring and the strongest part of the posterior wall lies behind the superficial ring. Hence, when pressure within the abdomen rises, the anterior and posterior walls of the canal are firmly opposed. In addition, when the abdominal muscles contract, the canal is compressed by the descent of fibres of internal oblique and transversus abdominis in its roof.

Fig. 4.19   External spermatic fascia and a strip of the external oblique aponeurosis have been removed to show the spermatic cord and ilioinguinal nerve within the canal.

Fig. 4.20   Lower fibres of internal oblique and part of the spermatic cord have been excised to reveal the posterior wall and floor of the canal.

Contents

In the male, the canal contains the spermatic cord (Fig. 4.19). In the female, it transmits the round ligament of the uterus (Fig. 4.22), a fibromuscular cord running from the body of the uterus to the subcutaneous tissues of the labium majus. Lymphatics from part of the body of the uterus accompany the round ligament and terminate in the superficial inguinal nodes (see Fig. 6.11).

In both sexes the ilioinguinal nerve (see Fig. 4.12) lies deep to the external oblique aponeurosis close to the inguinal ligament. The nerve runs medially in the anterior wall of the canal and emerges through the superficial ring (Figs 4.18 & 4.22).

Inguinal hernias

The inguinal canal is the most common site for an abdominal hernia. Two types of inguinal hernia are recognized. The direct type passes through the inguinal falx into the medial part of the canal. By contrast, the indirect (oblique) type traverses the deep ring and turns medially along the canal. Hernias of both types may emerge through the superficial ring and descend into the scrotum or labium majus. Direct and indirect hernias are distinguished by their relationships to the inferior epigastric vessels. A direct hernia lies on the medial side of these vessels while the indirect type enters the inguinal canal lateral to them.

In the male, an indirect hernia may pass along the canal within a patent processus vaginalis, giving rise to an 'infantile inguinal hernia'.

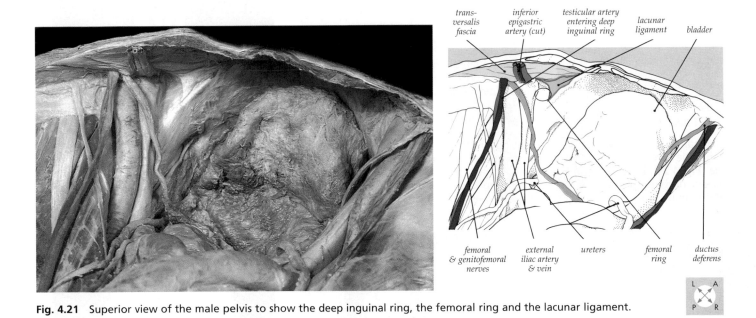

Fig. 4.21 Superior view of the male pelvis to show the deep inguinal ring, the femoral ring and the lacunar ligament.

Fig. 4.22 Superficial ring and inguinal canal in the female showing the round ligaments of the uterus.

continues upwards in the cord. When the upper part of the scrotum is palpated, the ductus can be distinguished from the accompanying testicular vessels by its firm consistency.

After traversing the inguinal canal, the ductus runs backwards across the pelvic brim and along the lateral wall of the pelvis (see Fig. 4.21) before terminating in the ejaculatory duct (see page 207).

PERITONEUM

The peritoneum is a serous membrane with parietal and visceral layers which encloses a space, the peritoneal cavity. The parietal peritoneum lines the walls of the abdomen and pelvis while the visceral layer covers many of the abdominal and pelvic organs. In the male the peritoneal cavity is a closed sac, but in the female it communicates with the interior of the uterus and vagina via a microscopic channel through each uterine tube. Normally, the peritoneal cavity contains only a few millilitres of serous fluid, but in certain diseases several litres of serous fluid can accumulate.

The peritoneal cavity comprises the greater and lesser sacs. The greater sac is very extensive and can be traced from the diaphragm above into the pelvic cavity below. The lesser sac (omental bursa) is located in the upper part of the abdomen behind the stomach and communicates with the greater sac through a narrow opening, the omental (epiploic) foramen.

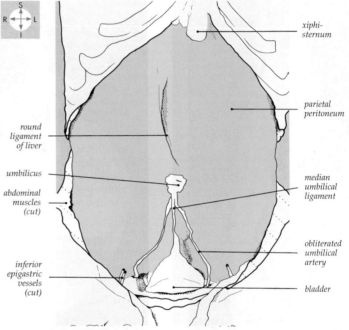

Fig. 4.28 Removal of muscles and fascia of the anterior abdominal wall reveals the parietal peritoneum and extraperitoneal structures.

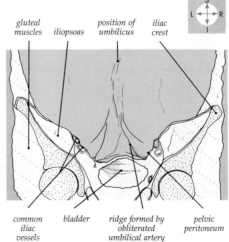

Fig. 4.29 Removal of the abdominal organs from a coronal section shows the parietal peritoneum from within.

Parietal peritoneum

The parietal peritoneum is applied to the inner aspect of the abdominal and pelvic walls (Fig. 4.28) and continues superiorly across most of the undersurface of the diaphragm. The peritoneum lining the anterior abdominal wall is raised into several folds or ridges. Below the umbilicus the median umbilical ligament often raises a midline ridge (median umbilical fold), on each side of which the obliterated umbilical artery (medial umbilical ligament) may produce a further peritoneal fold (medial umbilical fold) (Fig. 4.29). Above the umbilicus the round ligament of the liver (Fig. 4.28) is contained in a large fold of peritoneum, the falciform ligament, which attaches the liver to the anterior abdominal wall and the diaphragm (see Fig. 4.55).

Posteriorly the peritoneum covers several organs that lie on the muscles of the posterior abdominal wall (Fig. 4.30). These retroperitoneal organs include the ascending and descending parts of the colon, the kidneys, ureters and suprarenal glands, and most of the pancreas and duodenum. Also lying behind the peritoneum are the aorta and its branches, and the inferior vena cava and its tributaries.

Nerve supply

The parietal peritoneum of the abdominal wall is innervated by the lower thoracic and first lumbar nerves. The lower thoracic nerves also innervate the peritoneum covering the periphery of the diaphragm. Inflammation of this peritoneum consequently gives rise to pain in the lower thoracic wall and abdominal wall. By contrast, the peritoneum on the central part of the diaphragm receives sensory branches from the phrenic nerves (C3, C4 & C5) and irritation here may produce pain referred to the region of the shoulder (the fourth cervical dermatome; see page 20).

Visceral peritoneum and mesenteries

Most of the abdominal organs have a covering of visceral peritoneum and are suspended within the abdominopelvic cavity by mesenteries. Although organs possessing mesenteries are often termed 'intraperitoneal', they do not lie within the peritoneal cavity but merely project into it. Mesenteries consist of double layers of peritoneum containing the vessels and nerves of the 'intraperitoneal' organs. Most mesenteries attach to the posterior abdominal wall, where their peritoneal layers are continuous with the parietal peritoneum. Typical examples include the mesenteries of the small intestine (see Fig. 4.33) and the transverse mesocolon.

The mesenteries of the stomach (the omenta) do not attach to the abdominal wall but to other organs. The lesser curvature of the stomach is connected to the liver by the lesser omentum while the

Fig. 4.30 Transverse section at the level of the third lumbar vertebra showing parietal peritoneum and some retroperitoneal structures. Inferior aspect. Compare Fig. 4.108.

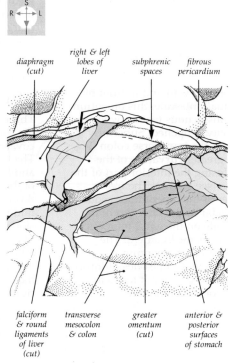

diaphragm (cut)   right & left lobes of liver   subphrenic spaces   fibrous pericardium

falciform & round ligaments of liver (cut)   transverse mesocolon & colon   greater omentum (cut)   anterior & posterior surfaces of stomach

Fig. 4.34   Supracolic compartment of the greater sac. After removal of most of the greater omentum, the greater curve of the stomach has been displaced upwards to show the position of the omental bursa (pink).

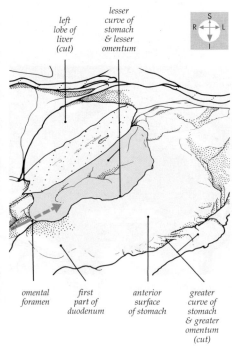

left lobe of liver (cut)   lesser curve of stomach & lesser omentum

omental foramen   first part of duodenum   anterior surface of stomach   greater curve of stomach & greater omentum (cut)

Fig. 4.35   Lesser omentum and omental foramen after removal of part of the left lobe of the liver.

Supracolic compartment of greater sac

The supracolic compartment lies above and in front of the transverse mesocolon (Fig. 4.34). Its superior part intervenes between the diaphragm and the liver and is divided by the falciform ligament into two subphrenic spaces. The compartment includes the deep recess between the right lobe of the liver and the right kidney (the hepatorenal recess) and extends across the midline below the left lobe of the liver and in front of the stomach.

Omental bursa (lesser sac)

The omental bursa is the small part of the peritoneal cavity behind the stomach (Figs 4.34 & 4.36). It communicates with the greater sac through a narrow opening, known as the omental or epiploic foramen, which lies between the first part of the duodenum and the undersurface of the liver (Fig. 4.35).

The omental bursa is isolated from the greater sac by the stomach and several peritoneal folds. One of these folds, the lesser omentum, connects the lesser curvature of the stomach to the posterior

surface of the liver (Fig. 4.35). Two further folds, the gastrosplenic and splenorenal ligaments, attach the spleen to the greater curvature of the stomach and the left kidney respectively (Fig. 4.36).

The omental bursa extends upwards behind the stomach and the caudate lobe of the liver as far as the diaphragm. On the left it continues to the hilum of the spleen, terminating between the gastrosplenic and splenorenal ligaments. Inferiorly the omental bursa usually extends a short distance below the greater curvature of the stomach between the gastric and colic attachments of the greater omentum.

- superior pole of right kidney
- right suprarenal gland
- liver
- inferior vena cava
- omental foramen
- portal vein, hepatic artery & bile duct
- spleen
- left suprarenal gland
- splenorenal ligament
- aorta & coeliac trunk
- gastrosplenic ligament
- greater curve of stomach
- lesser curve of stomach & lesser omentum

Fig. 4.36 Transverse section at the level of the disc between the twelfth thoracic and first lumbar vertebrae showing the omental bursa. In this specimen the left kidney lies lower than usual. Superior aspect.

STOMACH

The stomach is the dilated portion of the gut in which the early stages of digestion take place. It lies in the upper part of the abdomen beneath the left dome of the diaphragm (Fig. 4.37). Proximally the stomach joins the oesophagus at the cardiac orifice and distally it is continuous with the duodenum at the pylorus. Between these two relatively fixed points, the organ varies considerably in size, shape and location in response to its muscle tone, the quantity and nature of its contents and the position of the individual (Figs 4.39 & 4.40). Usually the loaded stomach is J-shaped and lies in the left hypochondrium, the epigastrium and umbilical region of the abdomen.

The oesophagus pierces the diaphragm and has a short intra-abdominal course before joining the stomach at the cardiac orifice. This lies a little to the left of the midline at about the level of the eleventh thoracic vertebra (Fig. 4.40).

Fig. 4.37 Stomach and some of its relations, seen after removal of the anterior half of the diaphragm and left lobe of the liver and dissection of the greater omentum.

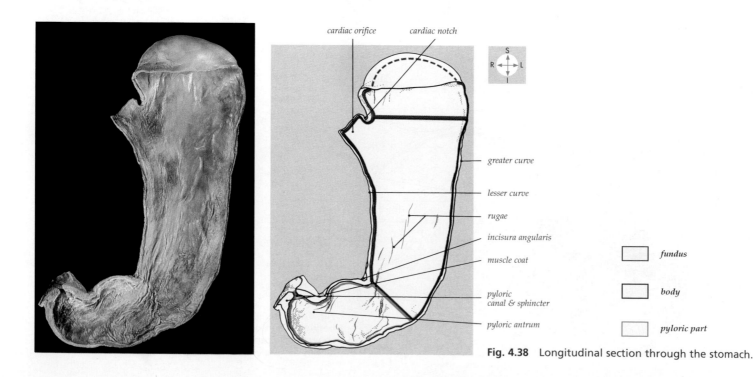

Fig. 4.38 Longitudinal section through the stomach.

The stomach has two surfaces, anterior and posterior, which meet at two curved borders, the curves or curvatures (Fig. 4.38). The lesser curve extends from the cardiac orifice downwards and to the right to reach the upper border of the pylorus. A notch, the incisura angularis, is usually present on the lesser curve towards its pyloric end. The greater curve is longer and begins at the cardiac notch on the left side of the cardiac orifice. It arches upwards and to the left before descending along the left and inferior aspects of the organ to reach the inferior border of the pylorus.

The pylorus is normally situated just to the right of the midline at the level of the first lumbar vertebra, on the transpyloric plane.

By convention the stomach is described as having three parts, the fundus, the body and the pyloric part (Fig. 4.38). The fundus lies above an imaginary horizontal plane passing through the cardiac orifice while the antrum lies to the right of the incisura angularis. The body lies between the fundus and the pyloric part and is the largest part of the stomach. In the pyloric part, the cavity of the pyloric antrum tapers to the right into a narrow passage, the pyloric canal.

The mucosal lining presents numerous longitudinal folds or rugae which are most prominent when the stomach is empty (Fig. 4.38). There is a well developed smooth muscle coat which is thickened around the pyloric canal and pylorus to form the pyloric sphincter.

Relations

The anterior surface of the stomach lies in contact with the diaphragm, the anterior abdominal wall and the left and quadrate lobes of the liver. Posterolateral to the fundus lies the gastric surface of the spleen (Fig. 4.37). The remainder of the stomach's relations are situated posteriorly and collectively form the stomach bed. This includes the diaphragm, left suprarenal gland, upper part of the left kidney, the splenic artery, pancreas, transverse mesocolon and sometimes the transverse colon (see Fig. 4.41). However, these structures are separated from the stomach by the omental bursa (see below).

oesophagus

gas in fundus

11th rib

12th rib

duodenum

pyloric part

Fig. 4.39 Anteroposterior radiograph following a barium meal. The subject is supine and most of the barium has pooled into the pyloric part of the stomach.

diaphragm

oesophagus

barium in fundus

cardiac orifice

pyloric canal

pyloric part

Fig. 4.40 Oblique radiograph of the same individual, now lying on his left side. The barium has flowed into the fundus of the stomach.

liver (cut)

anterior surface
of stomach

posterior surface
of stomach

pancreas
(deep to peritoneum)

right gastro-omental
vessels

transverse
mesocolon & colon

a short
gastric artery

gastrosplenic
ligament

left
gastro-omental
artery

spleen

Fig. 4.41 Omental bursa and stomach bed, seen after removal of the greater omentum and lifting the greater curve upwards.

Omenta and omental bursa

Peritoneum covers both surfaces of the stomach. Attached to the curves are double layers of peritoneum, which form the lesser and greater omenta.

The lesser omentum extends from the liver (see Fig. 4.35) to the lesser curve of the stomach and also attaches to the abdominal oesophagus and the commencement of the duodenum (see Fig. 4.37). Near the lesser curve it contains the left and right gastric vessels (Fig. 4.42), accompanied by lymphatics and autonomic nerves, while its free border encloses the portal vein, the bile duct and the proper hepatic artery.

The greater omentum hangs from the distal part of the greater curve and from the first part of the duodenum. Near the greater curve it contains the left and right gastro-omental (gastroepiploic) vessels (Fig. 4.41). To the left the greater omentum is continuous with the gastrosplenic ligament which connects the proximal part of the greater curve to the hilum of the spleen.

The omental bursa (lesser sac) lies behind the stomach and the lesser omentum (Fig. 4.41). Its opening (the omental foramen) lies above the first part of the duodenum, immediately posterior to the free border of the lesser omentum. From here the omental bursa extends to the left as far as the hilum of the spleen where it is limited by the gastrosplenic and splenorenal (lienorenal) ligaments. Superiorly it reaches the undersurface of the diaphragm behind the caudate lobe of the liver. Inferiorly the bursa extends a short distance below the greater curve between the two peritoneal folds that constitute the greater omentum.

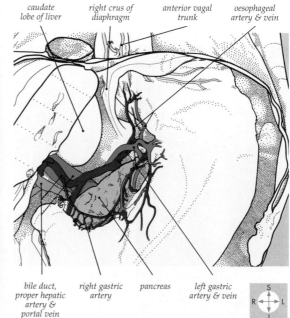

caudate
lobe of liver

right crus of
diaphragm

anterior vagal
trunk

oesophageal
artery & vein

bile duct,
proper hepatic
artery &
portal vein

right gastric
artery

pancreas

left gastric
artery & vein

Fig. 4.42 Dissection of the lesser omentum showing structures along the lesser curve of the stomach.

Arterial supply

The stomach is supplied by several arteries, which are all derived from branches of the coeliac trunk and which anastomose extensively with each other. The coeliac trunk (Fig. 4.43) is a short, wide vessel arising from the anterior aspect of the aorta just below the diaphragm. It divides into three branches: the left gastric, the common hepatic and the splenic arteries.

The left gastric artery is the smallest branch, passing upwards and to the left behind the omental bursa to reach the oesophagus, then descending along the lesser curve within the lesser omentum (Fig. 4.42). Its branches include two or three to the lower oesophagus which ascend through the oesophageal opening of the diaphragm. Other branches supply the cardiac region and lesser curve of the stomach.

The common hepatic artery gives rise to the right gastric and gastroduodenal arteries. The right gastric artery (Fig. 4.42) arises above the first part of the duodenum and runs to the left within the lesser omentum, supplying the lesser curve and anastomosing with the left gastric artery. One of the branches of the gastroduodenal artery is the right gastro-omental (gastroepiploic) artery (Fig. 4.41). This vessel runs to the left within the greater omentum, parallel to the greater curve, giving numerous branches to the pyloric part and body of the stomach.

The splenic artery is the largest branch of the coeliac artery (Fig. 4.43). It runs a tortuous course to the left along the superior border of the pancreas, initially behind the omental bursa and then within the splenorenal ligament, and terminates near the hilum of the spleen. It provides collateral branches to the pancreas and terminal branches to the spleen and stomach. There are several gastric branches, which pass to the greater curve by way of the gastrosplenic ligament. Most of these vessels supply the fundus of the stomach and are called short gastric arteries (Fig. 4.41). However, one branch, the left gastro-omental artery, continues downwards and to the right within the greater omentum. It follows the greater curve, supplies the body of the stomach and may anastomose with the right gastro-omental artery.

Venous drainage

The veins of the stomach accompany the gastric arteries and drain into the portal venous system, the portal vein itself receiving the right and left gastric veins. The splenic vein receives the short gastric and left gastro-omental (gastroepiploic) veins while the right gastro-omental vein usually enters the superior mesenteric vein. The oesophageal tributaries of the left gastric vein (Fig. 4.42) take part in an important portacaval anastomosis (see page 166) with tributaries of the azygos venous system within the thorax.

Nerve supply

In the thorax the vagus nerves form a plexus on the surface of the oesophagus. From this plexus emerge two principal nerves, the anterior and posterior vagal trunks, which enter the abdomen on the respective surfaces of the oesophagus. The anterior vagal trunk (Fig. 4.42), derived mostly from the left vagus nerve, gives branches to the anterior surface of the stomach including the pyloric region. Branches from the posterior trunk, whose origin is mainly from the right vagus nerve, pass to the posterior surface of the stomach and also to the coeliac plexus (see pages 178 & 179). The parasympathetic innervation of the stomach by the vagus nerves is important in relation to both secretion and motility of the organ.

oesophagus (cut)
left gastric artery (cut)
proper hepatic artery
gastroduodenal artery (cut)
portal vein
superior mesenteric artery & vein (cut)
pancreas (cut)

spleen
left crus of diaphragm
splenic vessels
coeliac trunk
inferior vena cava

Fig. 4.43 Stomach and most of the pancreas have been removed to reveal the coeliac trunk and its branches.

SPLEEN

The spleen is a lymphoid organ lying in the left hypochondrium posterior to the stomach. The fresh spleen is purple in colour, of soft and delicate consistency and rather variable in size and shape. Since it lies entirely behind the midaxillary line and under cover of the left lower ribs, the normal spleen cannot be palpated in the living subject, even during full inspiration.

Surface features

The spleen is oval in shape when viewed from its anterior aspect (Fig. 4.44) and its long axis lies parallel to the left tenth rib. The two extremities of the organ are

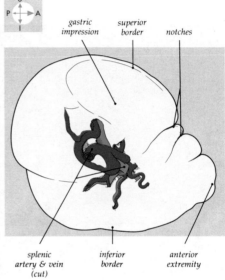

Fig. 4.44 Visceral surface of the spleen.

Fig. 4.45 Diaphragmatic surface of the spleen. This specimen has several well-defined notches on its superior border and a single notch on the inferior border.

connected by superior and inferior borders. The superior border often possesses one or more notches near its anterior end while the inferior border is usually smooth. The organ has two easily distinguishable surfaces. The diaphragmatic surface faces backwards and laterally and is smoothly convex (Fig. 4.45). The visceral surface faces anteromedially and is characterized by ridges and depressions. The centrally placed hilum is perforated by numerous blood vessels together with lymphatics and nerves. The depressions around the hilum accommodate adjacent organs.

Relations

The spleen is an intraperitoneal organ and most of its capsule is covered by peritoneum of the greater sac. However, there is a small bare area near the hilum which gives attachment to two peritoneal folds or ligaments. The splenorenal ligament runs medially to reach the left kidney while the gastrosplenic ligament connects the spleen to the greater curve of the stomach. Part of the omental bursa lies between these two ligaments and extends

to the left as far as the splenic hilum (see Fig. 4.36).

Arching above the spleen and descending posterior and lateral to it, the left dome of the diaphragm is responsible for movements of the organ during ventilation (Fig. 4.46). The diaphragm separates the spleen from the left lung and pleura, and from the ninth, tenth and eleventh ribs.

The depression on the visceral surface of the spleen above the hilum is termed the gastric impression since it accommodates part of the posterior surface of the stomach. Below the medial half of the hilum is the renal impression, which abuts the superior pole of the left kidney.

Near the lateral extremity of its visceral surface the spleen may possess a small colic impression which lies against the colic flexure. The tail of the pancreas extends laterally into the splenorenal ligament and its tip may reach the splenic hilum (Fig. 4.46).

Blood supply

The splenic artery is a direct branch of the coeliac artery. It follows a tortuous course

along the upper border of the pancreas, giving off several pancreatic branches. The artery traverses the splenorenal ligament and divides into its terminal branches near the hilum of the spleen. Several splenic branches enter the hilum, while the short gastric arteries and the left gastro-omental artery enter the gastrosplenic ligament to supply the fundus and greater curve of the stomach respectively.

Veins accompany the terminal branches of the splenic artery and unite adjacent to the hilum of the spleen to form the splenic vein. Running to the right, this vein lies posterior to the tail of the pancreas within the splenorenal ligament and continues retroperitoneally posterior to the body of the gland and inferior to the splenic artery. It then crosses the anterior aspects of the left kidney and renal vessels and receives several small tributaries from the pancreas. Posterior to the neck of the pancreas the splenic vein unites with the superior mesenteric vein to form the portal vein and, close to its termination, is usually joined from below by the inferior mesenteric vein.

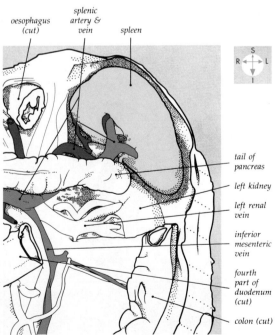

oesophagus (cut)

splenic artery & vein

spleen

tail of pancreas

left kidney

left renal vein

inferior mesenteric vein

fourth part of duodenum (cut)

colon (cut)

Fig. 4.46 Spleen and its vessels and relationship to the diaphragm, pancreas and left kidney. The stomach, and part of the colon and peritoneum have been removed.

DUODENUM

The duodenum, the proximal portion of the small intestine, begins at the pylorus and terminates at the duodenojejunal flexure. Deeply placed in the epigastric and umbilical regions of the abdomen, it curves round the head of the pancreas and is shaped like the letter C (Fig. 4.47). Unlike the remainder of the small intestine, the duodenum is mostly retroperitoneal and therefore relatively immobile. The duodenal lumen receives bile and pancreatic secretions via the bile duct and the pancreatic ducts.

Parts and structure

The duodenum is conventionally described as consisting of four parts (Fig. 4.47). The first (superior) part begins slightly to the right of the midline at the level of the first lumbar vertebra (on the transpyloric plane) and passes upwards, backwards and to the right. In clinical practice its initial segment is often termed the duodenal bulb or duodenal cap. The second (descending) part runs vertically to the level of the third lumbar vertebra. The third (inferior or horizontal) part runs transversely to the left across the midline, arching forwards across the inferior vena cava and aorta. The fourth (ascending) part slopes upwards and to the left and terminates at the level of the second lumbar vertebra by turning sharply forwards at the duodenojejunal flexure. Close to the pylorus the duodenal mucosa is smooth but in the second and subsequent parts of the organ it is raised to form numerous circular folds, the plicae circulares (Fig. 4.48).

The bile duct and main pancreatic duct approach the second part of the duodenum near its midpoint from the posteromedial aspect (Fig. 4.49). They usually pierce the duodenal wall in proximity and commonly open into a single chamber, the hepatopancreatic ampulla (ampulla of Vater). The ampulla raises a projection, the major duodenal papilla, on the internal aspect of the duodenum. Bile and pancreatic secretions enter the duodenal lumen through the tip of this papilla via a minute opening controlled by a ring of smooth muscle, the ampullary sphincter (of Oddi). Immediately above the major duodenal papilla there is often a prominent mucosal fold forming a hood (Fig. 4.48), which may serve as a guide to the location of the papilla, particularly during endoscopic examinations. The pancreas usually possesses a second and smaller

Fig. 4.47 Duodenum and some related structures. The liver and gall bladder have been slightly displaced.

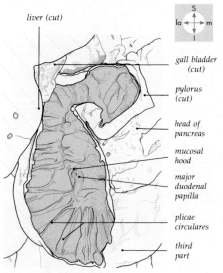

Fig. 4.48 First and second parts of the duodenum opened to show the plicae circulares and the major duodenal papilla.

duct, the accessory pancreatic duct, which enters the second part of the duodenum at the minor duodenal papilla, about 2 cm proximal to the major papilla.

Relations

Most of the duodenum is retroperitoneal. However, the initial 2 cm have peritoneal relationships similar to the stomach in that the lesser and greater omenta attach respectively to the superior and inferior borders. This short segment is relatively mobile and lies immediately inferior to the opening into the omental bursa (Fig. 4.47).

Anterior relations of the proximal portion of the duodenum include the liver and gall bladder. Crossing in front of the second part are the transverse colon and mesocolon (Fig. 4.47), below which lie coils of jejunum and ileum. Running obliquely across the third part of the duodenum are the superior mesenteric vessels (Fig. 4.47), contained in the root of the mesentery of the small intestine. Adjacent to the fourth part there are often folds of peritoneum which may form small recesses, the paraduodenal fossae.

Posteriorly the first part of the duodenum is related to the portal vein, the bile duct and the gastroduodenal artery (Fig. 4.50). The second part lies in front of the hilum of the right kidney and the right renal vessels while the third part crosses the right ureter and gonadal vessels, the inferior vena cava, aorta and origin of the inferior mesenteric artery (Fig. 4.50). The fourth part ascends in front of the left psoas muscle, the left gonadal and renal vessels and the inferior mesenteric vein.

Within the concavity of its C-shaped curve, all parts of the duodenum are related to the pancreas (Figs 4.47 & 4.50).

Blood supply

The gastroduodenal branch of the common hepatic artery descends behind the first part of the duodenum and divides into right gastro-omental and superior pancreaticoduodenal branches (Fig. 4.50). The latter vessel, which is often duplicated, runs in the interval between the duodenum and head of the pancreas and supplies the portion of the duodenum proximal to the major papilla.

The remainder of the duodenum is supplied by the inferior pancreaticoduodenal branch of the superior mesenteric artery (Fig. 4.50), given off as the superior mesenteric artery emerges from between the neck and uncinate process of the pancreas. The inferior pancreaticoduodenal artery runs to the right between the duodenum and pancreas, supplying both structures and anastomosing with the superior pancreaticoduodenal artery. The veins draining the duodenum follow the arterial supply and terminate in the portal venous system.

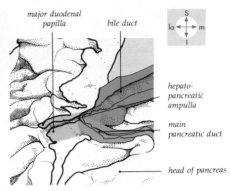

Fig. 4.49 Terminal portions of the bile and main pancreatic ducts and the hepatopancreatic ampulla have been opened.

Fig. 4.50 Arterial supply and some relations of the duodenum. The first part of the duodenum has been displaced laterally to reveal the gastroduodenal artery, bile duct and portal vein.

PANCREAS

The pancreas is both an exocrine and an endocrine gland. Most of its substance is involved in producing pancreatic juice which is conveyed by a duct system into the second part of the duodenum. In addition, microscopic clumps of endocrine tissue, the islets of Langerhans, are dispersed throughout the gland.

The pancreas is a long and narrow, lobulated organ, deeply located on the posterior abdominal wall. It lies approximately on the transpyloric plane (L1 vertebral level) and slopes slightly upwards from right to left. Its extremities lie in the right and left paravertebral gutters while the intermediate portion is thrust forwards in the midline by the prominence of the vertebral column and aorta.

The gland is divided into four parts, from right to left, the head, neck, body and tail (Fig. 4.51). The head is the broadest part and is surrounded by the loop of the duodenum. Projecting to the left from its lower portion is the uncinate process. The neck is indented posteriorly by the portal and superior mesenteric veins. The body, of fairly uniform width, extends to the left and is continuous with the tail, which tapers as it approaches the hilum of the spleen. The tail is contained within the splenorenal ligament but all other parts are retroperitoneal.

In cross-section the pancreas is triangular. It has well-defined superior and inferior borders and a blunt anterior border, to which is attached the transverse mesocolon. The inferior half of the gland is related to the infracolic compartment of the peritoneal cavity while the upper half lies in the floor of the omental bursa and contributes to the stomach bed.

Relations

Surrounded by the loop of the duodenum, the head of the pancreas lies anterior to the inferior vena cava, the right renal vessels and the terminal portion of the bile duct, which is sometimes embedded within the substance of this part of the gland (Fig. 4.52). The anterior surface of the head is related to the first part of the duodenum, the transverse colon and the gastroduodenal artery (Fig. 4.51). The uncinate process lies immediately superior to the third part of the duodenum. The superior mesenteric vessels cross the anterior surface of the uncinate process and separate it from the neck of the gland, which lies in front of the superior mesenteric vein and the commencement of the portal vein. The anterior surface of the neck is separated from the pylorus by the omental bursa.

neck of pancreas

proper hepatic artery
gastroduodenal artery

second part of duodenum

superior mesenteric
artery & vein

head of pancreas

body of pancreas

spleen

tail of pancreas

splenic vein

left kidney

uncinate process

third part of duodenum

Fig. 4.51 Principal relations and parts of the pancreas.

The body of the pancreas crosses the aorta and usually covers the origins of its ventral branches, the coeliac artery, whose common hepatic and splenic branches are related to the superior border of the gland (Fig. 4.53), and the superior mesenteric artery, which emerges at the lower border (Fig. 4.51). Further to the left the gland covers the left renal vessels and suprarenal gland, and the hilum of the left kidney. Immediately posterior to the body the splenic vein receives a major tributary, the inferior mesenteric vein (Figs 4.52 & 4.53). The inferior border of the body is related to the duodenojejunal flexure, coils of jejunum and the left colic flexure. Overlying the anterior surface of the body are the transverse mesocolon, the stomach and omental bursa, and part of the lesser omentum.

The tail of the gland lies within the splenorenal ligament and is accompanied posteriorly by the splenic vessels (Fig. 4.53). It lies anterior to the visceral surface and hilum of the spleen and posterior to the stomach and omental bursa.

Pancreatic ducts

The main pancreatic duct arises in the tail of the gland and traverses the body and neck to reach the head where it curves downwards and to the right to reach the medial wall of the second part of the duodenum (Fig. 4.52). The duct receives numerous tributaries and gradually increases in calibre from left to right. It pierces the intestinal wall at the greater duodenal papilla (see Fig. 4.49).

The main pancreatic duct and the bile duct usually enter the duodenal wall together and unite to form a common chamber, the hepatopancreatic ampulla (of Vater), in which pancreatic juice and bile may mix before entering the duodenal lumen. There is usually a second and smaller duct, the accessory pancreatic duct, which opens into the duodenum about 2 cm above the main duct, at the minor duodenal papilla.

Blood supply

This is derived from branches of the coeliac and superior mesenteric arteries. The head and uncinate process receive superior pancreaticoduodenal branches from the gastroduodenal artery (a branch of the hepatic artery; Fig. 4.51) and inferior pancreaticoduodenal branches from the superior mesenteric artery (see Fig. 4.50). The remainder of the gland is supplied by branches from the splenic artery (Fig. 4.52). The venous drainage of the pancreas passes into the portal system. Superior and inferior pancreaticoduodenal veins from the head of the gland pass respectively into the portal vein and the superior mesenteric vein. Veins from the remainder of the gland terminate in the splenic vein.

Fig. 4.52 Dissection of the pancreas to expose the terminal portions of the bile and main pancreatic ducts.

Fig. 4.53 Principal vascular relations of the body and tail of the pancreas.

LIVER

The liver is the largest organ in the body and lies in the upper part of the abdominal cavity just beneath the diaphragm and mostly under cover of the ribs. It fills the right hypochondrium and extends across the epigastrium into the left hypochondrium. The living organ is reddish-brown and very soft and delicate.

In the living subject the surface marking of the inferior margin of the liver coincides with the right costal margin as far anteriorly as the ninth costal cartilage and inclines across the abdomen to the eighth left costal cartilage. In life, a healthy liver is usually impalpable.

The liver has the shape of a wedge tapering towards the left (Fig. 4.54). Of its five surfaces the superior, the anterior and the right lateral merge with no distinct borders intervening. However, a sharp inferior margin separates the anterior from the inferior or visceral surface. The latter faces obliquely downwards, backwards and to the left. The posterior surface blends with the visceral and superior surfaces at indistinct borders. Most of the surface of the liver is clothed in peritoneum.

Surface features and relations

Anterior and lateral surfaces

The anterior and lateral surfaces of the liver are smoothly convex to conform with the diaphragm and the anterior abdominal wall (Fig. 4.55). A two-layered fold of peritoneum, the falciform ligament, connects the anterior surface to the abdominal wall and demarcates the right and left lobes of the organ. In the free lower border of this ligament runs the fibrous remnant of the umbilical vein, the round ligament (ligamentum teres) of the liver, passing from the umbilicus to the visceral surface of the liver.

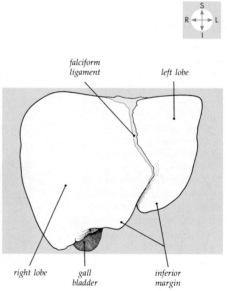

Fig. 4.54 Anterior view of the liver.

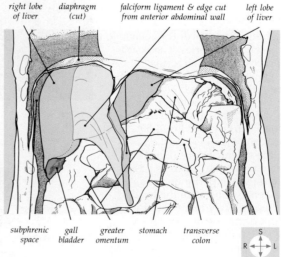

Fig. 4.55 Liver and some of its relations. In this specimen the greater omentum is adherent to the liver and stomach.

Superior surface

This surface is gently convex on each side of a shallow depression related to the central tendon of the diaphragm. Above the liver the two layers of the falciform ligament diverge. One layer passes to the right and continues as the superior layer of the coronary ligament (Fig. 4.56); the other extends to the tip of the left lobe where it forms the left triangular ligament. The posterior layer of this ligament, when traced to the right, is continuous with the lesser omentum.

Visceral surface

This surface (Fig. 4.57) is divided into three areas by two vertical features, the gall bladder and the fissure for the round ligament, the upper ends of which are linked by a horizontal cleft. This cleft is the porta hepatis through which pass the branches of the proper hepatic artery and portal vein and the hepatic ducts. The round ligament ascends along its fissure to reach the portal vein. To the left of the fissure the left lobe of the liver overlies the body of the stomach and lesser omentum.

To the right of the fissure is the small rectangular quadrate lobe, which is related to the anterior aspects of the pyloric region of the stomach and the first part of the duodenum. To the right of the quadrate lobe is the gall bladder, embedded in its fossa. An indentation to the right of the gall bladder accommodates the upper pole of the right kidney. This surface of the right lobe is also related to the right colic flexure and the second part of the duodenum.

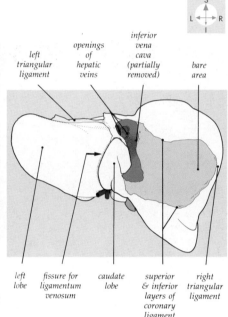

Fig. 4.56   Posterior view of the liver.

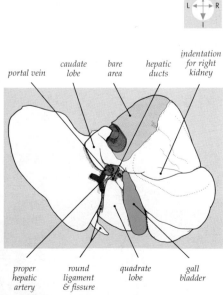

Fig. 4.57   Inferior view of liver and gall bladder showing porta hepatis and visceral surface.

Posterior surface

This surface is also divided into three areas (see Fig. 4.56). Extending upwards from the left end of the porta hepatis is the fissure in which lies the ligamentum venosum, the fibrous remnant of the fetal ductus venosus. The lesser omentum attaches to the liver in the depths of this fissure and around the margins of the porta hepatis (Fig. 4.58). The portion of the liver to the left of the fissure covers the front of the abdominal oesophagus and the fundus of the stomach.

To the right of the fissure lies the caudate lobe, facing into the superior recess of the omental bursa. To the right of this lobe lies the inferior vena cava, which usually grooves the liver deeply. Further to the right is the bare area (see Fig. 4.56), where the right lobe of the liver is in direct contact with the diaphragm and the right suprarenal gland with no

intervening peritoneum. The bare area is bounded above and below by the two layers of the coronary ligament which converge laterally to form the right triangular ligament.

Subphrenic and subhepatic spaces

The arrangement of the various peritoneal ligaments around the liver produces several clinically important spaces in which fluids may accumulate. Between the liver and the diaphragm are the subphrenic spaces (see Fig. 4.55), separated from each other by the falciform ligament and the superior layer of the coronary ligament. The subhepatic spaces lie below and behind the liver, adjacent to either the stomach or the right kidney.

Biliary apparatus

Ducts

Bile produced by the liver is collected by a system of canaliculi that drain into the right and left hepatic ducts. The two hepatic ducts emerge through the porta hepatis and soon unite to form the common hepatic duct. As this duct descends in the free border of the lesser omentum it is joined from the right by the cystic duct to form the bile duct (Fig. 4.59).

Initially the bile duct lies in the free edge of the lesser omentum, to the right of the hepatic artery and in front of the portal vein. It then passes behind the first part of the duodenum with the gastroduodenal artery and curves to the right behind the head of the pancreas, sometimes grooving the gland (see Fig. 4.52). The bile duct pierces the wall of the second part of the

Fig. 4.58 Posterior view of liver, stomach and lesser omentum. The spleen, left kidney, parts of the pancreas, aorta and inferior vena cava have been removed.

duodenum in company with the main pancreatic duct (see Fig. 4.49).

Gall bladder

This is a hollow, pear-shaped organ in which bile from the liver is concentrated and stored (see Fig. 4.57). It lies against the visceral surface of the liver, often partially buried in its substance, and usually projects beyond the inferior margin to end blindly in a rounded fundus. The fundus normally makes contact with the anterior abdominal wall where the lateral edge (linea semilunaris) of the right rectus abdominis muscle crosses the costal margin. The body of the gall bladder is its widest part and tapers superiorly into the neck, which continues as the cystic duct. This duct, through which bile enters and leaves, runs upwards towards the porta hepatis and then turns downwards to join the common hepatic duct. The undersurface of the gall bladder is covered by peritoneum continuous with that surrounding the liver.

The body is usually related to the proximal part of the duodenum and the fundus often makes contact with the transverse colon.

The arterial supply to the gall bladder is provided by the cystic artery, which usually springs from the right branch of the proper hepatic artery (Fig. 4.59) though its origin is variable. The cystic vein normally drains into the portal vein or its right branch.

Hepatic blood vessels

Blood is conveyed to the liver by the proper hepatic artery and the portal vein, both of which enter via the porta hepatis. Blood is drained by the hepatic veins embedded in the organ which enter the anterior aspect of the inferior vena cava immediately below the diaphragm (see Fig. 4.56). The common hepatic artery, a branch of the coeliac artery (Fig. 4.60), runs retroperitoneally downwards and to the right to the superior border of the first part of the duodenum (Fig. 4.59). Here the common hepatic artery

gives off the right gastric and gastroduodenal arteries and continues as the proper hepatic artery. The right gastric artery arises above the first part of the duodenum and runs to the left within the lesser omentum, supplying the lesser curve of the stomach. The larger gastroduodenal artery descends behind the first part of the duodenum alongside the bile duct. Its terminal branches are the superior pancreaticoduodenal artery (see Fig. 4.50) and the right gastro-omental artery (see Fig. 4.41). The proper hepatic artery ascends in the free border of the lesser omentum on the left of the bile duct and anterior to the portal vein. Near the porta hepatis it divides into right and left branches to enter the liver with corresponding branches of the portal vein. The left branches of the artery and vein are distributed to the left, quadrate and most of the caudate lobes. The right branches supply the remainder of the liver. The proper hepatic artery also supplies the gall bladder via the cystic artery (Fig. 4.59).

Fig. 4.59 Porta hepatis including the right, left and common hepatic ducts and the cystic artery, a branch of the hepatic artery.

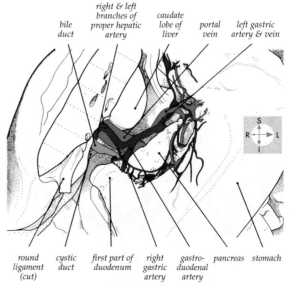

Fig. 4.60 Course and branches of the common hepatic artery. The lesser omentum has been removed.

PORTAL VENOUS SYSTEM

The hepatic portal venous system drains blood from most of the alimentary tract (including the abdominal oesophagus, stomach, small and large intestines), pancreas, and spleen. Blood from these organs is drained by the superior mesenteric and splenic veins which unite to form the portal vein (Fig. 4.75). This large vein approaches the porta hepatis with the proper hepatic artery, and branches of both vessels enter the liver and further subdivide. After traversing the liver, blood from both sources is drained by the hepatic veins, which enter the inferior vena cava.

Tributaries

The superior mesenteric vein (Fig. 4.76) receives blood from most of the small intestine and the proximal half of the large intestine. It drains the duodenum distal to the major papilla, the jejunum and ileum, the caecum and appendix, and the ascending and most of the transverse colon. The vein accompanies the superior mesenteric artery within the root of the mesentery and its tributaries generally correspond to the branches of the artery.

The splenic vein (Fig. 4.76) drains the spleen and parts of the pancreas and stomach. It arises at the hilum of the spleen and runs to the right in the splenorenal ligament behind the tail of the pancreas. The vein continues behind the body of the pancreas and usually receives the inferior mesenteric vein and other tributaries corresponding to the branches of the splenic artery.

The inferior mesenteric vein drains the upper part of the anal canal, the rectum, the sigmoid and descending parts of the colon and the distal part of the transverse colon. The vein initially accompanies the corresponding artery but in the latter part of its course it ascends the posterior abdominal wall independently, passing to the left of the duodenojejunal junction. The vessel usually terminates by joining the splenic vein behind the body of the pancreas (Fig. 4.75), but it may enter the superior mesenteric vein (Fig. 4.76).

liver (cut)

proper hepatic artery

portal vein

bile duct

duodenum (cut)

spleen

gastroduodenal artery (cut)

superior mesenteric vein & artery (cut)

splenic vein

inferior mesenteric vein

Fig. 4.75 Portal and splenic veins. Most of the pancreas has been removed and the first part of the duodenum turned aside.

Portal vein

The portal vein is formed behind the neck of the pancreas by the union of the superior mesenteric and splenic veins (Fig. 4.75). It runs upwards and to the right behind the gastroduodenal artery and the first part of the duodenum. The vein then enters the free border of the lesser omentum accompanied anteriorly by the bile duct and the proper hepatic artery (see Fig. 4.42). Near the porta hepatis the vein divides into left and right branches, which enter the liver. Several small veins enter the portal vein directly, including the left and right gastric veins and the cystic vein.

Portacaval anastomoses

There are numerous anastomoses between the tributaries of the portal venous system and those of the systemic venous system. In health, these portacaval anastomoses are microscopic; but if there is obstruction of blood flow through the portal vein or liver they may dilate and give rise to characteristic clinical features. For example, in the wall of the lowest part of the oesophagus, veins draining into the left gastric vein communicate with tributaries of the azygos venous system. Portal vein obstruction can cause gross swelling of these oesophageal veins (oesophageal varices), which may bleed profusely.

Similarly, paraumbilical veins accompanying the round ligament of the liver communicate with the portal vein at the porta hepatis and with veins of the anterior abdominal wall around the umbilicus. Portal vein obstruction, therefore, may result in dilatation of the subcutaneous veins of the abdominal wall. Other sites of portacaval anastomoses include the anal canal and retroperitoneal parts of the intestine.

Fig. 4.76 Tributaries of the portal vein. In this specimen the inferior mesenteric vein joins the superior mesenteric vein.

KIDNEYS AND SUPRARENAL GLANDS

Kidneys

The two kidneys lie behind the peritoneum on either side of the upper lumbar vertebrae (Fig. 4.77). They are embedded in fat in the paravertebral gutters of the posterior abdominal wall and are placed obliquely with their anterior surfaces directed slightly laterally (Fig. 4.78). The left kidney usually lies at a higher level than the right.

Each kidney is bean-shaped, flattened anteroposteriorly and approximately 11 cm long. The anterior and posterior surfaces are gently convex and the superior and inferior poles are rounded. The lateral border is convex while the indented medial border bears an aperture, the hilum (Fig. 4.79), which is traversed by the renal pelvis or ureter, the renal vessels, lymphatics and autonomic nerves. The hilum leads into a cavity within the kidney, the renal sinus, which is occupied by the calices and renal pelvis (Fig. 4.81), the renal blood vessels and a quantity of fat.

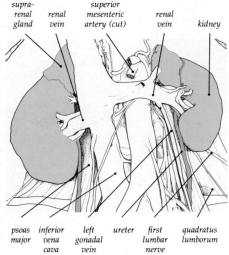

supra-
renal   renal   superior   renal
gland   vein   mesenteric   vein   kidney
                               artery (cut)

psoas   inferior   left   ureter   first   quadratus
major   vena   gonadal   lumbar   lumborum
          cava   vein   nerve

Fig. 4.77 Kidneys, suprarenal glands and some of the vessels associated with them.

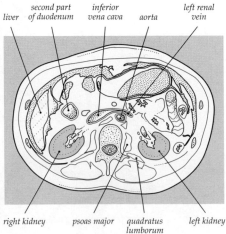

          second part   inferior
liver   of duodenum   vena cava   aorta   left renal
                                                            vein

right kidney   psoas major   quadratus   left kidney
                                    lumborum

Fig. 4.78 Transverse section at the level of the first lumbar vertebra showing some relations of the kidneys. The spleen is not evident in this specimen. Inferior aspect. Compare Fig. 4.107.

Covered by a thin capsule, the kidney comprises an outer cortex and an inner medulla. The medulla contains numerous pyramids whose apices project into the renal sinus as the renal papillae. Urine discharged from the papillae is collected by about ten trumpet-shaped chambers, the minor calices (Fig. 4.81), which unite to form two or three major calices. These fuse into the single, funnel-shaped renal pelvis, which lies posterior to most of the vessels and is continuous with the ureter.

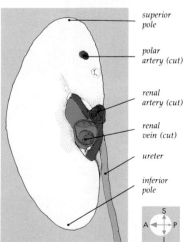

Fig. 4.79 Medial aspect of the right kidney showing the renal vessels passing through the hilum.

Fig. 4.80 Intravenous urogram showing detail of the pelvicaliceal system.

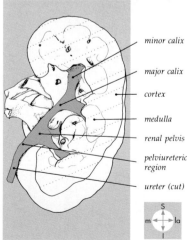

Fig. 4.81 Right kidney dissected from behind to show the renal pelvis and calices.

Perirenal tissues

Each kidney is surrounded by a layer of perinephric (perirenal) fat enveloped in a thin sheet of connective tissue, the renal fascia (Fig. 4.82). This fascia also encloses the suprarenal gland and the proximal part of the ureter. From the inferior pole of the kidney, the renal fascia tapers downwards into the iliac fossa. Around the fascia is a further layer of fat (paranephric or pararenal fat) lying against the posterior abdominal muscles and covered anteriorly by the peritoneum.

Relations of kidneys

The right and left kidneys have similar posterior relations (see Fig. 4.78). The superior poles lie against the diaphragm and the twelfth ribs, below which run the subcostal nerves and vessels. On the left the upper pole is also related, through the diaphragm, to the pleura and eleventh rib. The medial border of each kidney overlaps psoas major (see Fig. 4.77) while the inferolateral portion is related to quadratus lumborum and transversus abdominis, and to the first lumbar nerve.

The anterior relations of the kidneys are asymmetric. On the right, from above downwards, they include the bare area of the liver, the second part of the duodenum (see Fig. 4.78), the right flexure of the colon and coils of jejunum. The medial border of the right kidney is related to the inferior vena cava, the renal vessels and the upper part of the ureter (Fig. 4.82).

On the left, from above downwards, the anterior relations include the stomach and spleen, the splenic vessels, the tail of the pancreas, the left colic flexure and coils of jejunum. The medial border relates to the suprarenal gland, the renal and suprarenal vessels, the left gonadal vein and the proximal part of the ureter (see Fig. 4.85).

Renal vessels

At the level of the first lumbar vertebra the aorta usually supplies one renal artery to each kidney (Fig. 4.83). Each artery lies behind the corresponding vein, and the artery on the right crosses behind the inferior vena cava. However, there are often supernumerary (anomalous, aberrant or accessory) renal arteries arising from the aorta above or below the typical vessel. Regardless of its origin, each renal artery divides as it approaches the kidney and all the branches usually traverse the hilum. However, a polar artery may occasionally be found entering the medial border of the organ above or below the hilum (see Figs 4.79 & 4.85).

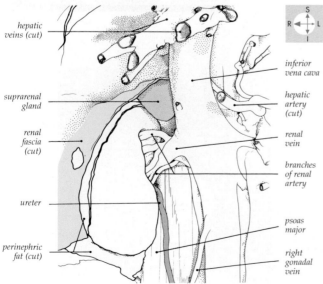

Fig. 4.82 Right kidney and suprarenal gland seen within the renal fascia and perinephric fat, part of which has been removed.

Fig. 4.83 Renal arteries exposed by removal of the renal veins and a portion of the inferior vena cava.

Several veins unite near the renal hilum, anterior to the arteries, forming the renal vein. On the right the vein runs a short course to terminate in the inferior vena cava. The left renal vein is longer and usually receives the suprarenal and gonadal veins before passing in front of the aorta to reach the inferior vena cava (see Fig. 4.77). Because of its termination, the left gonadal vein may become dilated if the renal vein is obstructed. In the male this can lead to swelling of the pampiniform plexus within the scrotum (varicocele).

Suprarenal glands

The suprarenal glands lie adjacent to the superior poles of the kidneys, embedded in the perinephric fat. On the right the gland is tetrahedral and occupies the angle between the superior pole of the kidney and the inferior vena cava (Fig. 4.84). The left gland is crescentic and is applied to the medial border of the kidney above the hilum (Fig. 4.85).

The blood supply to the suprarenal glands is provided by branches of the renal and inferior phrenic arteries and the aorta. The right suprarenal vein is very short and enters the inferior vena cava directly while that on the left descends to enter the left renal vein.

The medulla of each suprarenal gland is richly innervated by preganglionic sympathetic nerves from the adjacent part of the sympathetic trunk.

The blood supply to the abdominal part of the ureter is derived from branches of the renal artery, supplemented by minute peritoneal vessels.

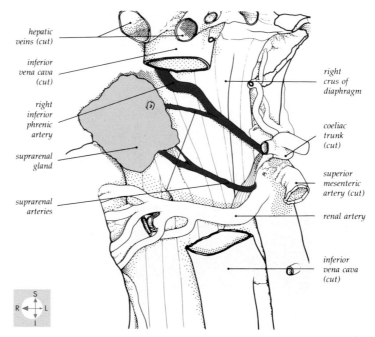

Fig. 4.84 Right suprarenal gland and its arteries exposed by removal of the renal vein and a portion of the inferior vena cava.

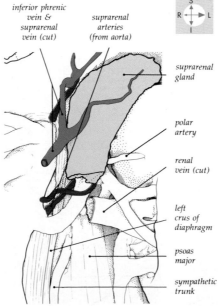

Fig. 4.85 Left suprarenal gland and its vessels. The renal vein and inferior tip of the gland have been excised to reveal the suprarenal arteries.

Abdominal parts of ureters

From the pelviureteric region each ureter descends through the retroperitoneal tissues of the posterior abdominal wall as far as the pelvic brim. Here it crosses in front of the external iliac vessels and continues down the lateral wall of the pelvis (see page 201). Within the abdomen the ureter lies on psoas major (Fig. 4.82), behind which are the lumbar transverse processes (see Fig. 4.80).

The right ureter commences behind the second part of the duodenum and is crossed by the root of the mesentery, the gonadal vessels and branches of the superior mesenteric artery and accompanying veins. This ureter is also related to coils of small intestine, and sometimes to the caecum and appendix. The left ureter is covered initially by the pancreas and is subsequently crossed by the gonadal vessels, branches of the inferior mesenteric artery and vein (see Fig. 4.74) and coils of small intestine and sigmoid colon. At the pelvic brim, it passes behind the root of the sigmoid mesocolon.

ABDOMINAL AORTA

The aorta enters the abdomen behind the median arcuate ligament of the diaphragm at the level of the twelfth thoracic vertebra. It descends behind the peritoneum, inclining slightly to the left of the midline to its bifurcation in front of the fourth lumbar vertebra (Fig. 4.87). Throughout its course the abdominal aorta is accompanied by lymph vessels and nodes and is surrounded by a plexus of autonomic nerves (see pages 176–179).

Posterior to the aorta lie the left lumbar veins, the anterior longitudinal ligament and the lumbar vertebral bodies. Anterior relations, from above downwards, include the body of the pancreas, the splenic and left renal veins, the third part of the duodenum, the root of the mesentery and coils of small intestine.

To the right of the aorta lie the right crus of the diaphragm and the inferior vena cava (Fig. 4.87). On the left are the left diaphragmatic crus, suprarenal gland and kidney.

Visceral branches

Three arteries arise from the anterior aspect of the aorta to supply the alimentary organs while three pairs of lateral branches pass to the suprarenals, kidneys and gonads respectively.

The coeliac and superior mesenteric arteries arise at the levels of the twelfth thoracic and first lumbar vertebrae respectively whilst the smaller inferior mesenteric artery takes origin at the level of the third lumbar vertebra (Fig. 4.87). For details of the course and distribution of each of these arteries see pages 147, 160 and 165.

The suprarenal branches of the aorta (Fig. 4.87) are small and variable and are often supplemented by branches from the inferior phrenic and renal arteries

Fig. 4.86 Right testicular vessels within the abdomen. Several lumbar vessels are also seen.

(see Fig. 4.84; see also Fig. 4.90). The renal arteries usually arise at the level of the first lumbar vertebra but variations are common (see page 170).

The long and slender gonadal (testicular or ovarian) arteries usually arise from the aorta just below the renal arteries (Fig. 4.87). The gonadal artery on the right crosses in front of the inferior vena cava, and the arteries of both sides incline downwards and laterally through the retroperitoneal tissues on the psoas major muscles (Fig. 4.86). Each artery is accompanied by one or more gonadal veins and crosses anterior to the ureters but posterior to blood vessels supplying the

intestines. Inferiorly the testicular artery follows the psoas major round the pelvic brim and enters the deep inguinal ring (see page 133). The ovarian artery crosses the external iliac vessels and pelvic brim to reach the ovary within the pelvis (see page 200).

Parietal branches

These vessels supply the diaphragm and the posterior walls of the abdomen and pelvis. The paired inferior phrenic arteries are the first branches of the aorta within the abdomen (Fig. 4.87; see Fig. 4.90) and often furnish small branches to the suprarenal

glands before arching upwards and laterally on the abdominal surface of the diaphragm.

Four pairs of lumbar arteries usually arise from the posterolateral aspect of the aorta and supply the posterior abdominal wall (Fig. 4.86; see Fig. 4.88). The arteries on the right cross behind the inferior vena cava to curve round the side of the corresponding vertebral body deep to psoas major.

A single small vessel, the median sacral artery, arises from the back of the aortic bifurcation and descends behind the left common iliac vein to reach the anterior surface of the sacrum (Fig. 4.88).

Fig. 4.87 Abdominal aorta and its branches, seen after removal of the renal veins and part of the inferior vena cava.

ILIAC VESSELS

Common and external iliac vessels

The aortic bifurcation gives rise to the two common iliac arteries, which incline downwards and laterally on the medial aspects of psoas major (Fig. 4.88). The vessels terminate in front of the sacroiliac joints by dividing into internal and external iliac arteries. The right common iliac artery crosses in front of the left common iliac vein, while that on the left is crossed by the inferior mesenteric vessels. The ureter crosses either the lower end of the common iliac artery or the commencement of its external branch (Fig. 4.88). The internal iliac artery begins at the bifurcation of the common iliac artery and descends on the lateral wall of the pelvis (see page 212).

The external iliac artery curves round the pelvic brim (Fig. 4.88) and, passing behind the inguinal ligament, enters the thigh as the femoral artery (see Fig. 6.19). The external iliac artery is accompanied on its medial side by the corresponding vein and posterolaterally by psoas major. The external iliac vessels are crossed by the ovarian vessels in the female and by the ductus deferens in the male. Near the inguinal ligament the artery gives off the inferior epigastric artery, which runs upwards and medially, medial to the deep inguinal ring (see Figs 4.17 & 4.21).

Each external iliac vein begins behind the inguinal ligament as the continuation of the femoral vein (Fig. 4.88). It receives the inferior epigastric vein, ascends on the medial side of the corresponding artery and joins the internal iliac vein (see page 213) to form the common iliac vein. The two common iliac veins continue upwards and medially, passing behind the right common iliac artery, by which they may be compressed, before uniting to form the inferior vena cava.

Fig. 4.88   Male pelvis and lower abdomen showing the common and external iliac vessels and some of their relations.

INFERIOR VENA CAVA

The inferior vena cava is formed at the level of the fifth lumbar vertebra, a little to the right of the midline (Fig. 4.89). It ascends the posterior abdominal wall and pierces the central tendon of the diaphragm to enter the thorax at the level of the eighth thoracic vertebra (see Fig. 2.61).

Behind the inferior vena cava lie the lumbar vertebral bodies, the anterior longitudinal ligament, the right sympathetic chain and right psoas major muscle. In addition, the right renal and right lumbar arteries cross behind the vena cava (see Figs 4.87 & 4.86) and most of the right suprarenal gland lies posterior to the vessel (Fig. 4.90).

Near its commencement the inferior vena cava is covered anteriorly by peritoneum and coils of small intestine. Superiorly it is crossed by the root of the mesentery, the right gonadal artery (see Fig. 4.86) and the third part of the duodenum (see Fig. 4.50). It continues behind the opening into the omental bursa (see Fig. 4.36) and then grooves the posterior surface of the liver (see Fig. 4.56) before piercing the diaphragm.

To the right of the vena cava lie the gonadal vessels, the ureter, the kidney and renal vessels (Fig. 4.89) and the right lobe of the liver. To the left lie the aorta with its associated lymph nodes, the right crus of the diaphragm and the caudate lobe of the liver.

Tributaries

The venous drainage of the suprarenal glands, the kidneys and the gonads is asymmetric. On the right each of these organs is drained by a vein that passes directly into the inferior vena cava (Figs 4.89 & 4.90) but on the left the renal vein receives the suprarenal and gonadal veins before crossing in front of the aorta to reach the vena cava. Immediately before its passage through the diaphragm the inferior vena cava receives several large hepatic veins (Fig. 4.90).

The parietal tributaries of the inferior vena cava drain the diaphragm and the posterior pelvic and abdominal walls. The lumbar and median sacral veins (see Figs 4.86 & 4.88) accompany the corresponding arteries, the upper lumbar veins often communicating with the renal, suprarenal, azygos and hemiazygos veins. Two or more inferior phrenic veins drain the undersurface of the diaphragm (Fig. 4.90).

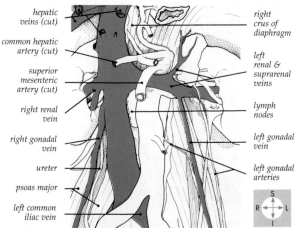

Fig. 4.89 Course and principal tributaries of the inferior vena cava.

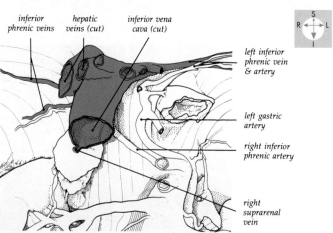

Fig. 4.90 Upper part of inferior vena cava showing its tributaries. In this specimen the left inferior phrenic artery arises from the left gastric artery.

LYMPHATICS OF ABDOMEN

The lymphatic vessels and nodes of the abdomen drain the abdominal and pelvic organs as well as the pelvic walls and the lower part of the abdominal wall. (The upper part of the abdominal wall is drained by the internal thoracic and axillary nodes; see page 132.) In addition, the abdominal lymphatics receive lymph from the lower limbs and the perineum.

ureter

testicular vein

external iliac lymph nodes & lymphatic vessel

external iliac artery & vein

common iliac node(s)

right & left common iliac arteries

peritoneum (cut)

Fig. 4.91   The common and external iliac arteries are accompanied by a chain of lymphatic vessels and nodes.

aortic lymph nodes

inferior vena cava

testicular vein

common iliac nodes

left gastric artery

common hepatic & splenic arteries (cut)

superior mesenteric artery (cut)

right testicular artery (cut)

aorta

inferior mesenteric artery

Fig. 4.92   Removal of the autonomic nerves and retroperitoneal connective tissues reveals the lymphatic vessels and nodes lying on the right side of the aorta.

Some lymph nodes are situated adjacent to the organs they drain and include those of the liver and spleen and in the hila of the kidneys. The lymphatic vessels draining most of the abdominal organs accompany blood vessels and pass to nodes grouped around the aorta. Often lymph passes through intermediate nodes situated along the courses of the arteries. Most of the lymph from the abdominal walls and viscera eventually drains into the thoracic duct.

Because of their deep position, most intra-abdominal lymph nodes are not palpable in the living subject, even when enlarged.

Iliac lymph nodes

The external iliac nodes (Fig. 4.91) receive lymph from the lower limb and perineum via the deep inguinal nodes. In addition, the iliac nodes drain the deeper layers of the abdominal wall below the level of the umbilicus via lymphatic vessels accompanying the inferior epigastric vessels. Lymph from the superficial tissues of the lower abdominal wall reaches the external iliac nodes, having passed first to superficial and then to deep inguinal nodes.

The internal iliac nodes drain the pelvic walls and floor and some of the pelvic organs, including the bladder, lower part of the rectum, prostate and uterus. However, lymph from most of the rectum, sigmoid colon and ovaries drains to the aortic nodes. From the external and internal iliac nodes lymph passes to nodes alongside the common iliac artery (Fig. 4.91) and subsequently to the aortic nodes.

Aortic nodes

The major abdominal lymphatic vessels and their associated nodes are arranged alongside the aorta (Fig. 4.92). The nodes on each side of the aorta receive lymph from the common iliac nodes, posterior abdominal wall, gonads, kidneys and suprarenal glands, while nodes lying immediately anterior to the aorta drain the digestive organs.

Nodes around the origin of the inferior mesenteric artery drain lymph from most of the rectum, and the sigmoid and descending parts of the colon. Nodes lying adjacent to the origins of the superior mesenteric and coeliac arteries drain the spleen, pancreas, liver, stomach, small intestine and the large intestine as far as the splenic flexure.

Cisterna chyli

Efferent lymphatics from the aortic nodes drain into the cisterna chyli (Fig. 4.93). This fusiform sac lies at the level of the upper two lumbar vertebrae, adjacent to the right crus of the diaphragm. It lies behind the right border of the aorta and opens superiorly into the thoracic duct. The duct ascends through the aortic opening of the diaphragm and continues through the thorax to drain into the great veins in the root of the neck (see page 61).

Fig. 4.93 Cisterna chyli, revealed by removal of parts of the crura and a segment of aorta.

AUTONOMIC NERVES OF ABDOMEN

The autonomic innervation to the abdominal viscera is provided by perivascular plexuses of nerves accompanying the arterial supply to each organ. The plexuses comprise sympathetic and parasympathetic fibres of both motor and sensory type. The autonomic nerves control glandular secretion, smooth muscle activity and vasomotor tone; they are also sensory, mediating the distension of hollow organs and the tension on mesenteries.

Parasympathetic nerves

Most of the parasympathetic supply is provided by the vagus (X cranial) nerves, but there are small contributions to the distal part of the colon from branches of the pelvic splanchnic nerves that arise from the sacral spinal nerves. The vagi and the pelvic splanchnic nerves carry preganglionic parasympathetic fibres which synapse with postganglionic fibres in the walls of the relevant organs.

From the oesophageal plexus (see page 61) two or more vagal trunks (gastric nerves) emerge and accompany the oesophagus through the diaphragm. The anterior trunk, derived mostly from the left vagus nerve (Fig. 4.94), enters the abdomen in front of the oesophagus and gives branches to the anterior surface of the stomach and to the liver. The posterior trunk, derived mostly from the right vagus, descends behind the oesophagus and supplies the posterior surface of the stomach and the coeliac plexus. From this plexus some vagal fibres pass inferiorly to the root of the superior mesenteric artery. The perivascular plexuses that accompany branches of the coeliac and superior mesenteric arteries convey these vagal fibres to all parts of the digestive system as far distally as the splenic flexure of the colon.

The remainder of the large intestine receives its parasympathetic supply from branches of the pelvic splanchnic nerves (nervi erigentes). These ascend through plexuses in the pelvis (see page 210) and cross the left common iliac vessels in the root of the sigmoid mesocolon to reach the root of the inferior mesenteric artery. By accompanying branches of this artery, parasympathetic fibres from the sacral segments of the spinal cord supply the descending and sigmoid parts of the colon and the rectum.

Sympathetic nerves

The sympathetic system in the abdomen comprises two ganglionated trunks and a network of nerves (the aortic or prevertebral plexuses) covering the surface of the aorta.

Each sympathetic trunk enters the abdomen behind the medial arcuate ligament of the diaphragm (Fig. 4.95) and descends along the medial border of psoas major, the trunk on the right lying posterior to the inferior vena cava. Each trunk passes behind the common iliac vessels and crosses the pelvic inlet at the ala of the sacrum.

Within the abdomen each trunk bears five lumbar ganglia. Only the upper two ganglia receive fibres from the central nervous system. These preganglionic sympathetic fibres are conveyed in white rami communicantes arising from the first and second lumbar spinal nerves. Some preganglionic fibres synapse in the sympathetic trunk while others pass into branches of the trunk and synapse nearer the target organs.

Each ganglion of the trunk gives a branch, a grey ramus communicans, to the corresponding spinal nerve. The postganglionic sympathetic fibres in the grey rami are distributed to the body wall and the lower limb. In addition, the ganglia supply branches (containing both pre- and postganglionic fibres) to the abdominal and pelvic organs. Branches from the upper ganglia reinforce the aortic plexuses whilst the lumbar splanchnic nerves descend from the lower ganglia and cross anterior to the common iliac vessels (Fig. 4.96). The lumbar splanchnic nerves from the right and left trunks unite below the bifurcation of the aorta to form the hypogastric plexus from which branches descend to reach the pelvic autonomic plexuses (see page 210).

Aortic plexuses

The dense network of autonomic nerves (both parasympathetic and sympathetic)

oesophageal plexus
oesophagus
inferior vena cava (cut)
branch to liver
liver (cut)
descending thoracic aorta
anterior vagal trunk
diaphragm (cut)
branch to anterior surface of stomach
lesser omentum
stomach

Fig. 4.94 Anterior vagal trunk, revealed by removal of part of the diaphragm and exposure of the lower oesophagus.

that invests the abdominal aorta (Fig. 4.96) has several component plexuses, which are named according to the larger branches of the aorta. These are the coeliac, aorticorenal, renal, superior mesenteric, intermesenteric and inferior mesenteric plexuses. From these perivascular plexuses nerves are distributed to the abdominal organs.

The parasympathetic fibres in the aortic plexuses are derived mainly from the posterior vagal trunk, which enters the abdomen on the wall of the oesophagus, while the sympathetic fibres are provided principally by the thoracic splanchnic nerves (see page 63). These branches of the thoracic portions of the sympathetic trunks

pierce the crura of the diaphragm to reach the coeliac plexus. Additional sympathetic fibres are provided by the upper ganglia of the lumbar sympathetic chain. Within the aortic plexuses are numerous small ganglia in which the pre- and postganglionic sympathetic fibres synapse.

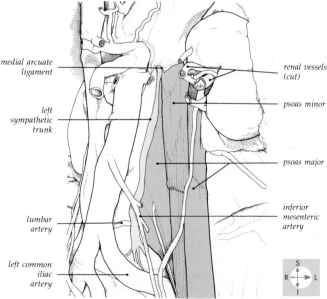

medial arcuate ligament

left sympathetic trunk

lumbar artery

left common iliac artery

renal vessels (cut)

psoas minor

psoas major

inferior mesenteric artery

Fig. 4.95 Lumbar portion of the left sympathetic trunk after removal of the aortic plexuses of nerves.

splenic & common hepatic arteries (cut)

superior mesenteric artery (cut) & plexus

inferior mesenteric artery & plexus

lumbar splanchnic nerves

left kidney & suprarenal gland

coeliac plexus

renal plexus

intermesenteric plexus

psoas fascia

Fig. 4.96 Aortic plexuses of autonomic nerves after removal of aortic nodes and lymph vessels.

POSTERIOR ABDOMINAL WALL

Posterior to the abdominal cavity lie the lumbar spine, the psoas, iliacus and quadratus lumborum muscles, and associated fasciae and nerves (Fig. 4.97). The posterior abdominal wall extends inferiorly to the pelvic brim and superiorly to the attachment of the diaphragm (see page 183) while laterally it merges with the anterolateral abdominal wall. The lumbar spine and the postvertebral muscles (erector spinae) are considered in Section 8.

Muscles

Psoas major

This long fusiform muscle (Fig. 4.97) attaches to the sides of the last thoracic and all five lumbar vertebral bodies, to the intervening discs and to the fronts of the lumbar transverse processes. At the side of each lumbar vertebral body, psoas major attaches to a fascial tunnel conveying a lumbar artery and vein (see Fig. 4.101). The muscle inclines downwards, passing behind the inguinal ligament to enter the anterior compartment of the thigh (Fig. 4.98). The psoas major tendon, which also

Fig. 4.97 Removal of the abdominal contents reveals the muscles and nerves of the posterior abdominal wall. On one side some iliac and psoas fasciae have been preserved.

Fig. 4.98 Iliacus and psoas major, seen after removal of the inguinal ligament and part of sartorius, attach to the lesser trochanter of the femur. The psoas minor tendon descends to the iliopubic eminence of the hip bone.

receives most of the fibres of iliacus, passes in front of the hip joint capsule, from which it is separated by a bursa, and attaches to the lesser trochanter of the femur.

Psoas major is innervated by the anterior rami of the upper lumbar nerves and its principal actions are flexion and medial rotation of the hip joint. In addition, the muscle flexes the lumbar spine both anteriorly and laterally. Within the substance of psoas major the anterior rami of the lumbar nerves form the lumbar plexus, whose branches emerge from the lateral, anterior and medial surfaces of the muscle.

Psoas minor

When present, this small muscle lies on the anterior surface of psoas major and gives way to a long narrow tendon (Fig. 4.98), which attaches to the iliopubic eminence of the hip bone.

Iliacus

This fan-shaped muscle attaches to the upper portion of the abdominal surface of the ilium and adjacent part of the sacrum (Fig. 4.98). Most of its fibres attach to the tendon of psoas major although some reach the femur below the lesser trochanter. The muscle is innervated by the femoral nerve (see Fig. 4.101) and assists psoas major in flexing the hip joint.

Quadratus lumborum

Quadratus lumborum is anchored inferiorly to the iliolumbar ligament and adjacent part of the iliac crest. Superiorly it reaches the medial part of the lower border of the twelfth rib. There are intermediate attachments to the transverse processes of the upper four lumbar vertebrae. This muscle is innervated by the subcostal nerve and anterior rami of the upper three lumbar nerves, and is a lateral flexor of the lumbar spine. When the diaphragm contracts during inspiration, quadratus lumborum stabilizes the twelfth rib.

Fasciae

The psoas and iliac fasciae form a continuous layer covering the anterior surfaces of their respective muscles (Fig. 4.97). The psoas fascia fuses superiorly with the diaphragmatic fascia and laterally and inferiorly with the transversalis fascia. Fascial thickenings over the upper parts of psoas major and quadratus lumborum form the medial and lateral arcuate ligaments (lumbocostal arches), which provide attachment for the diaphragm (see Fig. 4.101). Fascial layers covering the anterior and posterior surfaces of quadratus lumborum constitute part of the thoracolumbar fascia. These layers fuse at the lateral border of the muscle and give attachment to transversus abdominis.

Nerves

On each side of the midline the sympathetic trunk enters the abdomen behind the medial arcuate ligament of the diaphragm and descends on the medial border of psoas major (see Fig. 4.95). The anterior rami of the subcostal and lumbar nerves emerge through their respective intervertebral foramina and enter the substance of psoas major. All spinal nerves within psoas receive grey rami communicantes from the sympathetic trunk, but only the last thoracic and upper two lumbar nerves supply white rami to the trunk.

Subcostal (T12) nerve

This nerve follows the lower border of the twelfth rib and enters the abdomen behind the lateral arcuate ligament of the diaphragm. It crosses the anterior surface of quadratus lumborum and continues on the deep surface of transversus abdominis. The nerve pierces transversus to enter the neurovascular plane of the abdominal wall, and its subsequent course is similar to that of the lower intercostal nerves (see page 131).

Lumbar plexus

Within psoas major the anterior rami of the upper four lumbar nerves form the lumbar plexus, whose branches are distributed to the lower part of the abdominal wall, the lower limb and the sacral plexus in the pelvic cavity (see Figs 4.100 & 4.102).

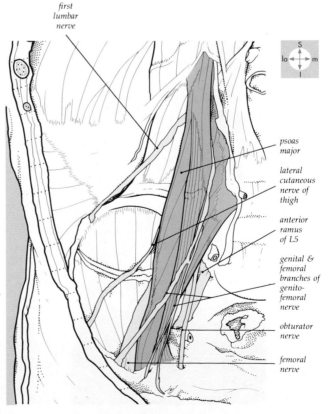

first lumbar nerve

psoas major

lateral cutaneous nerve of thigh

anterior ramus of L5

genital & femoral branches of genitofemoral nerve

obturator nerve

femoral nerve

Fig. 4.99 Branches of the lumbar plexus emerge from the substance of psoas major.

First lumbar nerve

Although a few first lumbar (L1) fibres contribute to the genitofemoral nerve (Fig. 4.100), most form a nerve that emerges from the lateral border of psoas major and crosses the anterior surface of quadratus lumborum (Fig. 4.101).

After a variable distance this nerve divides into iliohypogastric and ilioinguinal branches, which continue into the anterolateral abdominal wall. Their paths and distribution are considered on page 132.

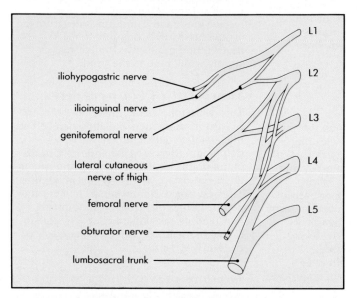

Fig. 4.100 Diagrammatic representation of the lumbar plexus to show the origins of each of its branches.

Genitofemoral (L1 & L2) nerve

This nerve emerges through the anterior surface of psoas major on which it descends, dividing into two branches (see Fig. 4.99). The genital branch enters the deep inguinal ring and innervates the cremaster muscle while the femoral branch passes behind the inguinal ligament to reach the subcutaneous tissue covering the femoral triangle (see Fig. 6.9).

Lateral cutaneous (L2 & L3) nerve of thigh

Emerging from the lateral side of psoas major, this nerve inclines across the anterior surface of iliacus (see Fig. 4.99). It passes behind or through the inguinal ligament close to the anterior superior iliac spine (a site of possible entrapment) and enters the subcutaneous tissue on the anterolateral aspect of the thigh (see Fig. 6.9).

Femoral (L2, L3 & L4) nerve

This large nerve appears at the lateral border of psoas major and descends in the gutter between this muscle and iliacus (see Fig. 4.99). It innervates iliacus (Fig. 4.101), passes behind the inguinal ligament lateral to the femoral artery and enters the anterior compartment of the thigh (see Fig. 6.8).

Obturator (L2, L3 & L4) nerve

Descending vertically within psoas major, this nerve emerges from the medial border of the muscle near the pelvic brim (Fig. 4.101; see Fig. 4.99). It passes behind the common iliac vessels and runs downwards and forwards on the lateral pelvic wall as far as the obturator canal (see page 211). Within the canal it divides into anterior and posterior branches, which enter the medial compartment of the thigh (see page 238).

Lumbosacral trunk

Fibres from the fourth lumbar anterior ramus join those of the fifth to form the lumbosacral trunk (Fig. 4.101). The trunk emerges from the medial side of psoas major and crosses the sacroiliac joint to enter the pelvis where it contributes to the formation of the sacral plexus (see page 211).

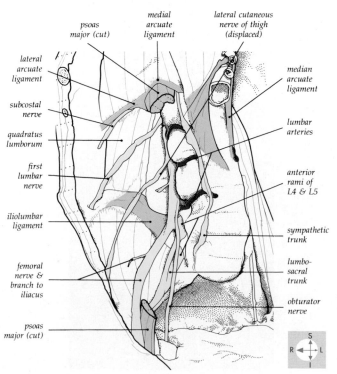

Fig. 4.101 Removal of most of psoas major and the genitofemoral nerve exposes the lumbar plexus.

DIAPHRAGM

The diaphragm is a musculotendinous partition separating the thoracic and abdominal cavities. Its periphery consists of skeletal muscle fibres, which merge centrally with an aponeurotic tendon (Fig. 4.102). The diaphragm has a pronounced convexity towards the thorax and has two domes or cupolas, the right usually lying at a higher level than the left (see Figs 4.103 & 4.104).

Musculature

Peripherally the diaphragmatic muscle is attached to the sternum, the costal margin and the vertebral column. The sternal attachment is by two small slips to the posterior surface of the xiphisternum. The costal attachment is to the inner surfaces of the lower six ribs and costal cartilages (see Fig. 4.103) by slips that interdigitate with those of transversus abdominis.

The diaphragm attaches to the vertebral column by two crura (pillars), one on each side of the abdominal aorta (Fig. 4.102). Both crura are anchored to the sides of the upper two lumbar vertebral bodies while the longer right crus is also attached to the third lumbar vertebra. The crura are linked in front of the aorta by the median arcuate ligament, the fibres interdigitating as they ascend towards the central tendon. Lateral to each crus the diaphragm attaches to the transverse process of the first lumbar vertebra by the medial arcuate ligament (lumbocostal arch) and to the twelfth rib by the lateral arcuate ligament.

A triangular gap, the lumbocostal trigone (Fig. 4.102), often exists between the fibres attaching to the last rib and those arising from the vertebral column.

Central tendon

The muscle fibres of the diaphragm converge on the margins of the central tendon, a V-shaped area of dense fibrous tissue with its apex directed towards the xiphisternum and its lateral parts running backwards into the domes (Fig. 4.102). The central tendon gives attachment to the fibrous pericardium and is pierced by the inferior vena cava (Figs 4.102 & 4.104).

central tendon

inferior vena cava (cut)

inferior phrenic arteries

right crus

medial arcuate ligament

sympathetic trunk

inferior phrenic vein

oesophagus (cut)

median arcuate ligament

abdominal aorta (cut)

vertebrocostal trigone

subcostal nerve

Fig. 4.102 Abdominal surface of the diaphragm after removal of peritoneum. The xiphisternum and anterior costal margin have been excised, including part of the anterior periphery of the diaphragm.

Structures passing between thorax and abdomen

Apertures in the diaphragm transmit the inferior vena cava and the oesophagus. The opening for the inferior vena cava (caval opening) lies to the right of the midline, and the oesophageal opening (hiatus) is slightly to the left (see Fig. 4.102). During quiet breathing these openings lie respectively at the levels of the eighth and tenth thoracic vertebrae. The caval opening pierces the central tendon and transmits the right phrenic nerve as well as the vena

cava. The oesophageal opening, which also transmits the vagal trunks and branches of the left gastric vessels, is surrounded by muscle fibres of the right crus (see Fig. 4.102). The left phrenic nerve pierces the left dome adjacent to the apex of the heart while on each side the thoracic splanchnic nerves pass through the crura to reach the coeliac plexus. The left crus may also be pierced by the hemiazygos vein.

The aorta enters the abdomen by descending behind rather than through the diaphragm and is accompanied by the thoracic duct and azygos vein (Fig. 4.105). The three vessels pass behind the median arcuate ligament and in front of the twelfth

thoracic vertebral body. The subcostal nerves and vessels enter the abdomen behind the lateral arcuate ligaments anterior to quadratus lumborum while the sympathetic trunks descend behind the medial arcuate ligaments anterior to psoas major (see Fig. 4.102). Close to the xiphisternum the superior epigastric vessels (branches of the internal thoracic vessels) pass between the sternal and costal slips of the diaphragm to enter the rectus sheath. Around the periphery of the diaphragm, intercostal nerves and vessels pass between the muscular slips to leave the lower intercostal spaces and reach the abdominal wall.

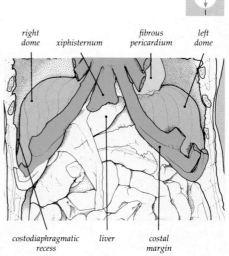

Fig. 4.103   The anterior chest and abdominal walls have been removed (except for the costal margins) to reveal the diaphragm. The abdominal organs are undisturbed but both lungs and the diaphragmatic pleura have been removed.

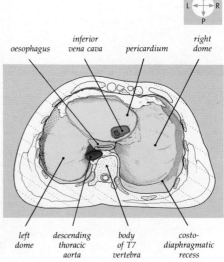

Fig. 4.104   Thoracic surface of the diaphragm. The parietal pleura remains in situ and the base of the fibrous pericardium has been retained.

Movements

The diaphragm is an important muscle of inspiration and also assists the muscles of the abdominal walls and pelvic floor in raising the pressure within the abdomen and pelvis. Thus, the diaphragm contracts during acts of lifting and straining (for example, defecation and childbirth).

The shape and position of the diaphragm vary according to body position and the phase of ventilation. During full inspiration the diaphragm contracts, pulling its central tendon downwards to approximately the level of the tenth thoracic vertebra. The descent of the diaphragm, which is enhanced by an upright body posture, enlarges the thoracic cavity. When the diaphragm relaxes during expiration, its central tendon is pushed superiorly by intra-abdominal pressure, compressing the thoracic contents. With the body recumbent or head downwards, this upwards displacement is accentuated by the weight of the abdominal organs.

Nerve supply

The right and left phrenic nerves provide the main motor and sensory supply to the diaphragm. The phrenic nerves arise in the neck, from the third, fourth and fifth cervical nerves (see page 293). Each nerve descends through the thorax (see page 59) and divides into terminal branches that pierce the diaphragm and innervate it from the abdominal surface.

Each phrenic nerve provides the motor supply to its own half of the diaphragm except the crus, which is innervated by the lower intercostal nerves. In addition, each phrenic nerve carries sensory fibres from the pericardium and from pleura and peritoneum covering the central portion of the diaphragm. Irritation of these sensory fibres may produce pain referred to the shoulder, because the skin covering this area is also supplied by the fourth cervical segment of the spinal cord. Sensory fibres from the peritoneum and pleura covering the periphery of the diaphragm are conveyed by the lower intercostal nerves.

Blood supply

The major blood supply is provided by the inferior phrenic arteries (see Fig. 4.102), which are usually direct branches of the aorta (see Fig. 4.90). The corresponding veins drain into the inferior vena cava. Also, the musculophrenic vessels (terminal branches of the internal thoracic vessels) supply the periphery of the diaphragm.

Relations

The inferior surface of the diaphragm is in contact with abdominal organs including the liver, kidneys, spleen and stomach. Its thoracic surface is related to the heart and lungs and their associated pericardium and pleura (Figs 4.103 & 4.104). Upward and downward excursions of the diaphragm cause corresponding movements of all the organs related to it. During the later stages of expiration the periphery of the diaphragm comes into contact with the chest wall as the costodiaphragmatic recesses deepen (Fig. 4.103).

Fig. 4.105 The aortic opening of the diaphragm has been opened by division of the median arcuate ligament and removal of parts of both crura. The aorta is accompanied by the azygos vein and thoracic duct.

PELVIC CAVITY

Although the pelvic cavity is in direct continuity with the abdominal cavity the two regions are delineated by an arbitrary plane, the pelvic inlet (pelvic brim). This lies at approximately 45 degrees to the horizontal and comprises the sacral promontory posteriorly, the arcuate and pectineal lines laterally and the pubic crests and upper border of pubic symphysis anteriorly (Fig. 5.4).

Below the pelvic inlet, the bony walls of the pelvis give attachment to two pairs of muscles. The obturator internus and piriformis muscles arise within the pelvis but their tendons pass out into the gluteal region to reach the femur. The fascia covering the medial surface of obturator internus is dense and provides attachment for the pelvic floor. The piriformis muscles spring from the anterior surface of the sacrum and are partially covered by the large nerves comprising the sacral plexuses (Fig. 5.4).

In both sexes the pelvic cavity contains the rectum and bladder along with the lower parts of the ureters and loops of small or large intestine. The remaining organs differ between the sexes. The male reproductive organs found within the pelvis (Fig. 5.5) are the prostate, seminal vesicles and ductus deferentes. Those of the female (Fig. 5.6) are the ovaries, uterine tubes, uterus and upper part of vagina.

Peritoneum

Peritoneum lines the lateral and posterior pelvic walls and covers most of the pelvic organs (Figs 5.5 & 5.6). In both sexes peritoneum passes from the anterior abdominal wall onto the upper surface of the bladder. In the male it descends on the posterior surface of the bladder and then passes onto the rectum, forming a recess, the rectovesical pouch (see Fig. 5.14). In the female, peritoneum is reflected from the bladder onto the anterior surface of the body of the uterus, forming the vesicouterine pouch (Fig. 5.6). It covers the fundus of the uterus and on each side passes over the uterine tube, forming the broad ligament. From the posterior surface of the uterus, peritoneum passes over the vault of the vagina onto the anterior wall of the rectum, forming the rectouterine pouch (of Douglas). Fluid may collect in the rectovesical pouch of the male or the rectouterine pouch of the female and, if infected, may form a pelvic abscess.

L5 vertebra

lumbosacral trunk (cut)

anterior rami of S1 & S2

piriformis

obturator internus

promontory & ala of sacrum

iliopectineal line

pelvic inlet

Fig. 5.4 Pelvis and lower abdomen after removal of all the organs and most of the vessels to demonstrate the pelvic inlet and cavity.

pubic symphysis   bladder   peritoneum   sigmoid colon

prostate   rectovesical septum   rectum   anal canal

Fig. 5.5 Median sagittal section through the male pelvis to show the peritoneum and the principal pelvic viscera.

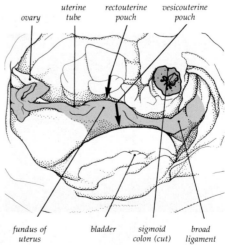

ovary   uterine tube   rectouterine pouch   vesicouterine pouch

fundus of uterus   bladder   sigmoid colon (cut)   broad ligament

Fig. 5.6 Superior view of peritoneum and organs within the female pelvis. The small intestine and most of the sigmoid colon have been removed.

RECTUM

The rectum is the distal portion of the large intestine and lies in the posterior part of the pelvic cavity. It is continuous with the sigmoid colon at the rectosigmoid junction in front of the third piece of the sacrum (Fig. 5.7), where there is often an acute angulation in the intestine which may hamper the passage of a colonoscope. The rectum curves downwards and forwards, lying first on the anterior surface of the sacrum and then on the upper surface of the pelvic floor. It deviates to either side of the midline and these lateral flexures become pronounced when the organ is distended. The lowest part of the rectum, the ampulla, is its most dilatable portion. Turning abruptly downwards and backwards, the rectum pierces the pelvic floor and terminates at the anorectal junction, where it is continuous with the anal canal (see Fig. 5.5).

Unlike the colon, the rectum is devoid of appendices epiploicae and has no taeniae, the longitudinal muscle being distributed uniformly around its circumference. The mucous membrane projects into the rectal lumen as three shelves, which form the horizontal folds.

Relations

The upper two-thirds of the rectum are related to the most inferior portion of the peritoneal cavity. The upper third of the organ is covered anteriorly and on both sides by peritoneum while the middle third, lying behind the rectouterine or rectovesical pouch, has peritoneum only on its anterior surface.

Posterior to the upper part of the rectum are the sacrum, coccyx and the piriformis muscles while its lower part rests on the levator ani muscles. Descending behind the organ are the superior rectal vessels (Fig. 5.7), the hypogastric plexus of autonomic nerves and, on each side of the midline, the sympathetic trunk and sacral plexus. Lateral to the rectum lie the pelvic plexuses of autonomic nerves and the ureters.

Anterior to the upper portion of the rectum lie those parts of the sigmoid colon and ileum that descend into the pelvic cavity. The anterior relations of the rectal ampulla are of clinical interest because they may be palpated on rectal examination. In the male these are the prostate (see Fig. 5.5), the base of the bladder, the seminal vesicles and ampullae of the ductus. These structures are separated from the rectum by the rectovesical septum. In the female the rectal ampulla lies adjacent to the posterior wall of the vagina, therefore rectal examination permits palpation of the cervix of the uterus.

Blood supply

The arterial supply to the rectum is derived principally from the superior rectal artery (Fig. 5.7), the continuation of the inferior mesenteric artery (see page 165). This supply may be supplemented by middle rectal branches from the internal iliac arteries. Venous blood drains into the portal venous system via the superior rectal vein and its continuation, the inferior mesenteric vein. In addition, middle rectal veins drain into the internal iliac veins. As the superior and middle rectal veins interconnect, the wall of the rectum is a site of portacaval anastomosis (see page 167).

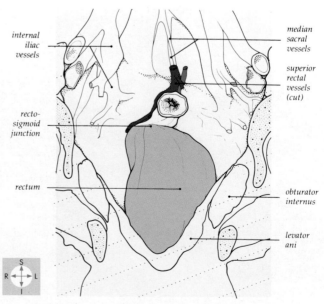

Fig. 5.7 Anterior aspect of rectum seen in a male pelvis sectioned coronally. All peritoneum has been removed.

FEMALE INTERNAL REPRODUCTIVE ORGANS

The female internal organs of reproduction include the uterus and vagina and the paired ovaries and uterine (fallopian) tubes. The uterus and ovaries are particularly affected by atrophy (shrinkage) after the menopause.

Uterus

The uterus is a pear-shaped organ approximately 8 cm in length. Its major component is the body (or corpus), which remains somewhat enlarged after pregnancy. Inferiorly the uterus tapers into the cylindrical neck or cervix, which protrudes into the upper part of the vagina (Fig. 5.9).

The uterus is most commonly positioned with its body lying on the superior surface of the bladder (Fig. 5.8). As the bladder fills and empties, the uterine body moves on the relatively immobile cervix. Thus, when the bladder is empty the uterine body is anteflexed (bent forwards on the cervix), but when the bladder is distended the uterus may become retroflexed.

Body

The uterine body possesses anteroinferior and posterosuperior surfaces. The right and left borders give attachment to the broad ligaments and superiorly give origin to the uterine tubes (Figs 5.8 & 5.11). The rounded upper end of the organ between the attachments of the tubes is called the fundus.

Fig. 5.8   Right ovary and broad ligament.

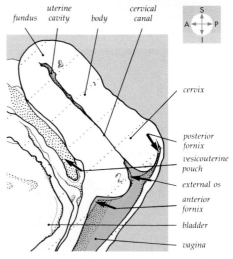

Fig. 5.9   Uterus and vagina in sagittal section.

BLADDER

The urinary bladder lies in the anterior part of the pelvic cavity. When distended the organ has an approximately spherical shape but when empty it assumes the form of a tetrahedron with four angles and four surfaces. The two posterolateral angles receive the ureters while the inferior angle, the bladder neck, is continuous with the urethra. The anterior angle gives attachment to a fibrous cord, the urachus (Fig. 5.16). This remnant of the fetal allantois ascends in the extraperitoneal tissues of the anterior abdominal wall to the umbilicus.

The superior surface and the two inferolateral surfaces expand considerably as urine accumulates but the comparatively small posterior surface or base remains relatively fixed. This surface lies between the entrances of the ureters and the bladder neck.

The wall of the bladder consists of smooth muscle (detrusor) whose thickness gradually decreases as the organ fills. Although the interior of the distended bladder is smooth, the mucosa becomes rugose when the organ empties (Fig. 5.16), except in the region of the trigone. This is the triangular area between the ureteric orifices and the internal urethral meatus (see Fig. 5.14). The ureters pierce the musculature of the bladder wall obliquely and open at slit-like orifices.

Relations

The superior surface of the bladder is covered with peritoneum (Fig. 5.16) on which rest coils of ileum and sigmoid colon. In both sexes the inferolateral surfaces lie against the obturator internus and levator ani muscles and their associated fascial coverings. Between the bladder and these muscles run the obturator nerve and vessels and the superior vesical vessels (Fig. 5.17). Anterior to the bladder is the retropubic space, filled with adipose tissue and veins (Fig. 5.16). The empty bladder lies behind the pubic bones but as it fills it rises above the level of the pubic crests and comes into contact with the lower part of the anterior abdominal wall. The distended bladder intervenes between the parietal peritoneum and the abdominal wall (see Fig. 4.28); surgical access to the organ can be made through an abdominal incision without opening the peritoneum.

In the male the seminal vesicle and the ampulla of the ductus deferens are applied to each side of the posterior surface. Peritoneum descends a short distance on this surface before being reflected onto the anterior surface of the rectum to form the rectovesical pouch (see Fig. 5.14). Below the level of this pouch the bladder is related to the rectovesical septum and the ampulla of the rectum. Inferior to the male bladder lie the prostate and the prostatic plexus of veins.

In the female the posterior part of the superior surface of the bladder is related to the body of the uterus (Fig. 5.16). Peritoneum passes from the superior surface of the bladder onto the uterine body, forming the vesicouterine pouch. Against the posterior surface of the female bladder lie the cervix of the uterus and the anterior wall of the vagina. The inferior angle of the bladder in the female lies at a lower level than in the male and is closely related to the two levator ani muscles.

Blood supply

The bladder is supplied by branches of the internal iliac arteries. On each side the superior vesical artery runs anteriorly along the lateral wall of the pelvis before turning medially to reach the bladder (Fig. 5.17). Anteriorly each superior vesical artery is continuous with a fibrous cord, the medial

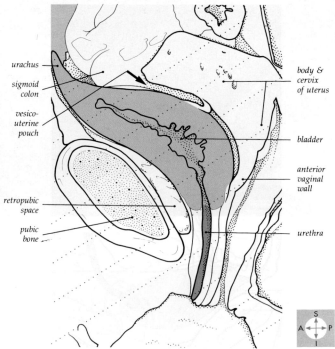

Fig. 5.16 Median sagittal section through the female pelvis to show the bladder and some of its relations.

umbilical ligament (remnant of the fetal umbilical artery), which continues upwards in the extraperitoneal tissues of the abdominal wall to the umbilicus (see Fig. 4.28). The bladder receives additional supply from the inferior vesical and obturator arteries. In the female the uterine and vaginal arteries also contribute to the vascular supply of the bladder.

Venous blood passes into an extensive network of veins, the vesical plexus, which communicates with the prostatic or vaginal plexus and drains into the internal iliac veins.

Nerve supply

The motor innervation to the detrusor muscle is by parasympathetic nerves conveyed in the pelvic splanchnic nerves and the pelvic plexus of autonomic nerves (see Fig. 5.29). In the male the smooth muscle surrounding the bladder neck (preprostatic sphincter) is innervated by sympathetic nerves derived from the hypogastric plexus. The parasympathetic motor innervation stimulates contraction of the bladder at the time of micturition while the sympathetic supply to the male bladder neck prevents reflux ejaculation.

FEMALE URETHRA

The female urethra is a fibromuscular tube 3–4 cm long and begins at the internal urethral meatus of the bladder. Embedded in the anterior wall of the vagina, it inclines downwards and forwards through the pelvic floor (Fig. 5.18) and terminates in the vestibule at the external meatus between the clitoris and the vaginal opening.

The urethra passes close to the posterior aspect of the pubic symphysis (Fig. 5.16), to which it is attached by the pubourethral ligaments. The middle third of the urethra is encircled by striated muscle fibres of the external urethral sphincter, whose tone is the principal factor in maintaining continence of urine. Occlusive force on the urethra is also provided by contractions of the levator ani muscles (Fig. 5.18). Micturition occurs when bladder pressure is higher than urethral pressure and is produced by contraction of the detrusor muscle of the bladder wall accompanied by relaxation of the external urethral sphincter.

The arterial supply to the urethra is provided by the inferior vesical arteries, and venous drainage is to the vesical plexus of veins. The mucosa receives its sensory nerve supply from the pudendal nerve, derived from the second, third and fourth sacral segments which also innervate the external urethral sphincter.

Fig. 5.17 Arterial supply and relations of the bladder in a female pelvis.

Fig. 5.18 Female urethra and its relationship to the vagina and the levator ani muscles.

MALE INTERNAL ORGANS OF REPRODUCTION

The organs of reproduction in the male comprise the paired testes, epididymides, ductus (vasa) deferentia, seminal vesicles, ejaculatory ducts and bulbourethral glands as well as the prostate and penis. The superficial organs (the external genitalia) include the penis (see page 217), and the testes and epididymides within the scrotum (see pages 136 & 137).

The reproductive organs described here are those that lie within the pelvis, namely the prostate, the seminal vesicles, the intrapelvic parts of the ductus deferentia (Fig. 5.22) and the ejaculatory ducts.

Prostate

The prostate is an approximately spherical organ lying immediately below the bladder (Fig. 5.23). The flattened superior surface (base) is applied to the neck of the bladder and is pierced by the urethra, which descends through the gland and emerges near the blunt apex. The part of the prostate behind the urethra and above and between the ejaculatory ducts (see below) is sometimes described as the median lobe (Fig. 5.24).

Anteriorly the prostate is anchored by the puboprostatic ligaments (see Fig. 5.19) to the inferior border of the pubic symphysis. Inferior to the organ lies the intermediate urethra (Fig. 5.23) surrounded by the external urethral sphincter, and posteriorly are the rectovesical septum and the ampulla of the rectum. On each side of the prostate is the medial border of levator ani.

With advancing age the gland often enlarges (benign prostatic hypertrophy) and may obstruct the prostatic part of the urethra, thus interfering with micturition.

Fig. 5.23 Coronal section of the pelvic walls and floor. Most of the bladder has been removed to reveal the prostate, the seminal vesicles and both ductus deferentes.

peritoneum (cut) of rectovesical pouch

seminal vesicle

internal urethral meatus

levator ani (cut)

intermediate urethra

ductus deferens & ampulla

neck of bladder

base & apex of prostate

ureters

ductus deferentes

bladder

left seminal vesicle

prostate

Fig. 5.22 Lateral view of the prostate, left seminal vesicle and both ductus deferentes.

Seminal vesicle

Each seminal vesicle is a sacculated gland approximately 3 cm long, lying lateral to the ampulla of the ductus deferens (Figs 5.24 & 5.25). The seminal vesicles lie in front of the rectum and rectovesical pouch of peritoneum (Fig. 5.23) and extend up the posterior wall of the bladder as far as the terminal parts of the ureters (Fig. 5.25).

Ductus (vas) deferens

Each ductus (vas) deferens begins at the tail of the epididymis in the scrotum, ascends within the spermatic cord and traverses the inguinal canal (see pages 133–135). After emerging from the deep inguinal ring the ductus runs along the lateral pelvic wall, covered by peritoneum, and passes medial to the superior vesical vessels and obturator nerve and vessels. The ductus then crosses above the ureter (Fig. 5.25) and turns downwards and medially posterior to the bladder (Fig. 5.23). The terminal part of the ductus is dilated to form the ampulla, which lies medial to the seminal vesicle. The ampulla is related posteriorly to the peritoneum of the rectovesical pouch and to the rectovesical septum and rectum.

Ejaculatory duct

The duct of each seminal vesicle joins the ampulla of the corresponding ductus deferens to form the ejaculatory duct (Fig. 5.24). The right and left ducts pierce the prostate and run downwards, forwards and medially through its substance to open into the prostatic urethra at slit-like orifices on the summit of the seminal colliculus.

Bulbourethral gland

The bulbourethral glands lie adjacent to the intermediate urethra and are described on page 204.

Blood supply

The artery to the ductus deferens is usually a small vessel which arises from the superior vesical artery and accompanies the ductus as far as the epididymis. The ampulla of the ductus, the seminal vesicle and prostate are supplied by the inferior vesical artery. From the internal reproductive organs, blood passes into the venous plexus (see Fig. 5.21) surrounding the prostate to drain into the internal iliac veins.

Ejaculation

Semen contains spermatozoa from the testes and secretions from the ampullae of the ductus, the seminal vesicles and prostate. Under the control of the sympathetic nervous system, contraction of smooth muscle in the ductus, seminal vesicles and prostate propels secretions into the prostatic urethra. Semen is then expelled from the urethra by contractions of the bulbospongiosus muscles, which compress the bulb of the penis (see page 218). Reflux of semen into the bladder is prevented by contraction of the smooth muscle in the wall of the bladder neck, the 'preprostatic sphincter'.

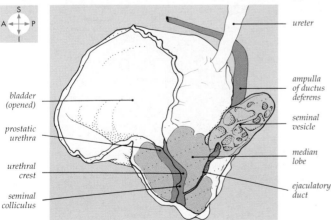

Fig. 5.24 Dissection of prostate and left seminal vesicle.

Fig. 5.25 Removal of the rectum and the posterior wall of the pelvis exposes the bladder, prostate, seminal vesicles and ductus deferentes.

PELVIC WALL AND FLOOR

The pelvic wall is formed by the bones of the pelvic girdle and their associated ligaments, muscles and fascia. The bony component comprises the right and left hip bones anterolaterally and the sacrum and coccyx posteriorly. The pelvic cavity is usually wider and shallower in females because of the differences in the shapes of the surrounding bones.

Hip bone

Only the medial or pelvic surface of the hip bone is considered here; the lateral surface is described on page 238. Each hip bone is formed by the fusion of three components: ilium, ischium and pubis (Fig. 5.26). The anterosuperior part of the ilium contributes to the abdominal wall and gives attachment to iliacus. The lower portion of the ilium extends below the pelvic inlet and contributes to the lateral wall of the pelvis. On the posterior part of the bone is the auricular surface, which articulates with the corresponding surface of the sacrum at the sacroiliac joint.

The ischium has a rounded tuberosity inferiorly, which bears body weight in the sitting position. Posteriorly is the pointed spine, which separates the greater and lesser sciatic notches, while anteriorly the ramus of the ischium ascends to fuse with the inferior pubic ramus.

The pubic bone has a superior ramus that merges with the ilium near the iliopubic eminence, and an inferior ramus which is continuous below the obturator foramen with the ramus of the ischium. The bodies of the right and left pubic bones articulate at the pubic symphysis.

The obturator foramen is a large aperture which is almost completely occluded by the obturator membrane (Fig. 5.26). Superiorly the membrane leaves a small gap, the obturator canal, which provides access between the pelvis and the medial compartment of the thigh.

Pelvic floor

The pelvic floor (or diaphragm) is a muscular partition separating the cavity of the pelvis above from the perineum below. It slopes downwards towards the midline, forming a trough that inclines downwards and forwards (Fig. 5.28). In the midline anteriorly, a narrow triangular gap between the muscle fibres transmits the urethra in both sexes and the vagina in the female (see Fig. 5.18). Posteriorly the pelvic floor is pierced by the anal canal.

The pelvic floor is formed principally by the right and left levator ani muscles, which are supplemented posteriorly by the coccygeus muscles (Fig. 5.28). The coccygeus muscle is applied to the medial surface of the sacrospinous ligament. Medially it attaches to the lateral border of the sacrum and coccyx, and laterally to the ischial spine.

Each levator ani muscle has a linear attachment to the pelvic wall. The attachment commences anteriorly on the pelvic surface of the body of the pubis and continues backwards as the tendinous arch along the obturator fascia as far as the ischial spine (Fig. 5.28). The levator ani muscle has two parts; the anterior part comprises pubococcygeus and the posterior part is iliococcygeus.

Pubococcygeus runs backwards and downwards. Its most anterior fibres lie near the midline and pass close to the urethra. In the male they support the prostate (see Fig. 5.23); in the female they attach to the vagina (see Fig. 5.18). The intermediate fibres of pubococcygeus reach the anal canal and either attach to its wall or loop behind the anorectal junction. The posterior fibres attach to the coccyx or fuse in the midline with fibres from the other side at the anococcygeal raphe.

The fibres of iliococcygeus pass downwards and medially below those of pubococcygeus and attach to the coccyx and to the anococcygeal raphe.

The levator ani muscles support the pelvic contents, actively maintaining the positions of the pelvic viscera. In particular, the pubococcygeus muscles compress the urethra and vagina and provide support for the bladder and uterus. The levator ani fibres that loop behind the anal canal help to maintain the angulation of the anorectal junction and play an important role in the continence of faeces. During defecation, the fibres attaching to the wall of the anal canal pull the organ upwards. Levator ani and coccygeus are innervated by the fourth sacral nerve. Weakening of these muscles, a common gynaecological problem, may result in the descent (prolapse) of the pelvic organs.

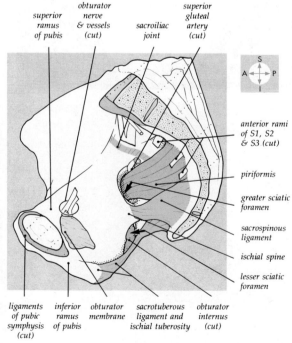

Fig. 5.26 Right hemipelvis showing the pubic symphysis, the obturator membrane, the ligaments and the foramina.

Joints

The pelvic girdle forms a stable ring because its constituent bones are bound together at the two sacroiliac joints and the pubic symphysis.

The symphysis is a secondary cartilaginous joint containing a pad of fibrocartilage (Fig. 5.27) that separates the bodies of the right and left pubic bones. The joint is stabilized by ligaments attached around the articular margins.

The sacroiliac joints allow very little movement because the articulating surfaces of their synovial cavities are irregular and behind each cavity is the thick posterior interosseous ligament. Each joint is further supported by the anterior and posterior sacroiliac ligaments and iliolumbar, sacrospinous and sacrotuberous ligaments. Body weight acting downwards through the lumbosacral disc tends to rotate the sacrum, tipping its lower part backwards, a movement prevented by the sacrospinous and sacrotuberous ligaments (Fig. 5.26).

The iliolumbar ligament attaches medially to the transverse process of the fifth lumbar vertebra and laterally to the iliac crest and front of the sacroiliac joint (see Fig. 8.23). The sacrospinous ligament passes from the lateral margins of the sacrum and coccyx to the ischial spine. The larger sacrotuberous ligament passes from the side and dorsum of the sacrum and the posterior surface of the ilium to the ischial tuberosity. These two ligaments convert the greater and lesser sciatic notches into the greater and lesser sciatic foramina (Fig. 5.26).

Muscles

Piriformis is a flat muscle attached to the pelvic surfaces of the second, third and fourth pieces of the sacrum (Fig. 5.26). Running laterally through the greater sciatic foramen, it enters the buttock and attaches to the upper part of the greater trochanter of the femur (see page 242). Piriformis rotates the hip joint laterally and is innervated by the first and second sacral nerves. Numerous vessels and nerves accompany the muscle through the greater sciatic foramen (Fig. 5.27).

Obturator internus is a fan-shaped muscle with an extensive attachment to the margins of the obturator foramen and the pelvic surface of the obturator membrane (Fig. 5.27). The muscle fibres converge on the lesser sciatic foramen to form a tendon, which turns laterally to enter the gluteal region. The tendon is attached to the medial aspect of the greater trochanter (see page 242). The muscle laterally rotates the hip joint. The nerve to obturator internus (L5, S1 & S2) enters the muscle within the perineum, having traversed the greater and lesser sciatic foramina.

Pelvic fascia

This term includes the fascial lining of the pelvic walls and the extraperitoneal connective tissue surrounding the pelvic viscera. The pelvic surfaces of obturator internus (Fig. 5.28), piriformis and levator ani are covered by fascia that is continuous superiorly with the transversalis and iliac fasciae. Between the pelvic organs, the pelvic fascia mostly comprises a loose meshwork of connective tissue. However, it is condensed anterior to the rectum to form the rectovesical septum; and some of the arteries to the pelvic organs, notably the uterine and vaginal vessels, are accompanied by thickened bands of fascia termed 'ligaments'. Radiating from the uterine cervix to the pelvic walls are the transverse cervical (lateral sacral) and uterosacral ligaments which provide support to the uterus.

Fig. 5.27   Right hemipelvis showing the pelvic attachment of obturator internus.

Fig. 5.28   Right levator ani and part of the anal canal, seen in a median sagittal section of the pelvis.

PELVIC NERVES

Autonomic nerves

The pelvic organs receive their autonomic innervation via the right and left pelvic plexuses, which lie adjacent to the internal iliac arteries and their branches (Fig. 5.29). Nerves pass from the plexuses to the bladder, reproductive organs and the rectum by accompanying the arteries to these organs. The plexuses and their branches contain efferent fibres from both the parasympathetic and sympathetic systems, which reach the pelvis from different parts of the spinal cord.

Parasympathetic nerves

The parasympathetic component of the pelvic plexuses is provided by the pelvic splanchnic nerves ('nervi erigentes'), which leave the spinal cord in the second, third and fourth sacral nerves. The parasympathetic fibres control micturition, dilation of the erectile tissues in both sexes, and defecation. The pelvic plexuses also provide the parasympathetic innervation of the descending and sigmoid parts of the colon. These fibres ascend into the abdomen in the hypogastric plexus and are distributed with the branches of the inferior mesenteric artery.

Sympathetic nerves

The sympathetic fibres destined for the pelvic autonomic plexuses arise from the lower thoracic and upper lumbar segments of the spinal cord and pass through the lumbar portions of the sympathetic trunks on the posterior abdominal wall. From here they descend in the hypogastric plexus to reach the pelvis. Sympathetic fibres innervate the smooth muscle of the reproductive organs in both sexes and in the male are responsible for coordinating ejaculation (see page 207).

The two sympathetic trunks pass from the posterior abdominal wall (see page 178) into the pelvis by crossing behind the common iliac vessels. Descending in front of the sacrum and piriformis muscles (Fig. 5.30), they incline towards the midline and fuse on the anterior surface of the coccyx. Each trunk bears three or four ganglia and provides grey rami communicantes, consisting of postganglionic fibres, to the sacral nerves. These fibres supply blood vessels and sweat glands in the areas innervated by the appropriate sacral nerves.

Fig. 5.29 Right pelvic plexus of autonomic nerves. This specimen has an abnormal obturator artery.

Spinal nerves

The lower lumbar and upper sacral spinal nerves are predominantly concerned with the innervation of the lower limb. However, a few fibres derived from these spinal nerves are distributed to the pelvic walls and floor and to the perineum.

Obturator nerve

This branch of the lumbar plexus (see page 182) emerges from the medial border of psoas major and enters the pelvis by crossing in front of the ala of the sacrum. It descends lateral to the common and internal iliac vessels and the ureter (Fig. 5.29) and reaches the medial surface of obturator internus. The nerve approaches the obturator vessels from above and continues with them through the obturator canal (Fig. 5.30) into the medial compartment of the thigh (see page 238).

Sacral and coccygeal nerves

The anterior rami of the first four sacral nerves emerge through the anterior sacral foramina and merge to form the sacral plexus (Fig. 5.30). The fifth sacral nerve and the coccygeal nerves are small and do not contribute to the plexus. All the sacral and coccygeal nerves receive grey rami communicantes from the sympathetic trunk.

Sacral plexus

This plexus lies on the posterior pelvic wall in front of piriformis (Fig. 5.30), covered anteriorly by the pelvic fascia. The plexus is formed by the anterior rami of the upper four sacral nerves and is supplemented by the lumbosacral trunk which carries fibres from the fourth and fifth lumbar nerves (see page 182). The branches of the sacral plexus are distributed to the lower limb, pelvic walls and floor, and perineum.

Those branches that leave the pelvis accompany piriformis through the greater sciatic foramen to enter the buttock (see pages 240 & 242). The nerve to obturator internus and the pudendal nerve then pass forwards through the lesser sciatic foramen to gain the perineum (see Fig. 5.27).

Fig. 5.30 Sacral plexus and pelvic portion of the sympathetic trunk.

PELVIC BLOOD VESSELS AND LYMPHATICS

The pelvic walls and floor and the pelvic organs receive most of their arterial supply from branches of the internal iliac artery, which also provides branches to the perineum and lower limb. The rectum, however, receives its principal supply from the superior rectal artery (see pages 165 & 196), while the posterior wall of the pelvis is supplied by the median sacral artery (see Fig. 5.30). The ovaries are supplied by the ovarian branches of the abdominal aorta (see page 200).

Internal iliac artery and branches

The internal iliac artery arises in front of the sacroiliac joint as one of the terminal branches of the common iliac artery (Fig. 5.31). The internal iliac artery runs downwards and backwards on the lateral pelvic wall, giving rise to visceral and parietal branches.

Visceral branches

The superior vesical artery runs forwards adjacent to the bladder, to which it gives one or more branches (see Fig. 5.17). The artery usually gives rise to the slender artery to the ductus deferens and continues as the obliterated umbilical artery to the umbilicus (see page 132).

The inferior vesical artery occurs only in the male and supplies the lower part of the bladder, the prostate, the seminal vesicle and the pelvic ureter. The uterine artery runs medially in the root of the broad ligament, crosses above the ureter (see Fig. 5.13) and supplies the vagina and the uterine cervix, body and tube. The artery follows the lateral border of the body of the uterus, then runs laterally in the broad ligament, close to the uterine tube, and terminates by anastomosing with the ovarian artery.

The vagina is supplied by branches of the uterine artery together with one or two small vaginal arteries from the internal iliac artery.

The middle rectal artery (Fig. 5.31) supplies the muscle coat of the rectum and in the male may give additional branches to the prostate and seminal vesicles.

Parietal branches

The obturator artery runs downwards and forwards, with the corresponding vein and nerve, to enter the obturator canal. It supplies the proximal part of the medial compartment of the thigh and the hip joint (see page 238). Occasionally the obturator artery takes origin from the inferior epigastric artery and descends into the pelvis to reach the obturator canal. Such a vessel, an 'abnormal obturator artery' (see Fig. 5.29), passes close to the femoral ring and may be damaged during femoral hernia operations.

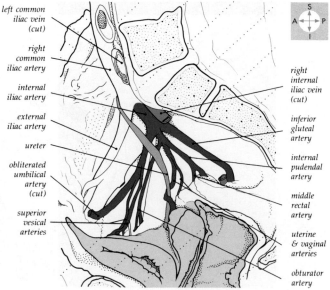

Fig. 5.31 Right internal iliac artery and some of its branches.

The superior and inferior gluteal arteries pass through the greater sciatic foramen into the buttock, the superior artery running above piriformis (see Fig. 5.30) and the inferior below (see page 242).

The internal pudendal artery provides the principal arterial supply to the perineum. The artery passes through the greater sciatic foramen into the gluteal region, curves round the ischial spine and then passes forwards through the lesser sciatic foramen into the perineum (see page 216).

The iliolumbar artery ascends the posterior abdominal wall to anastomose with the lower lumbar arteries.

The lateral sacral artery supplies the posterior wall of the pelvis and anastomoses with the median sacral artery.

Internal iliac vein and tributaries

The branches of the internal iliac artery are accompanied by veins that drain the buttock and perineum, the pelvic walls and most of the pelvic organs. These veins unite to form the internal iliac vein (Fig. 5.32), which ascends on the lateral pelvic wall posterior to the artery. The vein terminates by joining the external iliac vein to form the common iliac vein.

Most of the veins emerging from the pelvic organs anastomose freely, forming extensive venous plexuses (the vesical, prostatic, uterine and vaginal plexuses). While most blood from these plexuses passes into the internal iliac vein, some enters either the superior rectal vein via portacaval anastomoses or the vertebral venous plexus via the anterior sacral foramina.

Pelvic lymphatics

Lymph from the pelvis is drained by lymphatic vessels that accompany the arteries. Most of the lymph drains into nodes adjacent to the internal iliac artery and then into efferent vessels that pass to the common iliac nodes (see page 176). However, lymphatic vessels from the ovaries and the rectum pass directly to the aortic nodes, and some vessels from the body of the uterus accompany the round ligament through the inguinal canal to terminate in the superficial inguinal nodes.

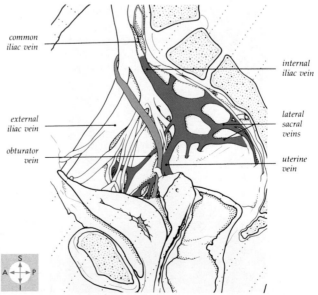

Fig. 5.32 Right internal iliac vein and tributaries.

PERINEUM

Below the pelvic floor lies the perineum, a superficial region traversed by the anal canal and the lower parts of the genital and urinary tracts. It is a diamond-shaped area, extending anteriorly to the pubic symphysis, posteriorly to the coccyx and laterally to the ischial tuberosities (Fig. 5.33). On each side the region is bounded by the conjoined rami of the ischium and pubis and by the sacrotuberous ligament, which is overlapped by the inferior border of gluteus maximus. Inferiorly the perineum is bounded by skin. By convention, the perineum is divided into two triangles by a line joining the ischial tuberosities. Posteriorly is the anal triangle, containing the anal canal and the ischioanal (ischiorectal) fossae, and anteriorly lies the urogenital triangle, containing the external genitalia.

Anal canal

The anal canal is the terminal part of the intestine and is approximately 4 cm long.

Beginning at the anorectal junction, it passes downwards and backwards as far as the anus (see Fig. 5.5). Its upper part is lined by mucous membrane bearing several longitudinal ridges, the anal columns, the lower part is lined by skin. The smooth muscle coat of the rectum continues into the wall of the anal canal and thickens to form the internal anal sphincter. Striated fibres from the levator ani muscles (Fig. 5.34) blend with the outer layers of the wall and continue as far as the perianal skin.

In addition, the lower two-thirds of the anal canal are encircled by the external anal sphincter (Fig. 5.35), composed of striated muscle fibres. This sphincter comprises three parts, of which the uppermost, the deep part, blends with the levator ani muscles. Inferior to this lies the superficial part, attached posteriorly to the coccyx and anococcygeal raphe and anteriorly to the posterior border of the perineal membrane. The most inferior component of the sphincter, the subcutaneous part, encircles the anal opening. Continence of faeces is not dependent on the external sphincter alone;

the fibres of the levator ani muscles that maintain the anorectal angulation play a major role.

The anal canal is supplied by inferior rectal branches (Fig. 5.35) from the pudendal nerve, which innervate the external sphincter and the cutaneous lining. The internal sphincter and the mucous membrane lining the upper part are innervated, like the rectum, by autonomic nerves (see page 208). The blood supply is provided by inferior rectal branches of the internal pudendal artery. The anal canal is a site of portacaval anastomosis because venous blood passes not only via inferior rectal veins to the internal iliac veins but also into the superior rectal vein, a tributary of the portal venous system (see page 166). Lymph drains from the upper part of the canal to the internal iliac nodes, but from the lower part it passes to the superficial inguinal nodes.

The cutaneous lining of the lower part of the anal canal has a rich nerve supply. Tears (fissures) in this skin are painful and produce reflex spasm of the external sphincter.

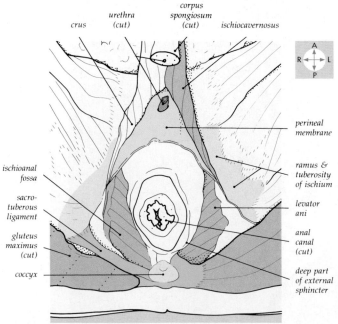

Fig. 5.33 Deep dissection of male perineum to show its boundaries. The bulb of the penis has been removed to expose the perineal membrane, and gluteus maximus on one side has been resected to reveal the sacrotuberous ligament.

ischial
tuberosity

fat in
ischioanal
fossa

rectum
(opened)

obturator
internus

levator
ani

anal canal

perianal
skin

Fig. 5.34 Coronal section through anal canal and ischioanal fossae.

anal
opening

scrotum

bulb of
penis

posterior
scrotal
nerve

hamstring
muscles

ischial
tuberosity

inferior rectal
nerve & artery

deep,
superficial &
subcutaneous
parts of external
anal sphincter

levator ani

gluteus
maximus

anococcygeal
raphe

Fig. 5.35 Oblique view of the anal triangle to show the parts of the external anal sphincter and the inferior rectal nerve and vessels.

Ischioanal (ischiorectal) fossa

On each side of the anal canal is a fat-filled space extending laterally as far as obturator internus, upwards to the levator ani muscle and downwards to the perianal skin (see Fig. 5.34). The fossae communicate behind the anal canal. Anteriorly each fossa tapers and continues above the perineal membrane and external urethral sphincter almost to the pubic symphysis. Entering each fossa from the gluteal region via the lesser sciatic foramen are the nerve to obturator internus, the pudendal nerve (Fig. 5.36) and the internal pudendal artery with its venae comitantes.

The nerve to obturator internus arises from the sacral plexus and supplies the muscle from within the ischioanal fossa (see Fig. 5.27).

The pudendal nerve and the internal pudendal vessels pass along the lateral wall of the fossa in a fascial tunnel, the pudendal canal. Branches from the nerve and artery traverse the upper part of the fossa to supply the anal canal and the posterior part of the scrotum or labium majus (see Fig. 5.35).

Internal pudendal artery

This vessel provides most of the arterial blood to the perineum. Arising from the internal iliac artery within the pelvis (see Fig. 5.31), it enters the buttock through the greater sciatic foramen and then traverses the lesser sciatic foramen to enter the ischioanal fossa. The artery runs forwards along the lateral wall of the fossa in the pudendal canal and gives off inferior rectal branches and posterior scrotal or labial branches. The artery continues above the perineal membrane, where it provides branches to the bulb of the penis (or vestibule) and crus of the penis (or clitoris), and terminates by dividing into deep and dorsal arteries of the penis (or clitoris). In the male the dorsal artery passes below the pubic symphysis and continues along the dorsum of the penile shaft (Fig. 5.36), lateral to the deep dorsal vein, and gives branches to the erectile tissue of the corpus cavernosum. The deep artery pierces the perineal membrane and supplies the erectile tissue of the corpus cavernosum. In the female there are comparable but smaller branches to the clitoris. The internal pudendal artery and its branches are accompanied by venae comitantes, which drain into the internal iliac vein.

Pudendal nerve

The pudendal nerve provides the principal innervation to the perineum. It arises from the sacral plexus (S2, S3 & S4) and accompanies the internal pudendal artery into the perineum. In the ischioanal fossa the nerve divides into the dorsal nerve of penis (or clitoris) and the perineal nerve (Fig. 5.36).

The perineal nerve supplies an inferior rectal branch to the anal canal and posterior scrotal (or labial) branches to the skin of the genitalia (see Fig. 5.35). On reaching the anterior part of the perineum, the perineal nerve gives branches to all muscles in the superficial perineal pouch as well as sensory branches to the urethra.

The dorsal nerve of the penis continues forwards with the internal pudendal artery above the perineal membrane and below the pubic symphysis. It runs along the dorsum of the penis, lateral to the dorsal artery (Fig. 5.38), and innervates the skin of the distal two-thirds of the organ. The dorsal nerve of the clitoris has a similar course and distribution.

Fig. 5.36 Left pudendal nerve, exposed by removal of the lateral wall of the pelvis.

MALE EXTERNAL GENITALIA

The male external genitalia comprise the scrotum and the penis. An account of the scrotum and its contents is given on pages 136 and 137. The penis consists of a shaft, which is free, and a root, which lies in the superficial perineal pouch, attached to the inferior surface of the perineal membrane.

Perineal membrane and pouches

The perineal membrane is a shelf of dense fascia spanning the triangular interval between the right and left ischial and pubic rami (see Fig. 5.33). The membrane has a long free posterior margin and a short anterior margin that is separated from the pubic symphysis by a small gap transmitting the deep dorsal vein of the penis. The central part of the membrane is pierced by the urethra and bulbourethral ducts.

At the root of the penis and around the neck of the scrotum the membranous layer of perineal subcutaneous tissue attaches laterally to the ischial and pubic rami. Posteriorly the fascia is anchored to the free edge of the perineal membrane. The space contained by the membranous layer of the penis and the scrotum is called the superficial perineal pouch. This pouch communicates with the subcutaneous tissues of the anterior abdominal wall but not with the ischiorectal fossae, the thighs or pelvic cavity. If the spongy part of the urethra is ruptured, urine may escape into the superficial pouch (superficial extravasation of urine).

On the pelvic aspect of the perineal membrane lie the external urethral sphincter and bulbourethral glands in a space often called the deep perineal pouch. The term 'urogenital diaphragm' is a misnomer sometimes applied to the deep perineal pouch and its boundaries.

Penis

The erectile tissue of the shaft of the penis consists of the paired corpora cavernosa lying in apposition and the midline corpus spongiosum.

The corpus spongiosum is uniform in diameter except at its extremity, where it expands into the glans (see Fig. 5.19), whose prominent margin forms the corona of the penis. Proximally the corpus spongiosum continues into the root of the penis to form the bulb, which is attached to the inferior surface of the perineal membrane (Fig. 5.37). The urethra pierces the perineal membrane, enters the bulb from above and curves downwards and forwards. It traverses the corpus spongiosum and glans (see Fig. 5.19) and terminates at the external urethral meatus near the apex of the glans.

Dorsal to the corpus spongiosum are the paired corpora cavernosa (Fig. 5.38), which extend distally as far as the concave proximal surface of the glans. Proximally the corpora cavernosa continue inferior to the pubic symphysis and diverge as the crura. Each crus tapers posteriorly and is attached to the inferior surface of the perineal membrane and the adjacent rami of the pubis and ischium (Fig. 5.37; see Fig. 5.33).

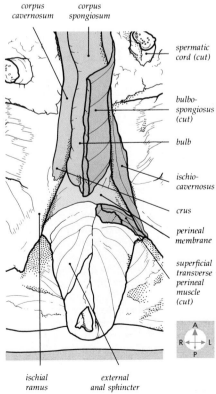

Fig. 5.37   Root of penis. On one side ischiocavernosus has been excised to reveal the crus and bulbospongiosus removed to expose half of the bulb.

Fig. 5.38   'Step' dissection of the shaft of the penis to show the three corpora and the dorsal vessels

Fascial layers and skin

The three corpora of the penis are enveloped by a sleeve of deep fascia, which also covers the dorsal vessels and nerves of the organ (see Fig. 5.38). Proximally the deep fascia is anchored to the front of the pubic symphysis by the suspensory ligament of the penis (see Fig. 5.36) while distally it terminates at the corona by fusing with the corpora. Covering the deep fascia is the superficial fascia.

The subcutaneous tissue of the penis is membranous, devoid of fat and traversed by superficial nerves and vessels (see Fig. 5.38). Proximally it is continuous with the subcutaneous tissue of the anterior abdominal wall and can be traced around the scrotum, where it contains smooth muscle, the dartos.

The cutaneous covering of the penis is freely mobile except over the glans to which it is adherent. The skin is reflected distally beyond the corona over the glans to form the hood-like prepuce or foreskin. This is attached to the undersurface of the glans by a vascular fold, the frenulum.

Muscles

Surrounding the bulb of the penis are the paired bulbospongiosus muscles (see Fig. 5.37). Their fibres attach to the perineal membrane and pass downwards and backwards to meet at a midline raphe and blend posteriorly with the external anal sphincter. The bulbospongiosus muscles contract during ejaculation and the terminal stages of micturition to compress the urethra and expel its contents.

Covering each crus is the ischiocavernosus muscle (see Fig. 5.37). From the posterior end of each crus a small superficial transverse perineal muscle runs medially to the penile bulb. All the penile muscles are innervated by the perineal branch of the pudendal nerve.

Vessels

The erectile tissues of the penis have a rich blood supply. Each internal pudendal artery (see Fig. 5.36) provides branches to the bulb and to the corresponding crus before terminating as the dorsal and deep arteries. The deep artery traverses the length of the corpus cavernosum while the artery to the bulb continues along the corpus spongiosum to reach the glans. The principal venous drainage is via the midline deep dorsal vein, which runs beneath the deep fascia (see Fig. 5.38). This vein is accompanied by the dorsal arteries and passes inferior to the pubic symphysis into the pelvic cavity, where it terminates in the prostatic venous plexus (see Fig. 5.21). From this plexus blood drains into either the internal iliac veins or the internal pudendal veins.

Erection of the penis is controlled by parasympathetic nerves (the pelvic splanchnic nerves or nervi erigentes) from the sacral segments of the spinal cord. Stimulation of these nerves causes arterial dilatation and simultaneous venous constriction. This results in engorgement of the erectile tissues leading to enlargement and stiffening of the penis.

The skin of the penis and the front of the scrotum are supplied by the external pudendal branches of the femoral arteries. The superficial veins of the penis and the anterior part of the scrotum drain via the external pudendal veins, which are tributaries of the great saphenous vein (see Fig. 6.11). The posterior part of the scrotum is supplied by posterior scrotal branches from the internal pudendal artery and venous blood passes into the internal pudendal veins.

Cutaneous innervation

The pudendal nerve supplies most of the penis and scrotum via its dorsal and posterior scrotal branches. However, the anterior part of the scrotum and the proximal part of the shaft of the penis are innervated by the ilioinguinal nerve, which descends from the superficial inguinal ring (see page 132).

Lymphatic drainage

Lymph from the superficial tissues of the penis and scrotum passes to the superficial inguinal nodes while that from the deeper tissues is conveyed via lymphatic vessels accompanying the internal pudendal artery and passes to the internal iliac nodes.

FEMALE EXTERNAL GENITALIA

Clitoris and bulbs of vestibule

The perineal membrane is thinner in the female than in the male and is pierced by both the vagina and the urethra. Attached to the inferior surface of the membrane is erectile tissue similar to that in the male, namely the crura of the clitoris and the bulbs of the vestibule covered by the thin ischiocavernosus and bulbospongiosus muscles respectively (Figs 5.39 & 5.40). The right and left crura attach to the medial margins of the ischial and pubic rami. Passing forwards and medially they merge beneath the pubic symphysis to form the shaft of the clitoris. This turns downwards and backwards towards the urethral opening and its tip is capped by the glans of the clitoris.

The paired bulbs of the vestibule surround the urethral and vaginal openings (Fig. 5.40). Anteriorly they taper and fuse into a midline structure that terminates as the glans of the clitoris. The posterior end of each bulb is expanded and covers the greater vestibular (Bartholin's) gland. This gland is approximately 1 cm in diameter and drains into a minute duct which opens into the vestibule lateral to the vaginal opening. Superficial transverse perineal muscles pass laterally from the bulbs of the vestibule to the ischial tuberosities.

Labia

The most superficial parts of the female external genitalia are the skin folds, the labia majora (see Fig. 5.39). These meet at the posterior commissure (fourchette) and anteriorly at the mons pubis. The mons is a pad of fat overlying the pubic symphysis and covering most of the clitoris. Between the labia majora lie the two labia minora, which become more prominent anteriorly. The labia minora fuse in the midline, forming two folds of skin around the glans of the clitoris. The hood-like anterior fold comprises the prepuce of the clitoris and the smaller posterior fold forms the frenulum.

Vestibule

The labia minora enclose a cleft, the vestibule, into which the vagina and urethra open (Fig. 5.40). The vaginal opening (introitus) is an anteroposterior slit, usually surrounded by a fringe of skin, the hymen. The external urethral meatus lies approximately 1 cm anterior to the vaginal opening.

The term 'vulva' is used to describe the mons pubis, the labia majora and minora, the clitoris and vestibule.

Cutaneous innervation and blood supply

The mons pubis and the anterior parts of the labia are innervated by the ilioinguinal nerves (see page 132). The posterior part of the vulva receives cutaneous innervation from the labial branches of the pudendal nerves, supplemented by branches of the posterior cutaneous nerves of the thighs and the perineal branches of the fourth sacral nerves.

The skin and subcutaneous tissues are supplied by the internal pudendal artery (see page 213) and the superficial and deep external pudendal branches of the femoral artery. Most of the venous blood passes into the venae comitantes of the internal pudendal artery, but anteriorly some blood drains by external pudendal veins into the great saphenous vein. Lymph from the skin and superficial tissues, including the vestibule and lower vagina, passes to the superficial inguinal nodes (see page 231), while lymphatics from deeper structures follow the course of the arteries to reach the internal iliac nodes.

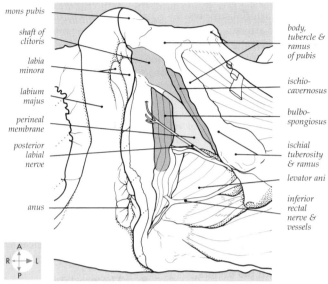

Fig. 5.39 Superficial dissection of one side of the female perineum, showing the muscles and cutaneous nerves.

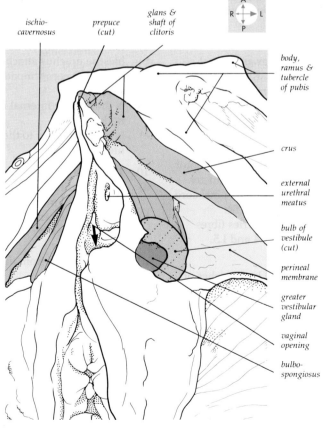

Fig. 5.40 Deeper dissection of the female perineum. The glans, shaft and left crus of the clitoris have been exposed. The left bulb of the vestibule has been cut to reveal the greater vestibular gland.

Identify the structures indicated. The answers are supplied at the foot of the page.

Fig. 5.45   Transverse section at the level of the pubic symphysis. Inferior aspect. Compare Fig. 5.42.

Fig. 5.46   Transverse section at the level of the ischiopubic rami. Inferior aspect.

Answers

Fig. 5.45   1 = obturator internus, 2 = femoral vein, 3 = spermatic cord, 4 = neck of bladder, 5 = pubis, 6 = pectineus, 7 = head of femur, 8 = greater trochanter, 9 = ischial tuberosity, 10 = levator ani, 11 = rectum (distended), 12 = ischioanal fossa, 13 = gluteus maximus.

Fig. 5.46   1 = tensor fasciae latae, 2 = femur, 3 = adductor muscles, 4 = crus of penis, 5 = corpora cavernosa, 6 = spermatic cord, 7 = sciatic nerve, 8 = bulb of penis, 9 = levator ani, 10 = anal canal, 11 = ischiopubic ramus, 12 = gluteus maximus, 13 = tendons of hamstring muscles.

6 LOWER LIMB

INTRODUCTION

The lower limb supports the body during standing and locomotion. The hip (coxal) bone (Fig. 6.1) provides attachment for muscles of the buttock and thigh, which link the limb to the trunk. The hip joint, between the acetabulum of the hip bone and the head of the femur, is multiaxial and provides versatility of movement.

The femur (Fig. 6.1) is surrounded by the muscles of the thigh and buttock. Its lower end with the patella and upper end of the tibia form the knee joint, a hinge joint. The tibia and fibula, surrounded by the leg muscles, form at their lower ends a socket which articulates with the talus at the ankle joint, also a hinge.

The foot contains three groups of bones: the tarsals posteriorly, the metatarsals more anteriorly and the phalanges within the toes. The skeleton of the foot is adapted for bipedal standing and walking.

The limb is covered by skin, subcutaneous tissue containing vessels and nerves, and by deep fascia. Intermuscular septa separate the muscles into different compartments (Figs 6.2 & 6.3). Each compartment contains muscles with common actions and is supplied by a neurovascular bundle. The thigh has anterior, posterior and medial compartments, whereas the leg has anterior, posterior and lateral compartments. The foot has only two: the dorsum and the sole.

The principal vessels and nerves enter the limb from the abdomen or pelvis by three different routes (Fig. 6.4): posterior to the inguinal ligament from the abdomen to the anterior compartment of the thigh; through the obturator canal between the pelvis and the medial compartment of the thigh; via the greater sciatic foramen, where the pelvis communicates with the gluteal region.

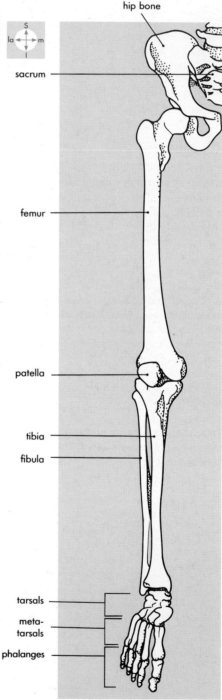

Fig. 6.1   The skeleton of the lower limb.

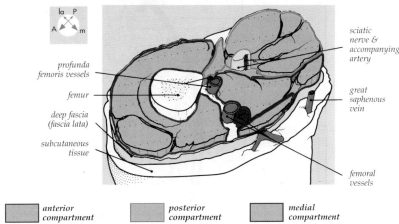

profunda
femoris vessels

femur

deep fascia
(fascia lata)

subcutaneous
tissue

sciatic
nerve &
accompanying
artery

great
saphenous
vein

femoral
vessels

| anterior compartment | posterior compartment | medial compartment |

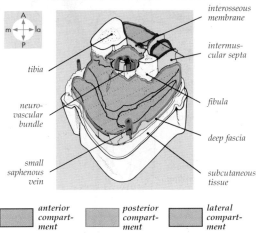

interosseous
membrane

intermus-
cular septa

tibia

neuro-
vascular
bundle

small
saphenous
vein

fibula

deep fascia

subcutaneous
tissue

| anterior compart-ment | posterior compart-ment | lateral compart-ment |

Fig. 6.2 'Step' dissection through the midthigh, showing the relationships of the compartments.

Fig. 6.3 'Step' dissection through the midcalf, showing the relationships of the compartments.

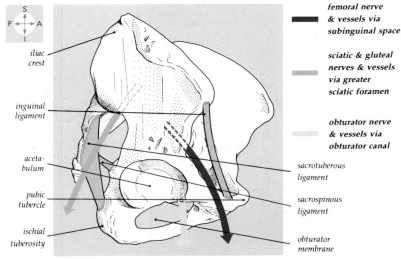

femoral nerve
& vessels via
subinguinal space

sciatic & gluteal
nerves & vessels
via greater
sciatic foramen

obturator nerve
& vessels via
obturator canal

iliac
crest

inguinal
ligament

aceta-
bulum

pubic
tubercle

ischial
tuberosity

sacrotuberous
ligament

sacrospinous
ligament

obturator
membrane

Fig. 6.4 Sites of access of the principal nerves and vessels from the abdomen and pelvis into the root of the lower limb.

cutaneous nerves of thigh:

L1, L2 & L3
T12 & L1
S1, S2 & S3
femoral branch of genitofemoral nerve
ilioinguinal nerve
obturator nerve

lateral
intermediate
medial

lateral cutaneous nerve of calf
saphenous nerve
sural nerve
superficial & deep fibular nerves
lateral & medial plantar nerves

Cutaneous nerves (Fig. 6.9) supply areas of skin which vary between individuals. The territories supplied by adjacent nerves overlap and therefore damage to a single nerve usually produces anaesthesia confined to the central part of the area supplied. The dermatome distribution is shown in Fig. 6.10. There is some overlap of dermatomes except along the axial lines.

- posterior rami
- lateral cutaneous branches of spinal nerves
- sciatic nerve (sacral plexus)
- posterior cutaneous nerve of thigh (sacral plexus)
- femoral nerve (lumbar plexus)
- other branches (lumbar plexus)

Fig. 6.9   Areas of distribution of cutaneous nerves in the lower limb.

S4
S3
L1
L2
S2
L3
L4
L5
S1

Fig. 6.10   The dermatomes of the lower limb.

ANTERIOR COMPARTMENT OF THIGH

The anterior compartment is the largest in the thigh, occupying the region between the inguinal ligament and the knee. Lateral and anteromedial intermuscular septa separate the contents from the posterior (hamstring) and medial (adductor) compartments respectively (see Fig. 6.2). The anterior compartment (Fig. 6.12) contains quadriceps femoris, sartorius and the tendon of iliopsoas, and is innervated by the femoral nerve. The femoral artery and vein, the principal vessels of the lower limb, traverse the compartment and leave via the opening in adductor magnus to gain the popliteal fossa.

Subcutaneous tissue (superficial fascia)

The subcutaneous tissue contains the great (long) saphenous vein and its tributaries with their accompanying arteries, superficial inguinal lymph nodes and cutaneous nerves. The great saphenous vein ascends on the medial side of the thigh (Fig. 6.11) and passes through the saphenous opening in the fascia lata to empty into the femoral vein. The great saphenous vein drains the superficial tissues of the entire limb except the lateral side of the leg and foot. Near its termination the vein receives tributaries which drain the buttock, the perineum and the abdominal wall below the umbilicus. These tributaries are accompanied by corresponding branches of the femoral artery.

The superficial inguinal lymph nodes, often palpable in the living, lie just distal and parallel to the inguinal ligament and adjacent to the termination of the great saphenous vein (Fig. 6.11). These nodes receive lymph from the same superficial tissues as those drained by the great saphenous vein and its tributaries. Efferent lymphatics from the superficial nodes pass through the fascia lata and drain into the deep inguinal nodes within the femoral triangle (see page 229).

Fig. 6.11 Great saphenous vein, its tributaries and the superficial inguinal lymph nodes lying in subcutaneous tissue.

Fig. 6.12 Muscles of the anterior compartment of thigh after removal of the skin and fascia lata.

The lateral cutaneous nerve of the thigh (L2 & L3) pierces the inguinal ligament close to the anterior superior iliac spine (see Fig. 6.17) and supplies skin as far as the knee. The intermediate and medial cutaneous nerves of the thigh arise from the femoral nerve and supply the anterior and medial surfaces of the thigh. Usually the obturator nerve gives a cutaneous supply to the medial side of the thigh. The femoral branch of the genitofemoral nerve (L1 & L2) passes beneath the inguinal ligament to supply skin over the femoral triangle, and the ilioinguinal nerve emerges through the superficial inguinal ring to supply the adjacent medial aspect of the thigh.

Fascia lata

The fascia lata (deep fascia) completely invests the thigh, providing attachment for muscles and associated intermuscular septa in the anterior compartment. It attaches superiorly to the inguinal ligament and iliac crest and inferiorly is continuous with the deep fascia of the leg. Below and lateral to the pubic tubercle is the saphenous opening, which transmits the terminal part of the long saphenous vein.

Over the lateral aspect of the thigh the fascia lata is particularly thick, forming the iliotibial tract. Gluteus maximus and tensor fasciae latae are attached to its upper part (see Fig. 6.30).

Muscles

Quadriceps femoris

The four parts of quadriceps femoris, namely rectus femoris, vastus lateralis, vastus intermedius and vastus medialis, cover the front and sides of the femur (Figs 6.12, 6.13 & 6.14). Rectus femoris is attached by a straight head to the anterior inferior iliac spine and by a reflected head to the ilium above the acetabulum.

Vastus lateralis attaches to the intertrochanteric line, the lateral lip of the linea aspera and the lateral supracondylar ridge of the femur (Figs 6.15 & 6.16). Vastus intermedius attaches to the upper two-thirds of the anterior and lateral surfaces of the femoral shaft, whilst vastus medialis anchors to the spiral line and medial lip of the linea aspera. Distally these four muscles form a common tendon which attaches to the upper border (base) of the patella. From the lower border (apex) of the patella the tendon continues as the ligamentum patellae (see Fig. 6.75) to attach to the tibial tubercle.

Quadriceps femoris is a powerful extensor of the knee joint during standing, walking and running. In addition, rectus femoris flexes the hip. The lower fibres of vastus medialis stabilize the position of the patella (see page 270). Quadriceps femoris is supplied by branches of the femoral nerve.

Sartorius

This strap-like muscle is attached proximally to the anterior superior iliac spine and descends obliquely across the thigh (see Fig. 6.12), crosses the posteromedial side of the knee and, with gracilis and semitendinosus, attaches to the upper end of the subcutaneous surface of the tibia (see Fig. 6.79). Sartorius flexes and laterally rotates the hip and flexes the knee. It is supplied by the femoral nerve.

Fig. 6.13 Quadriceps femoris. Vastus intermedius is partially revealed by removal of rectus femoris.

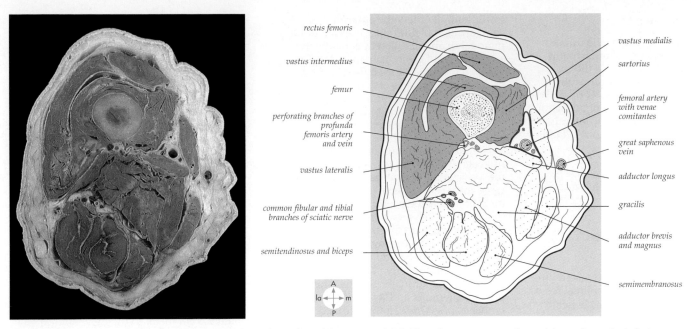

rectus femoris

vastus intermedius

femur

perforating branches of
profunda
femoris artery
and vein

vastus lateralis

common fibular and tibial
branches of sciatic nerve

semitendinosus and biceps

vastus medialis

sartorius

femoral artery
with venae
comitantes

great saphenous
vein

adductor longus

gracilis

adductor brevis
and magnus

semimembranosus

Fig. 6.14 Transverse section through the thigh to show the adductor canal (pink) and components of quadriceps femoris. Inferior aspect.

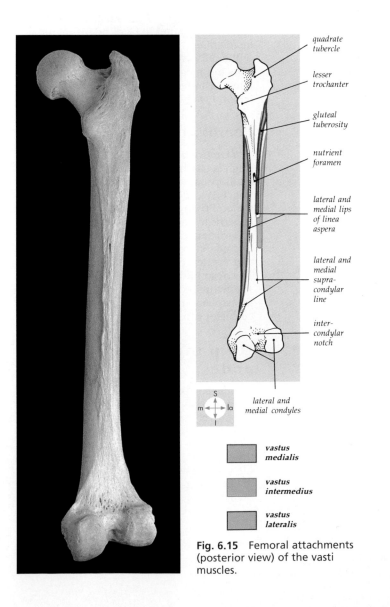

quadrate
tubercle

lesser
trochanter

gluteal
tuberosity

nutrient
foramen

lateral and
medial lips
of linea
aspera

lateral and
medial
supra-
condylar
line

inter-
condylar
notch

lateral and
medial condyles

vastus
medialis

vastus
intermedius

vastus
lateralis

Fig. 6.15 Femoral attachments
(posterior view) of the vasti
muscles.

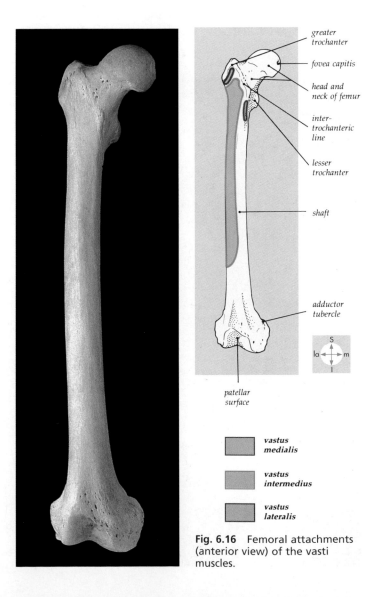

greater
trochanter

fovea capitis

head and
neck of femur

inter-
trochanteric
line

lesser
trochanter

shaft

adductor
tubercle

patellar
surface

vastus
medialis

vastus
intermedius

vastus
lateralis

Fig. 6.16 Femoral attachments
(anterior view) of the vasti
muscles.

Femoral triangle

The femoral triangle occupies the upper medial part of the anterior compartment of the thigh. Its upper boundary is the inguinal ligament; its lateral limit is the medial border of sartorius and its medial boundary is the medial border of adductor longus but some authors use the lateral border in their definition. The roof is fascia lata and the floor comprises iliopsoas, pectineus and adductor longus (Fig. 6.17). The triangle contains the femoral vessels and nerve, and the deep inguinal lymph nodes.

Adductor (subsartorial) canal

This canal is an intermuscular space linking the femoral triangle with the popliteal fossa. Triangular in cross-section, it lies beneath sartorius, occupying the groove between adductor magnus and vastus medialis. Through the canal run the femoral artery and vein, and nerve to vastus medialis and the saphenous nerve (Fig. 6.18).

Femoral vessels

The femoral artery, a continuation of the external iliac, is the main artery of the lower limb. It enters the anterior compartment behind the midpoint of the inguinal ligament where it is relatively superficial and easily palpable, descends through the femoral triangle (Fig. 6.19) and the adductor canal, and continues through the opening in adductor magnus as the popliteal artery (see page 246).

The femoral artery or its main branches supply all three compartments of the thigh. Subcutaneous branches of the artery traverse the saphenous opening or pierce the fascia lata to accompany the superficial veins in the groin (see Fig. 6.11). The largest deep branch is the profunda femoris artery (Fig. 6.20), which arises from the posterolateral aspect of the femoral artery about 4 cm below the inguinal ligament and runs distally behind the femoral artery, leaving the triangle by passing between pectineus and adductor longus. The profunda femoris and its perforating branches pass through the adductor muscles and contribute to the anastomosis in the posterior compartment of the thigh. One of the perforating arteries gives a large nutrient branch to the femur. Close to its origin the profunda femoris artery usually gives medial and lateral circumflex femoral branches (Fig. 6.20). The medial circumflex artery winds round the medial aspect of the femur between iliopsoas and pectineus to join the cruciate anastomosis (see page 238)

and the lateral circumflex artery encircles the femur, passing laterally deep to sartorius and rectus femoris.

The femoral vein is the continuation of the popliteal vein at the opening in adductor magnus. In the adductor canal it lies behind the femoral artery and continues through the femoral triangle lying medial to the artery (Fig. 6.19). Passing deep to the inguinal ligament the femoral vein becomes the external iliac vein. Tributaries of the femoral vein, except the great saphenous vein, correspond to the branches of the femoral artery.

Femoral sheath

The femoral artery and vein are invested in a thick fascial sleeve, the femoral sheath, derived from the transversalis and iliac fasciae. The sheath passes deep to the inguinal ligament and tapers inferiorly, blending with the adventitia of the vessels about 2.5 cm distal to the ligament.

Two vertical septa divide the sheath into three compartments. The femoral artery lies laterally while the femoral vein occupies the intermediate compartment. The medial compartment is called the femoral canal (Fig. 6.20) and contains fat and lymph nodes. The upper limit of the femoral canal is the femoral ring (see Fig. 4.21), an aperture bounded in front by the inguinal ligament and behind by the superior ramus of the pubis whilst laterally lies the femoral vein and medially the lacunar ligament. A femoral hernia descends through the femoral ring to enter the femoral canal.

Femoral nerve

The femoral nerve (L2, L3 & L4) enters the thigh beneath the inguinal ligament lying on iliopsoas lateral to the femoral sheath (Fig. 6.19). After a brief course in the femoral triangle, it divides into several superficial and deep branches. The superficial branches are the intermediate and medial cutaneous nerves of the thigh and the nerves to sartorius and pectineus. The deep branches include the nerves supplying rectus femoris and the vasti, and the saphenous nerve which enters the adductor canal.

Deep inguinal lymph nodes

The deep inguinal lymph nodes lie in the femoral triangle medial to the femoral vein. They receive lymph from the superficial inguinal nodes and from all parts of the limb deep to the investing fascia. They also drain the glans of the penis or clitoris. Efferent vessels pass proximally through the femoral canal to reach the external iliac nodes.

inguinal ligament

superficial inguinal ring

spermatic cord

iliopsoas

pectineus

lateral cutaneous nerve of thigh

sartorius

adductor longus

gracilis

adductor magnus

Fig. 6.17 Boundaries and floor of the femoral triangle.

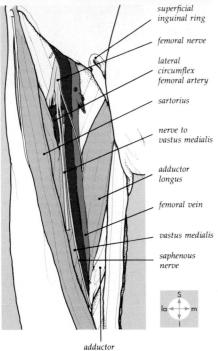

superficial
inguinal ring

femoral nerve

lateral
circumflex
femoral artery

sartorius

nerve to
vastus medialis

adductor
longus

femoral vein

vastus medialis

saphenous
nerve

adductor
magnus

Fig. 6.18 Contents and boundaries of the adductor canal, exposed by displacement of sartorius laterally.

inguinal
ligament

deep circumflex
iliac artery

femoral nerve
& cutaneous
branch

femoral canal

femoral vein
& artery

pectineus

branch to vasti

great saphenous
vein (cut)

branches
to sartorius

nerve to
vastus medialis

saphenous
nerve

lateral cutaneous   medial cutaneous
nerve of thigh   nerve of thigh

Fig. 6.19 Contents of the femoral triangle exposed by removal of its roof (fascia lata). The deep inguinal lymph nodes lie within the femoral canal.

femoral canal

femoral
nerve (cut)

lateral & medial
circumflex
femoral arteries

femoral artery
& vein (cut)

profunda femoris
artery & vein

vastus medialis

adductor longus

saphenous
nerve (cut)

Fig. 6.20 Profunda femoris vessels seen after removal of segments of the femoral artery and vein.

MEDIAL COMPARTMENT OF THIGH

The medial compartment of the thigh is wedge-shaped and lies between the anterior and posterior compartments. It contains pectineus, adductors longus, brevis and magnus, gracilis and obturator externus. The obturator nerve and vessels and the profunda femoris vessels, together with their perforating branches, supply the compartment.

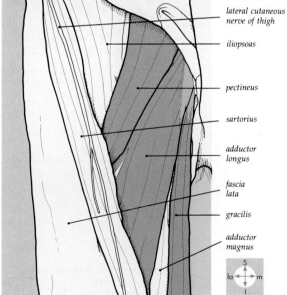

lateral cutaneous nerve of thigh

iliopsoas

pectineus

sartorius

adductor longus

fascia lata

gracilis

adductor magnus

Fig. 6.21   Anterior layer of muscles of the medial compartment of thigh.

pectineus

adductor longus (cut)

branches of anterior division of obturator nerve

adductor brevis

gracilis

adductor longus (cut)

adductor magnus

Fig. 6.22   Adductor brevis and branches of the anterior division of the obturator nerve, revealed by removal of part of adductor longus.

Muscles

The muscles are arranged in three layers. The anterior layer consists of pectineus, adductor longus and gracilis from lateral to medial (Fig. 6.21). Deep to these, forming the intermediate layer, is adductor brevis (Figs 6.22 & 6.23). The posterior layer consists of obturator externus and adductor magnus (Figs 6.24 & 6.25). The proximal attachments of these muscles lie on the outer surface of the bony pelvis between the superior pubic and ischial rami. In addition, obturator externus is attached to the obturator membrane.

pectineus (cut)

superior
pubic ramus

obturator
externus

posterior
& anterior
divisions of
obturator
nerve

adductor brevis

pectineus (cut)

adductor
magnus

quadriceps
femoris

gracilis

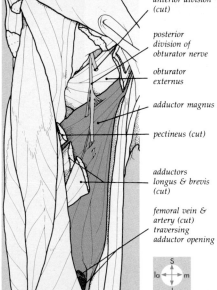

anterior division
(cut)

posterior
division of
obturator nerve

obturator
externus

adductor magnus

pectineus (cut)

adductors
longus & brevis
(cut)

femoral vein &
artery (cut)
traversing
adductor opening

iliopsoas (cut)

psoas bursa

capsule of hip
joint

anterior &
posterior
divisions of
obturator nerve
(cut)

obturator
externus

adductor
magnus (cut)

iliopsoas (cut)

sciatic nerve

hamstrings

adductor magnus
(cut)

Fig. 6.23 Division of the obturator nerve, revealed by removal of adductor longus and part of pectineus. In this specimen the posterior division lies in front of obturator externus.

Fig. 6.24 Adductor magnus and the posterior division of the obturator nerve. Adductor brevis has been removed.

Fig. 6.25 Obturator externus, completely revealed by removal of parts of iliopsoas and adductor magnus.

The more anterior muscles have higher attachments than those of the deeper layers (Fig. 6.26). Distally the muscles attach to the femur, except for gracilis (see Fig. 6.79), which descends below the knee to gain the proximal end of the subcutaneous surface of the tibia in company with sartorius and semitendinosus. Obturator externus passes laterally below and behind the capsule of the hip joint (see Figs 6.25 & 6.70) to the trochanteric fossa on the medial aspect of the greater trochanter. Pectineus and adductors longus, brevis and magnus slope downwards and laterally to attach in the region of the linea aspera, the sequence being related to the layer in which the muscle lies (Fig. 6.27). Adductor magnus has the longest attachment, extending from the gluteal tuberosity above to the adductor tubercle below.

All the muscles in the compartment except obturator externus adduct the hip joint. During walking they stabilize the femur whilst the abductors of the hip prevent tilting of the pelvis (see page 240). In addition, pectineus and adductor longus are medial rotators and obturator externus

a lateral rotator. Pectineus assists flexion at the hip joint and gracilis flexes and medially rotates the knee joint.

All the muscles in the medial compartment except pectineus are innervated by the obturator nerve. Pectineus usually has a supply from the femoral nerve but may also be supplied by the obturator nerve, and the ischial part of adductor magnus receives fibres from the sciatic nerve.

Obturator nerve

The obturator nerve gains the compartment through the obturator canal and promptly divides into anterior and posterior divisions (see Fig. 6.23). The former passes anterior to obturator externus whilst the posterior division usually pierces and supplies the muscle before emerging onto its surface. The two divisions then descend respectively anterior and posterior to adductor brevis. The anterior division supplies adductors longus and brevis and gracilis (see Fig. 6.22), and gives sensory branches to the hip joint and to skin on the

medial side of the thigh. The posterior division lies on and supplies adductor magnus (see Fig. 6.24) and gives sensory branches, which accompany the femoral artery through the opening in adductor magnus to supply the knee joint. Since the obturator nerve innervates the hip and knee joints, disease in one joint may cause referred pain in the other.

Vessels

The blood supply is derived from the profunda femoris artery and its perforating branches, supplemented by the obturator artery and other branches of the femoral artery. The obturator artery is small and forms an arterial circle around the margins of the obturator membrane, supplying the proximal parts of the muscles. An acetabular branch passes beneath the transverse acetabular ligament and accompanies the round ligament to the head of the femur. Venae comitantes accompanying the arteries in the compartment drain into the profunda femoris or internal iliac veins.

Fig. 6.26 Attachments of the muscles of the medial compartment of the thigh to the hip bone.

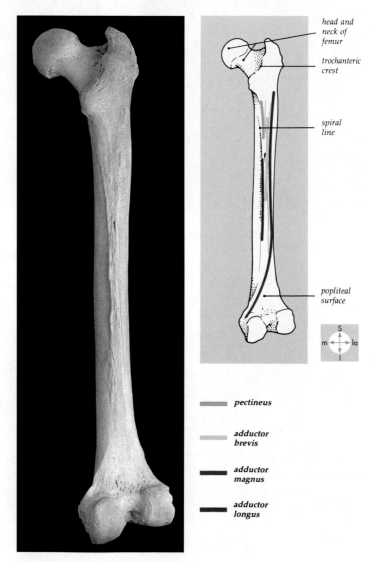

Fig. 6.27 Femoral attachments of the muscles of the medial compartment of the thigh.

GLUTEAL COMPARTMENT

The gluteal region or buttock forms part of the root of the limb. It overlies the dorsum of the ilium, ischium and sacrum and is continuous proximally with the lower trunk and distally with the posterior compartment of the thigh. Three substantial muscles (gluteus maximus, medius and minimus), covered by deep fascia and a thick layer of subcutaneous fat, form the bulk of the buttock and account for its surface contour. The gluteal fold, a prominent surface feature, lies at the junction of the buttock and thigh.

Gluteus maximus

This very large trapezoidal muscle is the most superficial in the buttock. Its fibres slope downwards and laterally (Fig. 6.28) and its lower edge passes obliquely across the gluteal fold. Some of the sensory nerves to the skin of the buttock penetrate the medial part of the muscle whilst others emerge around its upper and lower borders. Proximally the muscle has an extensive attachment: to the ilium behind the posterior gluteal line, to the lower part of the sacrum, to the coccyx, to the sacrotuberous ligament and to the thoracolumbar (lumbar) and gluteal fasciae. A synovial bursa is usually present where it crosses the ischial tuberosity. Distally some of the deeper fibres are attached to the gluteal tuberosity of the femur (Fig. 6.29), but most of the muscle is attached through the iliotibial tract (see Fig. 6.30) to the anterior surface of the lateral tibial condyle. The nerve supply is from the inferior gluteal nerve (L5, S1 & S2).

Fig. 6.28 The attachments of gluteus maximus include the thoracolumbar fascia and the iliotibial tract.

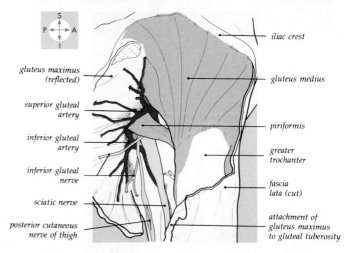

Fig. 6.29 Reflection of gluteus maximus exposes gluteus medius and neurovascular structures.

Gluteus maximus is a strong extensor of the thigh, especially during running and climbing, and also produces abduction at the hip joint. As an antigravity muscle it extends the trunk on the hip and through the iliotibial tract it extends and stabilizes the knee joint and the supporting limb during walking and standing.

Tensor fasciae latae

This small muscle is attached proximally to the ilium between the anterior superior iliac spine and iliac tubercle (Fig. 6.31) and distally to the anterior border of the iliotibial tract (Fig. 6.30) which it tenses. It is supplied by the superior gluteal nerve.

Structures deep to gluteus maximus

The arrangement of these structures is clarified by noting whether they enter the buttock above or below the piriformis muscle (see Fig. 6.29), which itself enters via the greater sciatic foramen (see Fig. 6.36).

Structures entering above piriformis

The superior gluteal nerve (L4, L5 & S1) arises within the pelvis from the lumbosacral plexus and enters the buttock through the greater sciatic foramen (see Fig. 6.36), running laterally between gluteus medius and gluteus minimus (Fig. 6.32). It supplies both muscles and terminates in tensor fasciae latae.

The superior gluteal artery arises from the posterior aspect of the internal iliac artery. It enters the buttock accompanying the corresponding nerve and divides into a superficial branch which supplies the overlying gluteus maximus (see Fig. 6.29) and two deep branches, an upper and lower, which supply gluteus medius and minimus (Fig. 6.32). The deep branches also contribute to anastomoses around the greater trochanter and anterior superior iliac spine. The accompanying veins form an extensive plexus between the muscles and drain into the internal iliac vein.

Gluteus medius and minimus

These fan-shaped muscles lie superior to piriformis. Gluteus medius (see Fig. 6.29) is attached proximally to the dorsum of the ilium between the posterior and anterior (middle) gluteal lines and to the gluteal fascia, which separates it from gluteus maximus. Distally it is attached to the lateral surface of the greater trochanter. Gluteus minimus lies immediately deep to gluteus medius and attaches proximally to the dorsum of the ilium between the anterior and inferior gluteal lines (Fig. 6.31) and distally to the anterior surface of the greater trochanter (Fig. 6.32). Both are supplied by the superior gluteal nerve.

Although both gluteus medius and minimus medially rotate the femur at the hip joint, their importance is in abduction. During walking, gluteus medius and minimus of the supporting limb contract to prevent tilting of the pelvis towards the unsupported side. Failure of this mechanism is the basis of Trendelenburg's sign of hip instability.

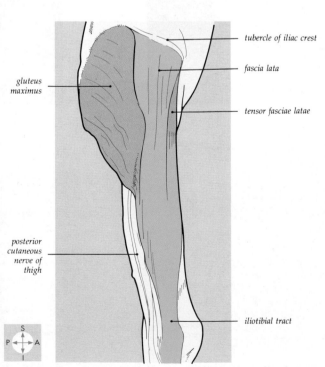

Fig. 6.30 Attachment of gluteus maximus and tensor fasciae latae to the iliotibial tract.

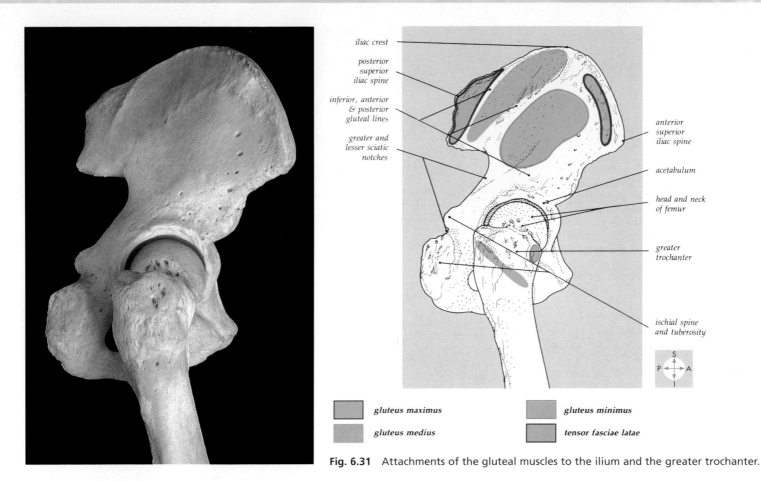

iliac crest

posterior
superior
iliac spine

inferior, anterior
& posterior
gluteal lines

greater and
lesser sciatic
notches

anterior
superior
iliac spine

acetabulum

head and neck
of femur

greater
trochanter

ischial spine
and tuberosity

	gluteus maximus		gluteus minimus
	gluteus medius		tensor fasciae latae

Fig. 6.31 Attachments of the gluteal muscles to the ilium and the greater trochanter.

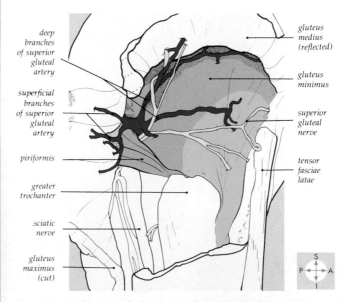

deep
branches
of superior
gluteal
artery

superficial
branches
of superior
gluteal
artery

piriformis

greater
trochanter

sciatic
nerve

gluteus
maximus
(cut)

gluteus
medius
(reflected)

gluteus
minimus

superior
gluteal
nerve

tensor
fasciae
latae

Fig. 6.32 Reflection of gluteus medius reveals gluteus minimus and the superior gluteal artery and nerve entering the buttock above piriformis.

Structures entering below piriformis

These are: three nerves laterally, the sciatic nerve, nerve to quadratus femoris and posterior cutaneous nerve of thigh; medially the internal pudendal artery, pudendal nerve and nerve to obturator internus; and in intermediate position, the inferior gluteal nerve and vessels.

The sciatic nerve (Fig. 6.33), the largest nerve in the lower limb, arises from the spinal nerves L4, L5, S1, S2 & S3 and supplies the entire limb, except for the gluteal structures and the medial and anterior compartments of the thigh. It leaves the greater sciatic foramen about halfway between the posterior superior iliac spine and ischial tuberosity and curves laterally and downwards, crossing the midpoint between the ischial tuberosity and greater trochanter. The nerve is separated from the capsule of the hip joint by obturator internus and the gemelli, quadratus femoris and the upper border of adductor magnus (Fig. 6.33). A branch of the inferior gluteal artery accompanies the nerve.

The nerve to quadratus femoris (L4, L5 & S1) lies deep to the sciatic nerve, obturator internus and the gemelli and supplies the inferior gemellus, quadratus femoris and the hip joint.

Superficial and medial to the sciatic nerve is the posterior cutaneous nerve of the thigh (Fig. 6.33), which arises from spinal nerves

S1, S2 & S3. Within the buttock its perineal branch runs forwards to supply the skin on the posterior part of the scrotum or labium majus. Other branches curl round the lower border of gluteus maximus to supply the skin over the buttock.

The inferior gluteal nerve and vessels occupy an intermediate position. The nerve turns immediately posteriorly to supply gluteus maximus.

The inferior gluteal artery, a branch of the internal iliac artery, accompanies the nerve and supplies gluteus maximus (see Fig. 6.29) and the short lateral rotators of the hip joint, and contributes to the trochanteric and cruciate anastomoses. Venae comitantes accompany the artery and drain into the internal iliac system.

The pudendal nerve (S2, S3 & S4), internal pudendal vessels, and nerve to obturator internus (L5, S1 & S2), also supplying the superior gemellus, enter beneath the medial part of piriformis (Fig. 6.33). Their course in the buttock is brief before turning forwards into the lesser sciatic foramen, crossing the sacrospinous ligament or ischial spine to enter the pudendal canal (see Fig. 6.36 and page 216).

Short muscles of buttock

The short muscles of the buttock are, from above downwards, piriformis, obturator internus with the gemelli, and quadratus

femoris (Fig. 6.33). Piriformis arises from the ventral surface of the sacrum (see page 209) and runs laterally through the greater sciatic foramen to converge on the medial border of the greater trochanter. It is innervated within the pelvis by the fifth lumbar and first and second sacral (L5, S1 & S2) nerves. Obturator internus attaches to the lateral wall of the pelvic cavity (see Fig. 6.72), including the obturator membrane, and runs backwards towards the lesser sciatic foramen where its tendon makes a right-angled turn to run laterally across the buttock to the medial aspect of the greater trochanter above the trochanteric fossa. The superior and inferior gemelli are small muscles arising from the upper and lower margins of the lesser sciatic notch to fuse with the obturator internus tendon.

Quadratus femoris attaches to the lateral margin of the ischial tuberosity and to the quadrate tubercle of the femur and the subjacent shaft. Being behind the hip joint, all the short muscles laterally rotate the hip.

Cruciate arterial anastomosis

The cruciate anastomosis lies at the lower border of quadratus femoris and receives contributions from: above, the inferior gluteal artery; below, the first perforating artery; and on each side the medial and lateral circumflex femoral arteries.

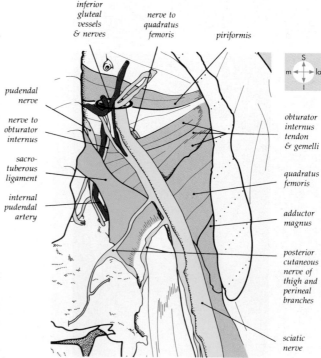

Fig. 6.33 Structures emerging below piriformis and the course and relations of the sciatic nerve.

POSTERIOR COMPARTMENT OF THIGH

The posterior compartment is enclosed within deep fascia, the fascia lata (Fig. 6.34), and extends from the gluteal region above to the popliteal fossa below. It contains the posterior cutaneous nerve of thigh, 'hamstring' muscles, sciatic nerve and terminal branches of the profunda femoris artery.

'Hamstring' muscles

These three muscles, semimembranosus, semitendinosus and biceps femoris (long head) (Fig. 6.35), attach proximally to the ischial tuberosity (see Fig. 6.36) and distally to the upper end of the tibia or fibula and are innervated by the sciatic nerve. They span the entire length of the femur and act on two joints, the hip for extension and the knee for flexion. After flexion of the trunk, the hamstrings act as antigravity muscles by pulling on the ischial tuberosities, thus extending the trunk into an upright position at the hip.

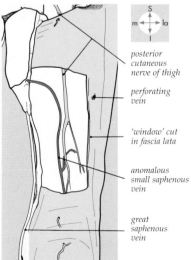

posterior cutaneous nerve of thigh

perforating vein

'window' cut in fascia lata

anomalous small saphenous vein

great saphenous vein

Fig. 6.34 Nerves and veins of the posterior compartment of thigh, seen through a 'window' cut in the fascia lata. This small saphenous vein continues proximally to terminate in the great saphenous vein.

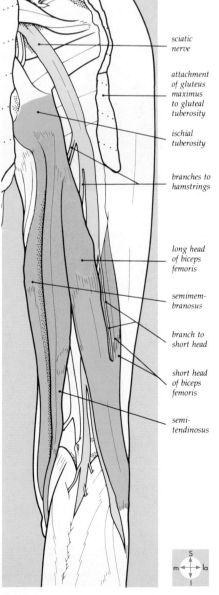

sciatic nerve

attachment of gluteus maximus to gluteal tuberosity

ischial tuberosity

branches to hamstrings

long head of biceps femoris

semimem-branosus

branch to short head

short head of biceps femoris

semi-tendinosus

Fig. 6.35 Principal contents of the posterior compartment of thigh, seen after removal of deep fascia.

Semimembranosus

This muscle is attached to the upper and lateral parts of the ischial tuberosity by a wide flat tendon, which is overlapped by the tendons of biceps and semitendinosus close to the tuberosity, and descends on the medial side of the popliteal fossa to its main attachment into a horizontal groove on the posteromedial aspect of the medial tibial condyle. Some of its fibres pass upwards and laterally behind the knee joint to form the oblique posterior ligament, others descend to reinforce the fascia over popliteus (see Fig. 6.39).

Semitendinosus

Proximally, semitendinosus is attached to the medial part of the ischial tuberosity. It descends on the medial side of the popliteal fossa, forming a narrow tendon which overlies semimembranosus, and attaches to the medial surface of the upper end of the tibial shaft close to the attachments of sartorius and gracilis (see Fig. 6.79). Besides contributing to the common actions of the hamstring group, semitendinosus and semimembranosus produce medial rotation of the leg at the knee.

Biceps femoris

This muscle has two heads. Proximally, the long head is attached to the medial part of the ischial tuberosity close to the semitendinosus and descends to the lateral side of the popliteal fossa where it fuses with the short head, which originates from the lateral lip of the linea aspera and lateral supracondylar ridge of femur (see Fig. 6.35). Inferiorly, the tendon of biceps is attached to the head of the fibula. In addition to the general actions of the hamstrings, biceps produces lateral rotation of the leg at the knee.

Sciatic nerve

The sciatic nerve emerges at the lower border of gluteus maximus lying just beneath the deep fascia, passes deep to the long head of biceps and descends in the midline of the limb. In the distal third of the thigh it usually divides into two terminal branches, the tibial and common fibular (common peroneal) nerves, which continue into the popliteal fossa (see Fig. 6.40). Division may occur more proximally in the thigh, within the buttock or even the pelvis. Proximally, fibres from the medial (tibial) part of the sciatic nerve supply the hamstrings (see Fig. 6.35) and the ischial head of adductor magnus. More distally, a branch from the lateral (common fibular) part of the nerve supplies the short head of biceps.

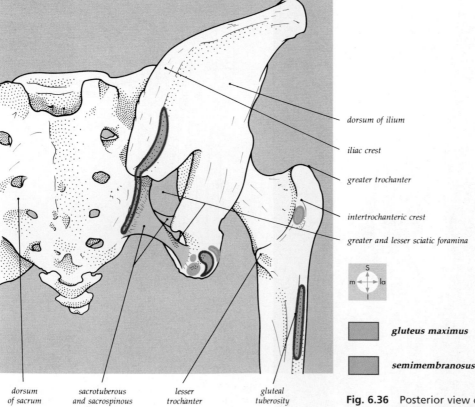

dorsum of ilium

iliac crest

greater trochanter

intertrochanteric crest

greater and lesser sciatic foramina

gluteus maximus

biceps and semitendinosus

semimembranosus

quadratus femoris

dorsum of sacrum

sacrotuberous and sacrospinous ligaments

lesser trochanter

gluteal tuberosity

Fig. 6.36 Posterior view of sacrum and bony pelvis showing sacrotuberous and sacrospinous ligaments with the greater and lesser sciatic foramina.

Posterior cutaneous nerve of thigh

The nerve enters the thigh superficial and slightly medial to the sciatic nerve and descends beneath the fascia lata to the upper part of the popliteal fossa (Fig. 6.37). Apart from branches arising near the lower border of gluteus maximus, the nerve gives sensory fibres to the skin on the back of the thigh.

Profunda femoris artery

Perforating branches of the profunda femoris artery penetrate adductor magnus and terminate in the posterior compartment. They anastomose with branches from the inferior gluteal artery above and the popliteal artery below.

POPLITEAL FOSSA

The popliteal fossa is a diamond-shaped space behind the knee joint. It contains the principal blood vessels and nerves passing between the thigh and the leg. It has a roof, four walls and a floor.

Roof

The roof is formed by the investing layer of deep fascia. In the subcutaneous tissue overlying the roof are the posterior cutaneous nerve of the thigh, which continues into the proximal part of the leg, and the small saphenous vein (Fig. 6.37). The vein usually penetrates the roof to drain into the popliteal vein but occasionally continues proximally to drain into the great saphenous vein (see Fig. 6.34).

Walls

The walls overhang the fossa. Superiorly they are formed by the diverging tendons of the hamstrings, namely semitendinosus and semimembranosus lying medially and biceps laterally. Inferiorly are the medial and lateral heads of gastrocnemius, which converge at the inferior angle (Fig. 6.38). Adjacent to the lateral head of gastrocnemius is the small plantaris muscle. On each side of the popliteal fossa the hamstring tendons overlap the heads of gastrocnemius and between the medial head of gastrocnemius and semimembranosus there is frequently a bursa (see Fig. 6.39).

Contents

The principal contents of the fossa are embedded in fat and comprise the popliteal artery and vein together with the two terminal branches of the sciatic nerve, the common fibular and tibial nerves (see Fig. 6.40). These vessels and nerves are responsible for the blood and nerve supply of most of the leg and foot.

Fig. 6.37 Removal of skin and subcutaneous tissue reveals the cutaneous nerves. The small saphenous vein and accompanying nerve pierce the roof of the popliteal fossa.

Fig. 6.38 Muscles forming the walls of the popliteal fossa.

The popliteal artery lies deepest and is the continuation of the femoral artery from the thigh. It enters through the opening in adductor magnus and descends vertically on the floor of the fossa to the inferior angle where it leaves beneath the fused heads of gastrocnemius. The artery is so deep that it is difficult to palpate unless the knee is flexed to relax the boundaries and roof of the fossa. The artery supplies the surrounding muscles and also forms a substantial plexus of articular branches anastomosing symmetrically around the knee joint (see Fig. 1.27).

The popliteal vein lies superficial to the artery and is formed at the inferior angle of the fossa by the union of the venae comitantes that accompany the tibial arteries in the leg. It continues proximally with the artery through the opening in adductor magnus to enter the adductor canal and become the femoral vein.

The tibial and common fibular nerves (Fig. 6.40), entering the fossa from the posterior compartment of the thigh, lie just beneath the roof, superficial to the popliteal vessels. The tibial nerve enters from beneath the hamstrings and descends vertically, bisecting the fossa, and leaves beneath the gastrocnemius at the inferior angle of the fossa, where it enters the posterior compartment of the leg. The tibial nerve is mainly motor in its distribution, supplying gastrocnemius, plantaris, popliteus and soleus. All these branches arise within the fossa. The nerve also gives sensory branches to the knee joint and a large cutaneous branch which passes into the calf to form the sural nerve. The common fibular nerve descends under cover of the tendon of biceps to reach the lateral angle of the fossa, where it enters the lateral (fibular or peroneal) compartment of the leg by winding around the neck of the fibula. It supplies sensory branches to the knee joint and two cutaneous nerves, one to the lateral side of the calf and the other, the lateral sural cutaneous nerve, joining the sural nerve in the calf.

The remaining contents of the popliteal fossa are the deeply placed popliteal lymph nodes which lie close to the popliteal artery. They drain the deep structures of the leg and foot and the knee joint, and receive superficial lymphatics which accompany the short saphenous vein from the lateral side of the foot and leg.

Floor

The floor of the fossa is formed, from above downwards, by the popliteal surface of the femur, the capsule of the knee joint reinforced by the oblique popliteal ligament, and popliteus (Fig. 6.39).

Popliteus

This muscle is attached to a triangular area on the posterior surface of the proximal end of the tibia above the soleal line. The tendon passes upwards and laterally, penetrating the capsule of the knee joint (see Fig. 6.77) to become attached to a pit below the lateral epicondyle of the femur.

Its action is to 'unlock' the knee joint by producing lateral rotation of the femur on the tibia during flexion of the joint from the fully extended position. Popliteus is supplied by the tibial nerve.

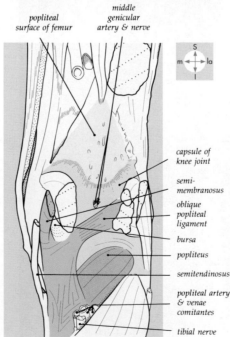

middle
popliteal   genicular
surface of femur   artery & nerve

capsule of
knee joint

semi-
membranosus

oblique
popliteal
ligament

bursa

popliteus

semitendinosus

popliteal artery
& venae
comitantes

tibial nerve

Fig. 6.39 Floor of popliteal fossa, seen after removal of walls and contents of the fossa.

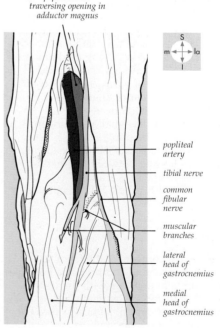

popliteal vein
traversing opening in
adductor magnus

popliteal
artery

tibial nerve

common
fibular
nerve

muscular
branches

lateral
head of
gastrocnemius

medial
head of
gastrocnemius

Fig. 6.40 Principal vessels and nerves of the popliteal fossa, revealed by removal of fat.

POSTERIOR COMPARTMENT OF LEG

The compartment extends from the popliteal fossa above to the ankle below. Gastrocnemius and soleus account for its bulk (Fig. 6.41) and the characteristic contour of the calf. Their common tendon is conspicuous as it passes towards the ankle. Deeper are tibialis posterior and the two long flexors of the toes, flexor hallucis longus and flexor digitorum longus, whose tendons all pass distally into the foot. The posterior tibial artery and its venae comitantes and the tibial nerve pass distally between soleus and the long flexors to enter the foot where they supply structures in the sole.

Superficial structures and deep fascia

The small (short) saphenous vein begins on the lateral side of the foot as a continuation of the dorsal venous arch. Passing behind the lateral malleolus (Fig. 6.42) it ascends in the midline of the calf and usually terminates by piercing the fascial roof of the popliteal fossa (see Fig. 6.37). The vein has frequent communications with the great saphenous vein and important communicating (perforating) veins which pierce the investing deep fascia to link up with the deep veins of the calf, particularly just above the ankle.

The sural nerve is formed principally from the cutaneous branch of the tibial nerve and descends from the popliteal fossa to pierce the deep fascia in the proximal part of the calf. Here it is joined by the sural communicating branch of the common fibular nerve and continues distally with the small saphenous vein posteroinferior to the lateral malleolus to reach the foot (Fig. 6.42). The nerve supplies skin over the lower two-thirds of the calf and on the lateral side of the ankle and foot.

The deep fascia is continuous proximally with the popliteal fascia and distally near the heel is thickened in two places. The first forms a thick band stretching between the tibia and fibula over which the tendo calcaneus passes, separated by a bursa. The second thickening, the flexor retinaculum, bridges the gap between the medial malleolus and the medial surface of the calcaneus, completing a fibro-osseous tunnel similar to the carpal tunnel of the wrist. It is the gateway into the sole of the foot for the tendons of the deep muscles of the compartment and the neurovascular bundle.

Fig. 6.41 'Step' dissection showing the muscle layers in the upper third of the leg and the location of principal nerves and vessels.

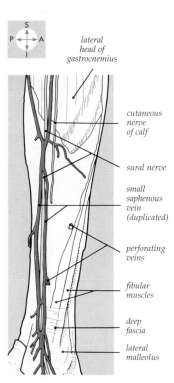

Fig. 6.42 Small saphenous vein and sural nerve. Perforating veins pierce the deep fascia to connect with deep veins in the calf muscles.

Superficial muscles

Gastrocnemius

The muscle has medial and lateral heads attached to the respective femoral condyles. The medial head is the larger and its fibres extend more distally. The two heads share a common aponeurosis which overlies that of the subjacent soleus (Fig. 6.43). The long parallel fibres of gastrocnemius provide a large range of movement and are used especially during walking and running.

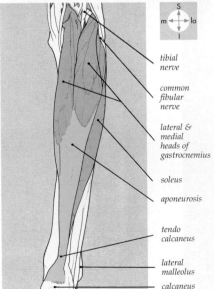

Fig. 6.43 Removal of the deep fascia reveals the superficial flexor muscles, gastrocnemius and soleus.

Because of its femoral attachments it is a weak flexor of the knee joint.

Soleus

This muscle attaches to the soleal line on the posterior border of the tibia, from where it arches across to the posterior aspect of the head and upper shaft of the fibula (Figs 6.44 & 6.45). Its short multipennate fibres are continually in action during standing.

The aponeuroses of gastrocnemius and soleus form the tendo calcaneus (Achilles) which is attached to the middle third of the posterior surface of the calcaneus, separated from the upper part of the bone by a bursa. The two muscles are the principal plantar flexors of the foot at the ankle joint.

Plantaris

This muscle attaches to the lower end of the femur close to the lateral head of gastrocnemius. Its long thin tendon passes deep to the medial head of gastrocnemius (see Fig. 6.45) between the aponeuroses of gastrocnemius and soleus to insert into the posterior surface of the calcaneus medial to the tendo calcaneus. It is a weak flexor of the knee and ankle joints.

Gastrocnemius, soleus and plantaris are supplied by the tibial nerve in the popliteal fossa (see Fig. 6.40). Soleus is further supplied by the tibial nerve as it passes beneath the soleal arch.

Neurovascular structures

Posterior tibial artery

At the lower border of popliteus the popliteal artery divides into two terminal branches, the anterior tibial artery (see page 260) and the larger posterior tibial artery. The latter, accompanied by its venae comitantes, passes deep to the soleal arch and descends on the fascia of tibialis posterior (see Fig. 6.41) between flexor digitorum longus and flexor hallucis longus. Near the ankle the artery lies on the distal end of the tibia and the capsule of the ankle joint, where its pulsations are easily felt. Passing beneath the flexor retinaculum it gives calcaneal branches to the superficial tissues of the heel and then divides into medial and lateral plantar arteries. It provides branches to the muscles in the calf and also a large nutrient artery to the tibial shaft.

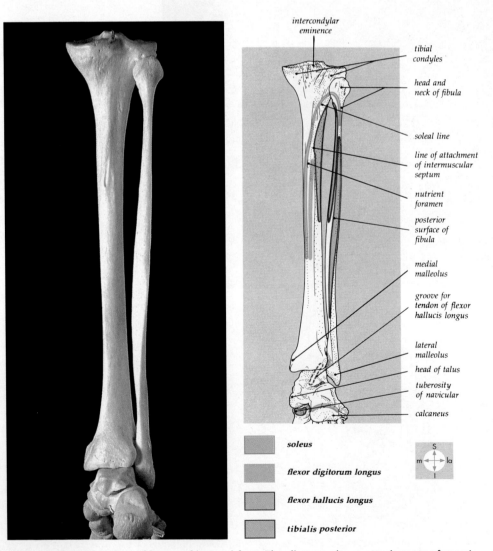

Fig. 6.44 Posterior view of bones of leg and foot. The diagram shows attachments of muscles of posterior compartment.

The most conspicuous branch, the fibular (peroneal) artery, arises just beyond the soleal arch (Fig. 6.46) and passes distally and laterally deep to flexor hallucis longus and upon the fascia of tibialis posterior. It gives muscular branches and a nutrient branch to the fibula. The fibular artery terminates behind the lateral malleolus as lateral calcaneal branches supplying the tissues of the heel. In the lower leg a communicating artery links the fibular and posterior tibial arteries.

A perforating branch of the fibular artery passes forwards through the interosseous membrane into the anterior compartment of the leg. When the anterior tibial artery is small, this perforating artery may substitute for it distally, continuing into the foot as the dorsalis pedis artery.

Tibial nerve

The tibial nerve enters the compartment from the popliteal fossa by passing beneath the soleal arch. Usually the posterior tibial artery lies medially as it descends through the calf on the fascia of tibialis posterior and on the distal end of the tibia (Fig. 6.46). Like the artery, as it enters the foot it often terminates beneath the flexor retinaculum as two branches, the medial and lateral plantar nerves. It supplies soleus and the deep leg muscles and gives sensory branches to skin over the ball of the heel.

Deep muscles

Lying deep to soleus are flexor digitorum longus, flexor hallucis longus and tibialis posterior (Figs 6.41 & 6.46). Proximally their attachments are limited by the origin of soleus from the tibia and fibula. Their tendons enter the foot beneath the flexor retinaculum.

Flexor digitorum longus arises from the posterior surface of the tibia (Fig. 6.44) and from the fascia covering tibialis posterior. In the foot the tendon divides into four slips, which are attached to the bases of the terminal phalanges of the lateral toes. The muscle flexes the toes and assists in plantar flexion of the ankle joint.

Flexor hallucis longus has extensive attachments to the posterior surface of the shaft of the fibula (Fig. 6.44), the posterior intermuscular septum and the fascia covering tibialis posterior. Its muscle fibres characteristically extend almost as far as the ankle (Fig. 6.46) and give way to a tendon which passes beneath the flexor retinaculum to insert into the base of the distal phalanx of the great toe. It is a powerful flexor of the hallux, especially in forward propulsion of the foot at the take-off point during walking. Plantar flexion at the ankle joint is also assisted.

Tibialis posterior is the deepest muscle in the compartment and attaches to the posterior surface of the tibia (Fig. 6.44), to the medial surface of the fibula and to the upper two-thirds of the interosseous membrane. Passing under the flexor retinaculum, the tendon enters the foot to attach principally to the tuberosity of the navicular and by small slips to the other tarsal bones. Together with tibialis anterior its action is to invert the foot. It is also a weak plantar flexor of the ankle joint.

All three deep muscles of the calf are supplied by the tibial nerve. Further details of their tendons in the sole of the foot are given on page 252.

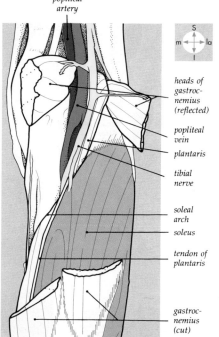

popliteal
artery

heads of
gastroc-
nemius
(reflected)

popliteal
vein

plantaris

tibial
nerve

soleal
arch

soleus

tendon of
plantaris

gastroc-
nemius
(cut)

Fig. 6.45 Partial removal of the two heads of gastrocnemius reveals soleus and the neurovascular bundle passing beneath the soleal arch to enter the calf.

fibula   soleus

tibialis
posterior

posterior
tibial artery

fibular
artery

tibial nerve

flexor
hallucis
longus

flexor
digitorum
longus

tendon of
tibialis
posterior

flexor
retinaculum

Fig. 6.46 Removal of the superficial flexor group shows the deep muscles of the compartment and the main neurovascular bundle.

Abductor digiti minimi traverses the lateral border of the sole (Fig. 6.49) and is attached posteriorly to the medial and lateral calcaneal tubercles. Entering the little toe, its tendon attaches to the lateral side of the proximal phalanx. The muscle is supplied by the lateral plantar nerve.

Long flexor tendons and associated intrinsic muscles

This layer includes the tendons of two long flexor muscles which arise in the leg, namely flexor hallucis longus and flexor digitorum longus. Attached to the tendon of flexor digitorum longus (Fig. 6.52) are quadratus plantae (flexor accessorius) and the four lumbricals.

The tendon of flexor hallucis longus grooves the posterior surface of the talus and curves forwards inferior to the sustentaculum tali and the spring (plantar calcaneonavicular) ligament. It passes deep to the tendon of flexor digitorum longus, to which it is usually attached. The tendon of flexor hallucis longus continues forwards inferior to the head of the first metatarsal, where it passes between the sesamoid bones in the two tendons of the flexor hallucis brevis (see below), and enters the fibrous flexor sheath of the great toe to reach its attachment to the base of the distal phalanx (Fig. 6.52). The actions and innervation of flexor hallucis longus are described on page 249,

The tendon of flexor digitorum longus passes forwards medial to the sustentaculum tali and divides into four tendons, one for each of the lateral four toes (Figs 6.51 & 6.52). Each tendon enters its fibrous flexor sheath and passes through the flexor digitorum brevis tendon before attaching to the base of the terminal phalanx. The actions and innervations of flexor digitorum longus are considered on page 249.

Quadratus plantae (flexor accessorius) (Figs 6.51 & 6.52) is quadrangular and is anchored posteriorly to the medial and lateral tubercles of the calcaneus. Anteriorly the muscle attaches to the tendons of flexor digitorum longus. By pulling on these tendons it can flex the toes irrespective of the position of the ankle. Its nerve supply is from the lateral plantar nerve.

The lumbricals are four small muscles attached proximally to the tendons of flexor digitorum longus (Fig. 6.52). Distally, each slender tendon winds around the medial side of the appropriate digit to attach to the extensor expansion and base of the proximal phalanx. The lumbricals extend the lateral four toes but flex the metatarsophalangeal joints. The first lumbrical is supplied by the medial plantar nerve and the remainder by the lateral plantar nerve.

Deep intrinsic muscles

The three muscles in this layer are located in the anterior part of the foot (Fig. 6.53), adjacent to the metatarsals. Flexor hallucis brevis and adductor hallucis lie medially and are attached to the great toe whilst flexor digiti minimi brevis lies laterally and acts on the little toe.

Flexor hallucis brevis lies along the medial side of the foot and is attached posteriorly to the cuboid and the three cuneiforms. Passing forwards on either side of the flexor hallucis longus tendon (see Fig. 6.52), the muscle gives rise to two short tendons, which lie inferior to the first metatarsophalangeal joint. Each tendon contains a sesamoid bone and enters the great toe to attach to the appropriate side of the base of the proximal phalanx. Flexor hallucis brevis flexes the proximal phalanx and is innervated by the medial plantar nerve.

Adductor hallucis (Fig. 6.53) consists of an oblique head which is attached to the bases of the second, third and fourth metatarsals, and a transverse head which lies across the anterior part of the sole, attached to the deep transverse metatarsal ligaments and the lateral three metatarsophalangeal joints. The two heads converge and attach to the lateral tendon and sesamoid of flexor hallucis brevis. Adductor hallucis assists flexor hallucis brevis and may help to support the transverse arch of the foot. It is supplied by the lateral plantar nerve.

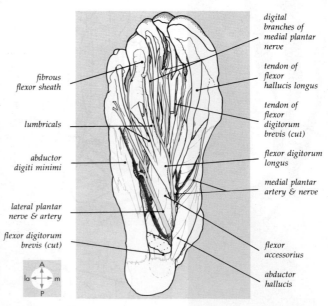

fibrous flexor sheath

lumbricals

abductor digiti minimi

lateral plantar nerve & artery

flexor digitorum brevis (cut)

digital branches of medial plantar nerve

tendon of flexor hallucis longus

tendon of flexor digitorum brevis (cut)

flexor digitorum longus

medial plantar artery & nerve

flexor accessorius

abductor hallucis

Fig. 6.51 Removal of flexor digitorum brevis has revealed the plantar nerves and arteries, which enter the sole deep to abductor hallucis.

Flexor digiti minimi brevis lies along the plantar surface of the fifth metatarsal (Fig. 6.53), attaching posteriorly to the base of the bone and anteriorly to the lateral side of the base of the proximal phalanx of the little toe. The muscle flexes the proximal phalanx and is innervated by the lateral plantar nerve.

Fig. 6.52 Tendons of flexor digitorum longus, flexor hallucis longus, quadratus plantae and the lumbricals, after removal of medial and lateral plantar nerves and the tendons of flexor digitorum brevis.

Fig. 6.53 Deep intrinsic muscles, revealed by removal of long flexor tendons and abductors of the great and little toes.

plantar
metatarsal
arteries

deep
transverse
metatarsal
ligament

plantar
inter-
osseous
muscles

dorsal
inter-
osseous
muscles

plantar
arch

adductor
hallucis
(cut)

lateral &
medial
plantar
arteries

Fig. 6.54   Interosseous muscles and the plantar arterial arch, exposed by removing adductor hallucis.

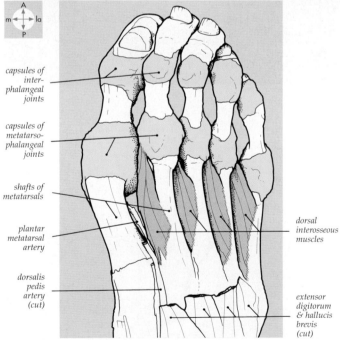

capsules of
inter-
phalangeal
joints

capsules of
metatarso-
phalangeal
joints

shafts of
metatarsals

plantar
metatarsal
artery

dorsalis
pedis
artery
(cut)

dorsal
interosseous
muscles

extensor
digitorum
& hallucis
brevis
(cut)

Fig. 6.55   Dorsal aspect of the foot showing the dorsal interosseous muscles after partial removal of extensor digitorum brevis. Extensor expansions have been removed to show joint capsules.

Interossei and tendons of fibularis (peroneus) longus and tibialis posterior

Lying deeply in the sole, attached to the metatarsals, the three plantar interosseous muscles (Fig. 6.54) attach by single heads to the plantar borders of the third, fourth and fifth metatarsals. The four dorsal interossei (Fig. 6.55) are bicipital and attach to contiguous surfaces of the shafts of the metatarsals. The tendons pass forwards dorsal to the deep transverse metatarsal ligaments and attach to the bases of the proximal phalanges and dorsal extensor expansions. These muscles are supplied by the lateral plantar nerve. They assist extension of the phalanges and flexion of the metatarsophalangeal joints. Their attachments indicate that plantar interossei should adduct and dorsal should abduct the toes, but these movements are often poorly developed, especially in the shod foot.

The tendons of fibularis (peroneus) longus and tibialis posterior (Fig. 6.56) pass deeply into the sole to reach their attachments on tarsal and metatarsal bones. The fibularis longus tendon enters the lateral side of the sole and is retained in a groove inferior to the cuboid by the long plantar ligament. The tendon passes forwards and medially to reach the lateral aspect of the base of the first metatarsal and adjacent medial cuneiform (compare with tibialis anterior, page 258). The tendon of tibialis posterior enters the medial aspect of the foot deep to the flexor retinaculum (Figs 6.48 & 6.56), attaches to the tuberosity of the navicular and sends additional slips to other tarsal bones and the metatarsal bases. These two tendons may help to support the medial longitudinal arch. The other actions of fibularis longus and tibialis posterior and their innervation are considered on pages 249 and 260.

Blood supply

Deep to the flexor retinaculum, the tibial artery divides into medial and lateral plantar branches (see Fig. 6.51). Passing forwards, the medial plantar artery runs deep to the superficial intrinsic muscles, gives off plantar cutaneous branches which pass between abductor hallucis and flexor digitorum brevis, and terminates by supplying digital branches to the medial (and occasionally lateral) side of the great toe. The larger lateral plantar artery passes forwards and laterally (Fig. 6.54) deep to the superficial intrinsic muscles towards the base of the fifth metatarsal. Here the artery inclines medially and deeply to form the plantar arch, lying on the interossei and bases of the metatarsals. A perforating branch between the first and second metatarsals usually links the arch with the dorsalis pedis artery (see page 260). From the arch, plantar metatarsal arteries (see Fig. 6.54) pass distally to the webs of the toes where they divide into digital branches. Venae comitantes accompany medial and lateral plantar arteries and their branches.

Nerve supply

Cutaneous branches of the tibial nerve supply the skin over the heel. Deep to the flexor retinaculum the tibial nerve divides into medial and lateral branches, which supply their respective sides of the sole (see Figs 6.48 & 6.51). The larger medial plantar nerve accompanies the corresponding artery and gives cutaneous branches to the medial three and one-half digits, including the nail beds. The nerve also supplies abductor hallucis, flexor hallucis brevis, flexor digitorum brevis and the first lumbrical.

The lateral plantar nerve accompanies the corresponding artery (see Fig. 6.51) supplying quadratus plantae and abductor digiti minimi and giving cutaneous branches to the sole. Near the base of the fifth metatarsal it divides into superficial and deep branches which supply the remaining muscles of the sole. The deep branch accompanies the plantar arch and terminates in adductor hallucis. In addition to muscular branches, the superficial branch also gives cutaneous branches to the lateral one and one-half toes.

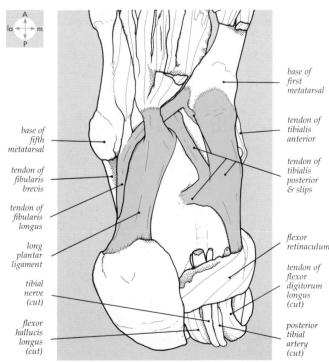

Fig. 6.56 Deep dissection of sole to show long plantar ligament and tendons of fibularis longus and tibialis posterior.

ANTERIOR AND LATERAL COMPARTMENTS OF LEG AND DORSUM OF FOOT

Anterior compartment of leg and dorsum of foot

The anterior compartment of the leg contains muscles that extend the ankle joint and toes and evert and invert the foot. Its neurovascular bundle comprises the anterior tibial artery and its venae comitantes and the deep fibular nerve (Fig. 6.57). The cutaneous branches of the superficial fibular nerve are also present.

On the dorsum of the foot are the long extensor tendons, the dorsalis pedis artery, the dorsal venous arch and, more laterally, the bellies of extensor digitorum brevis and extensor hallucis brevis. The medial and lateral malleoli lie on each side of the ankle.

Superficial structures

The dorsal venous arch (Fig. 6.58) drains blood from the toes and sole of the foot. From its medial end the great saphenous vein passes in front of the medial malleolus where it is palpable and accessible, and then ascends to the posteromedial aspect of the knee. From the lateral side of the arch the small saphenous vein passes behind the lateral malleolus and ascends to the popliteal fossa (see page 245). The saphenous nerve accompanies the great saphenous vein (Fig. 6.59), supplying skin on the medial side of the leg and medial border of the foot as far as the ball (metatarsophalangeal joint) of the great toe. The sural nerve accompanies the small saphenous vein (Fig. 6.58) and supplies skin along the lateral border of the foot and little toe.

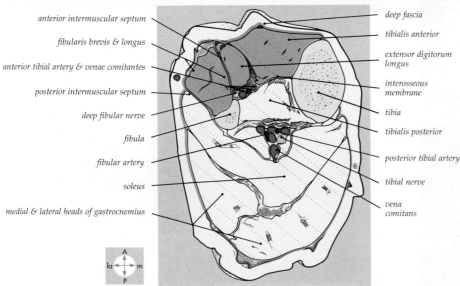

anterior intermuscular septum
fibularis brevis & longus
anterior tibial artery & venae comitantes
posterior intermuscular septum
deep fibular nerve
fibula
fibular artery
soleus
medial & lateral heads of gastrocnemius

deep fascia
tibialis anterior
extensor digitorum longus
interosseous membrane
tibia
tibialis posterior
posterior tibial artery
tibial nerve
vena comitans

Fig. 6.57   Transverse section through the leg showing anterior and lateral compartments and their contents. Inferior aspect.

The superficial fibular (superficial peroneal) nerve enters the anterior compartment of the leg from the lateral (fibular or peroneal) compartment at the anterior border of fibularis longus (see Fig. 6.60). Shortly after piercing the deep fascia it divides into medial and lateral branches which supply the skin of the leg and dorsum of the foot (Fig. 6.58). On reaching the toes the medial branch supplies the medial side of the great toe and the contiguous aspects of the second and third toes while the lateral branch innervates the adjacent sides of the third, fourth, and fifth toes. Thus, all of the digital skin is innervated by the superficial fibular nerve except for the cleft between the great and second toes (supplied by the deep fibular (peroneal) nerve) and the lateral aspect of the little toe (supplied by the sural nerve).

The skin and subcutaneous tissues over the anteromedial surface of the tibia are comparatively thin and have a sparse blood supply. As a consequence, lacerations in this region may heal relatively slowly.

saphenous nerve

great saphenous vein

superficial fibular nerve

saphenous nerve

lateral malleolus

medial malleolus

origin of great saphenous vein

origin of small saphenous vein

sural nerve

perforating vein

dorsal venous arch

terminal branch of deep fibular nerve

digital veins

Fig. 6.58 Superficial nerves and veins on the dorsum of the ankle and foot.

superficial fibular nerve

medial malleolus

saphenous nerve

Fig. 6.59 Superficial veins and nerves on the medial surface of the leg and foot.

Deep fascia

In the region of the ankle and foot there are thickenings of the investing deep fascia forming retinacula (Fig. 6.60) which prevent bowstringing of the long extensor tendons during muscular contraction. As the tendons pass beneath the retinacula to reach the foot they are enveloped in synovial membrane. By convention, superior and inferior extensor retinacula are described (see Fig. 6.64). The superior retinaculum forms a broad band passing between the anterior borders of the tibia and fibula. The inferior retinaculum is Y-shaped, with its stem attached to the upper surface of the calcaneus.

Muscles

The muscles in the anterior compartment are tibialis anterior, extensor hallucis longus, extensor digitorum longus and fibularis (peroneus) tertius. All are supplied by the deep fibular nerve. Tibialis anterior is the most medial (Figs 6.57 & 6.60), attaching to the lateral condyle and anterolateral surface of the shaft of the tibia, the adjacent interosseous membrane and the deep fascia overlying the muscle. Distally its tendon crosses the anterior border of the lower end of the tibia and attaches to the base of the first metatarsal and adjacent part of the first cuneiform bone (Fig. 6.61). The muscle inverts the foot and dorsiflexes the ankle joint.

The other three muscles all attach to the narrow anterior surface of the fibula and adjacent interosseous membrane. Extensor digitorum longus (see Fig. 6.57) is attached to the proximal three-quarters of the bone, fibularis tertius (when present) to the distal quarter, and extensor hallucis longus overlaps them medially at midshaft level. In addition, extensor digitorum longus attaches to the anterior intermuscular septum and overlying deep fascia.

The proximal part of extensor hallucis longus is overlapped by adjacent muscles, but in the lower part of the leg its tendon emerges lateral to that of tibialis anterior. As it descends towards the ankle the tendon crosses from the lateral to the medial side of the neurovascular bundle. In the foot the tendon of extensor hallucis longus runs forwards to the great toe (Fig. 6.62), where it attaches to the base of the distal phalanx. It is a powerful extensor of the toe, dorsiflexor (extensor) of the foot and assists inversion. Lateral to extensor hallucis longus, the muscle belly of extensor digitorum longus gives way distally to four tendons which pass to the dorsal aspects of the lateral four toes. Each tendon forms an extensor expansion that divides into three slips. The central slip attaches to the base of the middle phalanx whilst the two lateral slips combine to insert into the base of the distal phalanx (Fig. 6.62). Extensor digitorum longus extends the lateral four toes and dorsiflexes the foot. Fibularis tertius is a continuation of the belly of extensor digitorum longus. It attaches to the lateral border of the fifth metatarsal

(Fig. 6.62) and everts the foot and dorsiflexes the ankle.

The muscles of the anterior compartment of the leg are active during walking in both the supporting and swing phases. In the weight-bearing limb they help to incline the leg forwards while the foot remains stationary on the ground. In the swinging

fibularis longus

tibialis anterior

sub-cutaneous surface of tibia

extensor digitorum longus

fibularis brevis

superficial fibular nerve (cut)

fibularis tertius

extensor retinaculum

tendons of extensor digitorum longus

tendons of extensor hallucis longus

tendon of tibialis anterior

extensor digitorum brevis

tendon of fibularis tertius

sural nerve

tendons of extensor digitorum brevis

Fig. 6.60 Muscles of the anterior compartment of the leg and tendons on the dorsum of the foot, seen after removal of deep fascia. The extensor retinaculum has been retained.

limb the muscles maintain the ankle in dorsiflexion, thereby preventing the foot from dropping.

On the dorsum of the foot extensor digitorum brevis and extensor hallucis brevis (Fig. 6.62) are attached to the upper surface of the calcaneus and overlying stem of the inferior extensor retinaculum.

Extensor digitorum brevis gives rise to three short tendons, which pass deep to the long extensor tendons of the lateral three toes (Fig. 6.62) and attach to the dorsal extensor expansions of the second, third and fourth toes. The tendon of extensor hallucis brevis attaches to the base of the proximal phalanx of the great toe. The

muscles assist extension of the toes, particularly when the long extensors are flexing the leg forwards on the foot just before it is lifted from the ground during walking. The nerve supply is the deep fibular nerve.

Fig. 6.61 Anterior view of bones of leg and foot showing attachments of muscles of anterior compartment.

tibialis anterior

extensor digitorum longus

extensor hallucis longus

fibularis tertius

quadriceps femoris

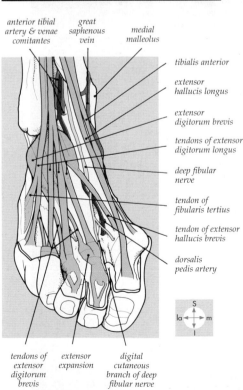

Fig. 6.62 Principal structures on the dorsum of the ankle and foot seen after removal of the extensor retinaculum.

Neurovascular bundle

This comprises the deep fibular nerve and the anterior tibial artery with its venae comitantes (see Fig. 6.57). The artery, a terminal branch of the popliteal artery

(see page 248), reaches the anterior compartment after passing through the interosseous membrane. It then descends on the anterior surface of the membrane (Fig. 6.63) and at the ankle lies midway between the two malleoli. It continues distally as the dorsalis pedis artery on the lateral side of the extensor hallucis longus tendon (see Fig. 6.62), where its pulsations are palpable in the living foot.

At the proximal end of the first intermetatarsal space the dorsalis pedis artery gives a deep branch which passes between the two heads of the first dorsal

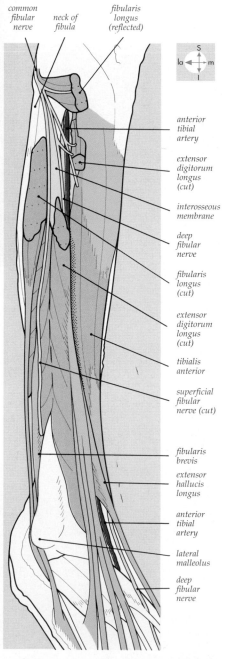

Fig. 6.63 The common fibular nerve and its branches and the anterior tibial artery, seen after deep dissection of both compartments.

interosseous muscle to join the plantar arch (see page 255). This arrangement provides an anastomosis between the anterior and posterior tibial arteries. The dorsalis pedis artery terminates as the first dorsal metatarsal artery, supplying the great toe and adjacent border of the second toe, and the arcuate artery. It turns laterally beneath the extensor tendons across the bases of the metatarsals and gives metatarsal arteries, which divide to supply adjacent borders of the remaining three digits.

The deep fibular (peroneal) nerve, a terminal branch of the common fibular nerve, winds around the neck of the fibula deep to fibularis (peroneus) longus (Fig. 6.63). The nerve accompanies the anterior tibial vessels into the foot and supplies all muscles in the anterior compartment. In the foot the nerve is close to the dorsalis pedis artery, usually lying lateral to the artery but sometimes medial to it (see Fig. 6.62). It gives a branch to extensors digitorum and hallucis brevis and the tarsal joints, and terminates by supplying the skin between the great and second toes (see Fig. 6.62).

Lateral compartment of leg

The lateral (fibular or peroneal) compartment of the leg extends from the head of the fibula above to the lateral malleolus below. Its principal contents are the fibularis longus and brevis muscles (Fig. 6.64). Fibularis (peroneus) longus is attached to the upper two-thirds of the lateral surface of the fibula and fibularis (peroneus) brevis to the lower two-thirds, with brevis being the more anterior. Both muscles are attached to the two crural intermuscular septa and the overlying deep fascia. On reaching the ankle the tendons pass behind and then below the lateral malleolus, restrained by the superior and inferior fibular retinacula and surrounded by synovial membrane (Fig. 6.64). The tendon of fibularis brevis passes forwards above the fibular trochlea of the calcaneus to attach to the base of the fifth metatarsal. The fibularis longus tendon passes forwards below the fibular trochlea and turns medially into the sole of the foot where it lies in a groove on the cuboid bone (Fig. 6.65). It attaches to the lateral side of the base of the first metatarsal and the adjacent first cuneiform.

Fibularis longus and brevis are evertors of the foot and weak plantar flexors of the ankle joint. Their nerve supply is the superficial fibular nerve, a terminal branch of the common fibular nerve, which enters the lateral compartment by winding around the neck of the fibula where it is palpable and may sometimes be compressed.

Branches of the fibular artery, which arises from the posterior tibial artery (see page 249) pierce the posterior intermuscular septum to supply fibularis longus and brevis.

gastrocnemius

fibularis longus

soleus

fibularis brevis

tendo calcaneus

superior & inferior
extensor retinacula

extensor digitorum brevis

tendon of fibularis longus

tendon of fibularis
brevis

Fig. 6.64 Lateral aspect of the leg and foot showing
fibularis longus and brevis.

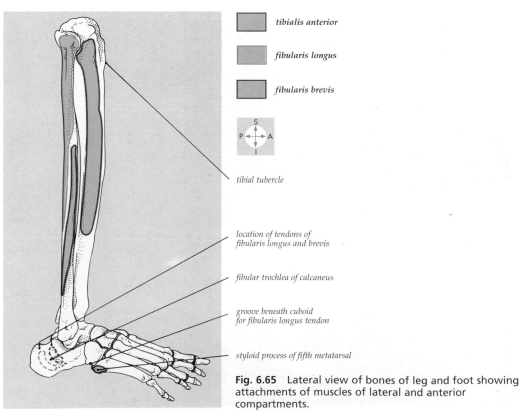

tibialis anterior

fibularis longus

fibularis brevis

tibial tubercle

location of tendons of
fibularis longus and brevis

fibular trochlea of calcaneus

groove beneath cuboid
for fibularis longus tendon

styloid process of fifth metatarsal

Fig. 6.65 Lateral view of bones of leg and foot showing
attachments of muscles of lateral and anterior
compartments.

HIP JOINT

The hip joint is a synovial ball-and-socket joint between the head of the femur and the acetabulum of the hip bone (Fig. 6.66).

Articular surfaces

The femoral head, covered by hyaline cartilage, forms two-thirds of a sphere and has a central pit (fovea; Fig. 6.66) giving attachment to the round ligament (ligamentum teres). The head surmounts the femoral neck, whose base abuts the medial side of the greater trochanter. The acetabulum is a deep socket with a C-shaped articular area covered with hyaline cartilage and a fat-filled non-articular area (acetabular fossa), whose margins give attachment to the base of the ligamentum teres (Fig. 6.67). The acetabulum is deficient inferiorly at the acetabular notch (Fig. 6.66), where blood vessels, bridged by the transverse acetabular ligament, enter the joint. A fibrocartilaginous labrum, attached to the margins of the acetabulum and the transverse ligament, helps to deepen the socket.

Capsule

Medially the fibrous capsule is attached to the outer margin of the labrum; laterally the capsule attaches to the intertrochanteric line (Figs 6.66 & 6.68) at the root of the femoral

Fig. 6.66   Articular surfaces of the hip joint comprise the acetabulum of the hip bone and the head of the femur.

Fig. 6.67   Internal features, revealed by disarticulation of the joint after cutting the ligaments and joint capsule.

neck and to the femoral shaft just above the lesser trochanter. From the femoral attachment of the capsule, retinacular fibres derived from the deep part of the capsule (Fig. 6.67) are reflected medially over the neck to the margins of the head. Posteriorly the line of attachment of the capsule is such that only the upper (medial) half of the femoral neck lies within the joint.

Ligaments

The iliofemoral, pubofemoral and ischiofemoral ligaments are capsular thickenings that spiral downwards and laterally from the hip bone to the femur. The strong iliofemoral ligament (Fig. 6.68) is an inverted Y shape, the stem attaching to the anterior inferior iliac spine and the limbs to the upper and lower ends of the intertrochanteric line.

The pubofemoral ligament (Fig. 6.68) passes from the iliopubic eminence to the femoral neck just above the lesser trochanter. The ischiofemoral ligament lies posteriorly (see Fig. 6.70) and reaches the root of the greater trochanter.

Within the joint is the ligamentum teres (Figs 6.67 & 6.69), which has the form of a flattened cone, the base attaching to the margins of the acetabular fossa and transverse acetabular ligament and the apex to the fovea on the femoral head.

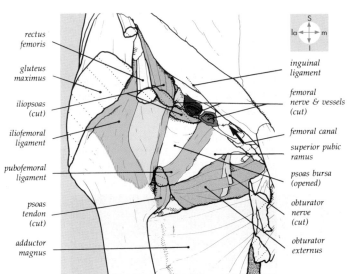

Fig. 6.68 Anterior surface of the joint capsule, its associated ligaments and immediate relations.

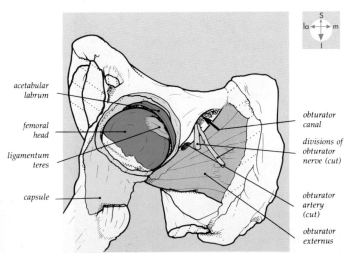

Fig. 6.69 Joint capsule opened anteriorly to show the interior of the joint. The femur has been abducted and externally rotated.

Synovial membrane and bursae

Synovial membrane lines the interior of the capsule and the non-articular surfaces of the joint, clothes the ligamentum teres and is reflected over the retinacular fibres and the femoral neck as far as the head. The iliopsoas tendon and anterior aspect of the capsule are separated by a large bursa (see Fig. 6.68), which often is in communication with the joint cavity.

The tendon of obturator externus is separated from the capsule by a smaller bursa, which may also communicate with the joint.

Movements

The hip joint is multiaxial and permits flexion, extension, abduction, adduction, medial and lateral rotation, and circumduction.

Flexion is produced by iliopsoas, assisted by sartorius, rectus femoris and pectineus. Gluteus maximus and the hamstrings are extensors. Abductors of the hip include gluteus medius and minimus while adduction is produced by adductors longus, brevis and magnus, pectineus and gracilis. Medial rotation is produced by iliopsoas, tensor fasciae latae and the anterior fibres of gluteus minimus and medius. Lateral rotation is produced by piriformis, quadratus femoris, obturator externus and internus and the gemelli.

Stability

The hip joint is very stable, largely because of its bony morphology and the deep fit of the femoral head into the acetabulum. Other important factors include the ligaments and the tone of the muscles crossing the joint. The ilio-, pubo- and ischiofemoral ligaments all limit extension and medial rotation. The iliofemoral ligament, in particular, prevents hyperextension, especially in the upright posture when body weight acts behind the transverse axis of the hip joint and tilts the pelvis backwards. The ligamentum teres limits adduction of the hip.

Relations

The joint is deeply placed behind the midpoint of the inguinal ligament. Laterally the greater trochanter covers the neck of the femur and is palpable on the lateral side of the thigh. Medially only the thin bone of the acetabular fossa (Figs 6.71 & 6.72) separates the head of the femur from structures within the pelvis that are vulnerable following acetabular fracture accompanied by medial displacement of the femoral head. Posteriorly lie structures of the gluteal region (Fig. 6.70), including the sciatic nerve, which may be damaged in posterior dislocation. Anteriorly the joint is covered by the iliopsoas and the femoral vessels and nerve. Obturator externus and the adductor muscles lie inferiorly (Fig. 6.72) whilst superiorly are gluteus medius and minimus.

Blood supply

The arterial supply of the hip joint, especially that of the head and neck of the femur, is of particular clinical importance. The joint receives branches from the obturator artery, superior and inferior gluteal arteries, and medial and lateral circumflex femoral arteries, either directly or from the trochanteric anastomosis they form. From this anastomosis (Fig. 6.70), nutrient arteries travel in the retinacular fibres to enter foramina on the upper part of the femoral neck and terminate in the head. As only the upper half of the neck is covered posteriorly by the joint capsule, fractures at this site may be classified as either intra- or extracapsular. Intracapsular fractures that tear the retinacular fibres may deprive the head of the femur of much of its blood supply. Additional blood supply comes from a branch of the obturator artery conveyed in the ligamentum teres to the femoral head, and from one of the perforating branches of the profunda femoris artery via a nutrient artery that enters the shaft to supply the femoral neck and head.

Nerve supply

Nerves to the joint include the nerve to rectus femoris from the femoral nerve, branches from the anterior division of the obturator nerve, and the nerve to quadratus femoris from the sacral plexus.

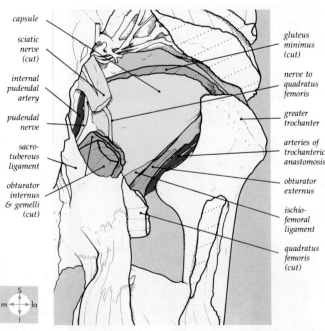

Fig. 6.70 Posterior surface of the joint capsule, the ischiofemoral ligament and close relations.

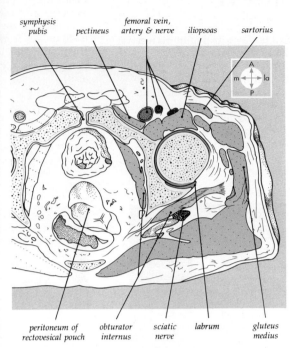

symphysis pubis

pectineus

femoral vein, artery & nerve

iliopsoas

sartorius

peritoneum of rectovesical pouch

obturator internus

sciatic nerve

labrum

gluteus medius

Fig. 6.71 Transverse section through the hip joint showing its relations. Superior aspect. Compare Fig. 5.42.

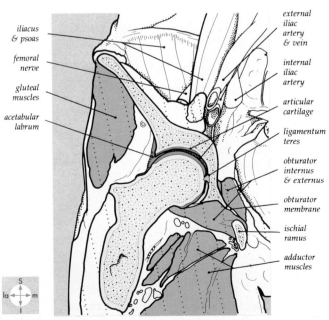

iliacus & psoas

femoral nerve

gluteal muscles

acetabular labrum

external iliac artery & vein

internal iliac artery

articular cartilage

ligamentum teres

obturator internus & externus

obturator membrane

ischial ramus

adductor muscles

Fig. 6.72 Coronal section through the hip joint showing its relations.

KNEE JOINT

The knee joint is a synovial joint between the distal end of the femur, proximal end of the tibia and posterior aspect of the patella (Fig. 6.73). It is a hinge joint with a wide range of flexion and extension and limited lateral and medial rotation. The joint is relatively superficial anteriorly and laterally where some of its bony features are palpable but posteriorly is inaccessible, being deeply placed in the floor of the popliteal fossa (Fig. 6.74).

Anteriorly the ligamentum patellae (Fig. 6.75) passes from the apex of the patella to the tibial tubercle. It is easily palpable and is used clinically for the stretch reflex (knee jerk).

Articular surfaces

The medial and lateral condyles of the femur have articular surfaces, covered by hyaline cartilage, which extend over their inferior and posterior aspects and articulate with the respective condyles on the tibia (Fig. 6.73). On the front of the femur lies the patellar articular surface while posteriorly a deep intercondylar fossa separates the two condyles. The articular areas on the tibial condyles are separated by the intercondylar eminence, the lateral articular area being flatter and smaller than the medial area (Fig. 6.73).

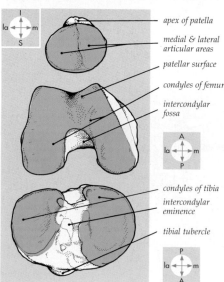

- apex of patella
- medial & lateral articular areas
- patellar surface
- condyles of femur
- intercondylar fossa
- condyles of tibia
- intercondylar eminence
- tibial tubercle

Fig. 6.73 Articular surfaces of the patella, femur and tibia.

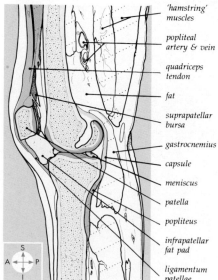

- 'hamstring' muscles
- popliteal artery & vein
- quadriceps tendon
- fat
- suprapatellar bursa
- gastrocnemius
- capsule
- meniscus
- patella
- popliteus
- infrapatellar fat pad
- ligamentum patellae

Fig. 6.74 Sagittal section through the knee joint showing the articular surfaces and relations.

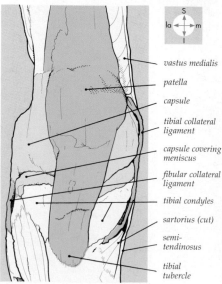

- vastus medialis
- patella
- capsule
- tibial collateral ligament
- capsule covering meniscus
- fibular collateral ligament
- tibial condyles
- sartorius (cut)
- semi-tendinosus
- tibial tubercle

Fig. 6.75 Superficial dissection from the anterior aspect to show patellar ligament, capsule, and collateral ligaments.

Capsule

The capsule is thin anteriorly and posteriorly but is reinforced on each side by strong collateral ligaments. On the sides of the femur the capsule attachment extends up to the epicondyles. Posteriorly it attaches along the superior margins of the condyles (Figs 6.76 & 6.78) and the intercondylar line whilst anteriorly it extends proximally (Fig. 6.75; see Figs 6.79 & 6.81) to accommodate the synovial membrane that forms the suprapatellar bursa (pouch).

On the sides of the tibia the capsule attaches close to the articular margins. Those parts of the capsule on each side of the joint that loosely anchor the outer borders of the menisci to the femur and tibia are called the coronary ligaments. Posteriorly the capsular attachment inclines downwards to include the posterior part of the intercondylar area whilst anteriorly the attachment deviates inferiorly as far as the tibial tubercle. On the patella the capsule is attached close to the articular margins.

Posteriorly part of the insertion of semimembranosus forms the oblique posterior ligament, which passes upwards and laterally (Figs 6.76 & 6.77), reinforcing the capsule. Where the posterior part of the capsule is pierced by popliteus, it thickens to form the arcuate ligament (Fig. 6.76).

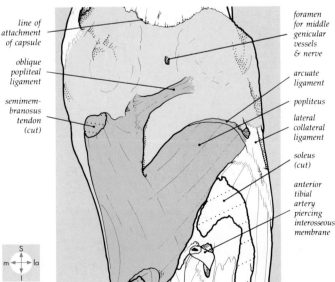

line of attachment of capsule

oblique popliteal ligament

semimem-branosus tendon (cut)

foramen for middle genicular vessels & nerve

arcuate ligament

popliteus

lateral collateral ligament

soleus (cut)

anterior tibial artery piercing interosseous membrane

Fig. 6.76 Posterior aspect of joint showing capsule, popliteus and semimembranosus insertion.

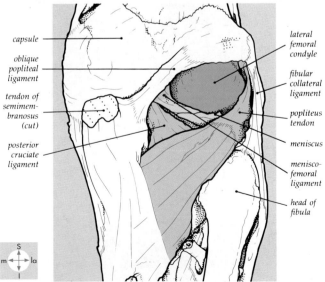

capsule

oblique popliteal ligament

tendon of semimem-branosus (cut)

posterior cruciate ligament

lateral femoral condyle

fibular collateral ligament

popliteus tendon

meniscus

menisco-femoral ligament

head of fibula

Fig. 6.77 Partial removal of capsule to reveal the meniscofemoral and posterior cruciate ligaments and the tendon of popliteus.

Collateral ligaments

On the medial side of the joint the thick tibial collateral ligament (Fig. 6.79) broadens as it descends from the medial femoral epicondyle to the upper part of the subcutaneous surface of the tibia. Its deep aspect is attached to the outer margin of the medial meniscus (Fig. 6.78), which diminishes mobility of the meniscus, making it more susceptible to tears. On the lateral side the cord-like fibular collateral

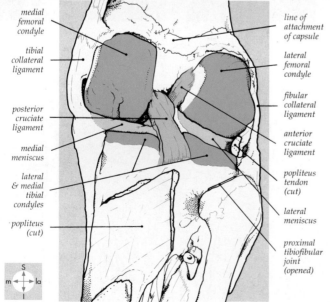

medial femoral condyle

tibial collateral ligament

posterior cruciate ligament

medial meniscus

lateral & medial tibial condyles

popliteus (cut)

line of attachment of capsule

lateral femoral condyle

fibular collateral ligament

anterior cruciate ligament

popliteus tendon (cut)

lateral meniscus

proximal tibiofibular joint (opened)

Fig. 6.78   The posterior part of the capsule has been removed to show the cruciate ligaments and menisci.

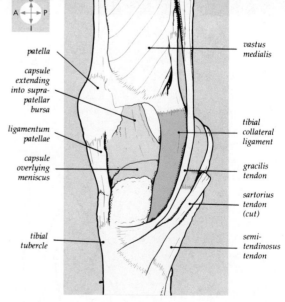

patella

capsule extending into supra-patellar bursa

ligamentum patellae

capsule overlying meniscus

tibial tubercle

vastus medialis

tibial collateral ligament

gracilis tendon

sartorius tendon (cut)

semi-tendinosus tendon

Fig. 6.79   Superficial dissection from the medial aspect showing the tibial collateral ligament, capsule and insertions of sartorius, gracilis and semitendinosus.

ligament (Fig. 6.80) descends from the lateral epicondyle of the femur to the styloid process and head of the fibula, separated from the lateral meniscus by the popliteus tendon (Fig. 6.78).

Intracapsular ligaments

The intracapsular ligaments comprise the anterior and posterior cruciate ligaments and the meniscofemoral ligament.

The cruciate ligaments (Fig. 6.78) are named according to their attachment to the intercondylar eminence of the tibia (see Fig. 6.82). The anterior ligament passes upwards, backwards and laterally to attach to the medial surface of the lateral condyle of the femur. The posterior ligament passes upwards, forwards and medially (Fig. 6.78) to attach to the lateral surface of the medial femoral condyle. The meniscofemoral ligament is adjacent to the posterior cruciate ligament (see Fig. 6.77) and attaches the posterior border of the lateral meniscus close to the femoral attachment of the posterior cruciate ligament. It stabilizes the meniscus during rotation of the femur on the tibia. Although within the capsule, the cruciate and meniscofemoral ligaments are covered by reflections of synovial membrane and are therefore not within the synovial cavity.

Menisci

The medial and lateral menisci are C-shaped (see Fig. 6.82) with their anterior and posterior horns attached to the intercondylar eminence of the tibia and their outer borders to the joint capsule (coronary ligaments). The menisci differ in size and shape, the medial being narrower though slightly larger so that its horns embrace those of the lateral meniscus. Also, the medial is attached to the medial collateral ligament and in cross-section is deeper than the lateral meniscus. A transverse ligament (see Fig. 6.82) connects the anterior horn of the medial meniscus with the anterior aspect of the lateral meniscus.

Infrapatellar fat pad

Deep to the ligamentum patellae is a quantity of fat (see Fig. 6.74), which bulges the synovial membrane into the interior of the joint. Folds of synovial membrane, the alar folds (Fig. 6.81), extend on either side from the main pad. Another fold, the ligamentum mucosum, lies in the midline between the anterior part of the intercondylar notch and the lower margin of the patella.

Synovial membrane and bursae

Synovial membrane lines the interior of the capsule but does not cover the menisci. On the femur it is attached to the margins of the intercondylar notch and covers the front

and sides of the cruciate ligaments. Synovial membrane also covers the infrapatellar fat pad and the tendon of popliteus.

The suprapatellar bursa (Fig. 6.81; see also Fig. 6.74) is a large pouch of synovial membrane, passing a hand's breadth proximal to the upper border of the patella, deep to quadriceps. Part of vastus intermedius attaches to it. Since the bursa is continuous with the synovial cavity of the joint, it provides a route for injecting fluid into or withdrawing fluid from the joint. After injuries to the joint, fluid accumulates

(effusion) in the suprapatellar bursa, causing typical fullness around the knee. Several other bursae lie near the knee joint and may enlarge, causing swellings. Bursae between the capsule and the two heads of gastrocnemius often communicate with the knee joint while that beneath the medial head may also communicate with the overlying semimembranosus bursa. Other bursae, which do not communicate with the joint, are the pre- and infrapatellar bursae beneath the skin covering the patella and ligamentum patellae respectively.

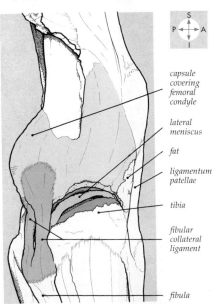

Fig. 6.80 Lateral aspect of joint showing the collateral ligament and the meniscus, revealed by removing part of the capsule.

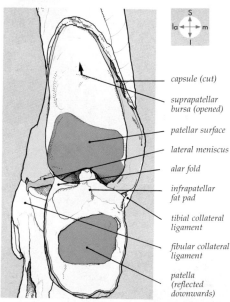

Fig. 6.81 Interior of joint, revealed by opening the capsule anteriorly and reflecting the patella downwards.

Popliteus

From its tibial attachment the popliteus passes upwards and laterally (see Fig. 6.76), penetrating the posterior aspect of the capsule of the knee joint deep to the arcuate ligament. Within the joint its tendon, covered by synovial membrane, attaches to the posterior border of the lateral meniscus and to the femur (see Fig. 6.77) immediately below the lateral epicondyle. Popliteus is supplied by the tibial nerve and its actions are considered below.

Movements

The principal movements of the knee joint are flexion and extension. Flexion is produced mainly by the hamstrings (semimembranosus, semitendinosus and biceps) assisted by the two heads of gastrocnemius. Extension is produced by quadriceps femoris acting through the ligamentum patellae. Gluteus maximus, acting through the iliotibial tract, maintains stability of the knee in the extended position.

Because of the shape of the articular surfaces, the femur rotates medially during the later stages of extension. The lateral condyle and meniscus (moving in unison because of the meniscofemoral ligament) glide forwards on the lateral tibial condyle whilst the medial condyle completes its movement of extension on the medial meniscus. Full extension is achieved with completion of medial rotation and further movement is prevented by tension in the collateral and oblique posterior ligaments. During the early stages of flexion, lateral rotation of the femur on the tibia is produced by popliteus, which also pulls the lateral meniscus posteriorly. During flexion and extension the patella glides over the patellar surface of the femur.

Slight active rotation of the tibia on the femur can occur when the knee is in a flexed but non-weight-bearing position. Sartorius, gracilis and semitendinosus rotate medially while biceps femoris rotates laterally.

Stability

The knee joint is very stable. The most important factors are muscle tone, especially in quadriceps, and the ligaments. The cruciate ligaments stabilize the femur on the tibia, preventing excessive anteroposterior movement. The collateral ligaments assist medial and lateral stability while the iliotibial tract stabilizes the knee during extension. All of these ligaments, together with the oblique posterior ligament, prevent hyperextension.

Owing to angulation of the femur relative to the tibia, contraction of quadriceps femoris tends to displace the patella laterally. This displacement is prevented by firstly the lowest fibres of vastus medialis, which insert into the medial patellar border and whose active contraction resists lateral movement of the patella, and secondly by the large size and prominence of the lateral femoral condyle making lateral patellar movement mechanically difficult.

Innervation

Branches from the femoral, obturator and sciatic nerves supply the joint, sensory fibres from the femoral nerve travelling with the branches to the vasti and sartorius. Genicular branches from the tibial and common fibular divisions of the sciatic nerve, together with fibres from the posterior division of the obturator nerve, also supply the joint.

Blood supply

The knee joint receives its blood supply from the extensive genicular anastomosis derived mainly from branches of the popliteal, anterior and posterior tibial arteries.

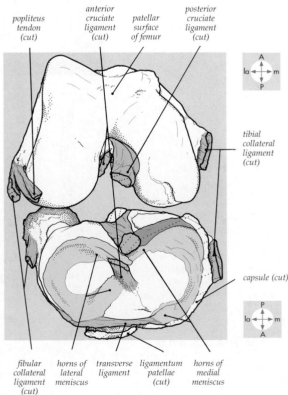

Fig. 6.82 Disarticulation of joint reveals menisci and attachments of cruciate ligaments.

TIBIOFIBULAR JOINTS

The tibia and fibula articulate at proximal and distal tibiofibular joints and are also connected by an interosseous membrane (Fig. 6.83), which unites the interosseous borders of the bones and separates the flexor and extensor compartments of the leg.

The proximal tibiofibular joint is a plane synovial articulation between the lateral condyle of the tibia and head of the fibula, and is supplied by the common fibular nerve. The capsule is reinforced by anterior and posterior ligaments, and the synovial cavity does not communicate with the knee joint.

The opposed triangular surfaces at the lower ends of the tibia and fibula are bound together by an interosseous ligament, forming the fibrous distal tibiofibular joint, which is strengthened by anterior and posterior tibiofibular ligaments. The transverse ligament, an inferior extension of the posterior ligament, contributes to the articular socket of the ankle joint (see Fig. 6.85), whose cavity frequently extends for a short distance between the tibia and fibula. The ankle is stabilized by the ligaments of the distal tibiofibular joint, which prevent separation of the malleoli. Innervation is by the deep fibular and tibial nerves.

Very little movement occurs at the tibiofibular joints, but slight rotation of the fibula may accompany flexion and extension of the ankle.

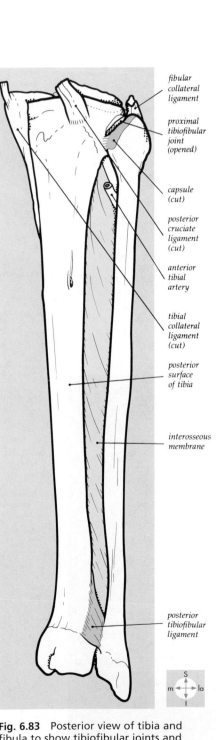

*fibular
collateral
ligament*

*proximal
tibiofibular
joint
(opened)*

*capsule
(cut)*

*posterior
cruciate
ligament
(cut)*

*anterior
tibial
artery*

*tibial
collateral
ligament
(cut)*

*posterior
surface
of tibia*

*interosseous
membrane*

*posterior
tibiofibular
ligament*

Fig. 6.83 Posterior view of tibia and fibula to show tibiofibular joints and interosseous membrane. The lower part of the tibiofibular ligament has been removed.

Fig. 6.84   Bones of the ankle joint showing their articular surfaces.

Labels (top to bottom): fibula; inferior surface of tibia; lateral and medial malleolus; superior surface of trochlea; body of talus; lateral and medial surfaces; neck; head

ANKLE JOINT

The ankle joint is a synovial **hinge** joint between the lower ends of the tibia and fibula and the upper part of the talus (Fig. 6.84), and all the articular surfaces are covered by hyaline cartilage. The proximal articular surface comprises the distal end of the tibia and the medial and lateral malleoli, which together form a deep socket (Fig. 6.85), completed posteriorly by the transverse tibiofibular ligament (see below). The socket is wider anteriorly than posteriorly and is completely congruous with the upper part of the talus, which is reciprocally wedge shaped (Fig. 6.86). The articular surface on the lateral side of the talus is more extensive than that on the medial side.

Capsule and synovial membrane

The fibrous capsule attaches to the margins of the articular surfaces, but anteriorly extends forwards onto the neck of the talus (Fig. 6.86). The capsule is thin anteriorly and posteriorly, but is reinforced on each side by ligaments. Synovial membrane lines the capsule internally and covers the intracapsular part of the neck of the talus.

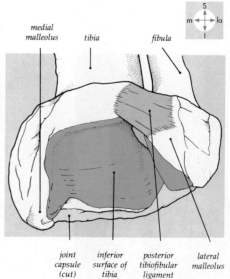

Labels: medial malleolus; tibia; fibula; joint capsule (cut); inferior surface of tibia; posterior tibiofibular ligament; lateral malleolus

Fig. 6.85   Oblique inferior view of the wedge-shaped articular socket of the ankle joint.

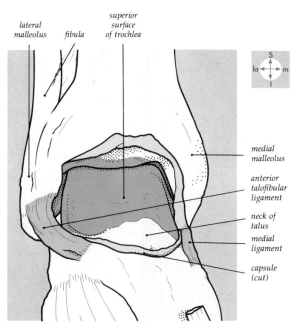

Fig. 6.86 Anterior view of the ankle joint showing articular surfaces, revealed by removal of the capsule.

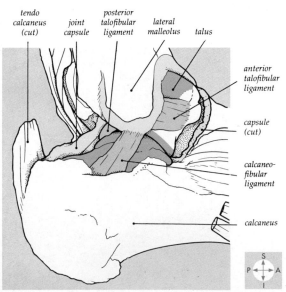

Fig. 6.87 Lateral aspect of joint to show lateral collateral ligament.

Ligaments

The transverse tibiofibular ligament spans the gap between the distal ends of the tibia and fibula, contributing to the articular socket posteriorly (see Fig. 6.85). There are two collateral ligaments. The medial (deltoid) ligament (Fig. 6.89) is attached by its apex to the tip of the medial malleolus. Its deeper fibres descend to the margin of the articular surface on the medial side of the talus and its longer superficial fibres attach to the tuberosity of the navicular, the medial border of the spring (plantar calcaneonavicular) ligament and the sustentaculum tali.

The lateral ligament has three components: the anterior and posterior talofibular and the calcaneofibular ligaments (Figs 6.87 & 6.88). All attach to the lateral malleolus. The anterior talofibular ligament passes forwards to the lateral side of the neck of the talus, the posterior talofibular ligament medially to the posterior tubercle of the talus, and the calcaneofibular downwards and backwards to the side of the calcaneus.

Movements

Only extension (dorsiflexion) and flexion (plantar flexion) occur at the ankle joint, around a transverse axis between the malleoli. Plantar flexion is produced by soleus and gastrocnemius, assisted by tibialis posterior, flexors hallucis longus and digitorum longus, and fibularis longus and brevis. Extension (dorsiflexion) is produced by tibialis anterior, extensors hallucis longus and digitorum longus, and fibularis tertius.

Stability

The joint is very stable due to the wedge shape of the articulating surfaces and the strong collateral ligaments. During standing and walking, body weight tends to displace the tibiofibular socket forwards so that it becomes closely packed against the wider

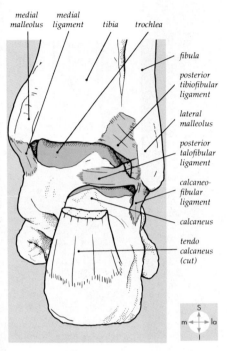

Fig. 6.88 Posterior view of the ankle joint showing the articular surface of talus after removal of the capsule.

Fig. 6.89 Medial collateral ligament of the ankle joint.

anterior part of the talus, which further enhances stability during dorsiflexion. Excessive forward displacement of the tibia and fibula on the talus is prevented by the posterior fibres of the medial (deltoid) ligament and by the calcaneofibular and posterior talofibular ligaments. However, in plantar flexion the narrow part of the talus articulates with the wider anterior part of the socket, allowing some side-to-side movement. In this position, forced inversion of the foot may damage the anterior talofibular ligament, one form of 'sprained ankle'.

Blood and nerve supply

Branches of the anterior and posterior tibial arteries, including the fibular, anastomose at the level of the malleoli and supply the joint. Innervation is from the deep fibular and tibial nerves.

Relations

The sides of the joint, the bony malleoli, are superficial (Fig. 6.90) and easily palpable. Passing subcutaneously in front of the joint are branches of the superficial fibular nerve and, just anterior to the medial malleolus, the saphenous nerve and great saphenous vein. On a deeper plane are the tendons of tibialis anterior and extensor hallucis longus, the dorsalis pedis artery, the deep fibular nerve, and the tendons of extensor digitorum longus and fibularis tertius (Fig. 6.91).

Posteriorly the tendo calcaneus (Achilles) lies separated from the joint capsule by a bursa and pad of fat. Behind the medial malleolus are the tendons of tibialis posterior, flexor digitorum longus and flexor hallucis longus (Fig. 6.90), accompanied by the tibial nerve and posterior tibial artery (Fig. 6.91). Passing below the medial malleolus, they enter the foot beneath the flexor retinaculum. Passing superficially behind the lateral malleolus are the small saphenous vein and sural nerve and, more deeply, the tendons of fibularis longus and brevis.

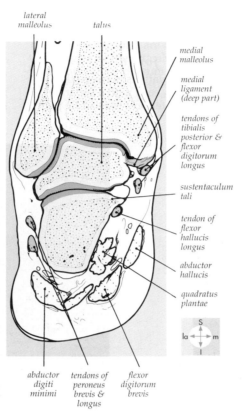

Fig. 6.90 Coronal section through ankle and talocalcaneal joints showing their relations.

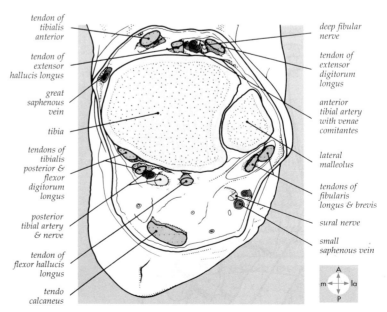

Fig. 6.91 Transverse section immediately above the ankle joint cavity showing relations.

Roof

The roof of the anterior triangle (Fig. 7.10) is formed by the investing fascia of the neck in a manner similar to that of the posterior triangle. Superficial to the fascia are platysma (see page 297) and the anterior jugular vein. This vessel pierces the roof and passes deep to sternocleidomastoid to drain into the external jugular vein just before its termination in the subclavian vein. The cutaneous innervation of the skin over the triangle has already been described (see page 288).

Floor

The floor of the anterior triangle is composed of the pretracheal fascia and posterolaterally the carotid sheath. The thyroid gland (Fig. 7.13) is enclosed by the pretracheal fascia whilst the larynx and trachea lie deep to it. Laterally the carotid arteries, internal jugular vein and vagus (X) nerve all lie within the carotid sheath.

Contents

The contents of the anterior triangle (Fig. 7.11) comprise infrahyoid or strap muscles (sternohyoid, sternothyroid, thyrohyoid and omohyoid) and their immediate nerve supply. The sternohyoid is the most superficial strap muscle and is attached inferiorly to the deep surface of the manubrium. Superiorly it is attached to the lower border of the body of the hyoid bone. Deep to sternohyoid are both sternothyroid and thyrohyoid. Sternothyroid extends from the manubrium to the oblique line on the lamina of the thyroid cartilage. In the same plane thyrohyoid runs from the thyroid cartilage to the inferior edge of the body of the hyoid bone. Omohyoid consists of two bellies linked by an intermediate tendon. The inferior belly is attached to the suprascapular ligament and the adjacent part of the scapula. It is this belly which crosses the posterior triangle and ends deep to sternocleidomastoid in the intermediate tendon. The tendon is anchored to the clavicle by a loop of investing fascia. The superior belly continues almost vertically to its attachment on the lower border of the hyoid bone lateral to the other muscles.

All four muscles are supplied segmentally by branches from the first three cervical spinal nerves. Thyrohyoid is supplied by fibres from C1 that have travelled with the hypoglossal (XII) nerve; the remaining muscles are supplied via the ansa cervicalis. Functionally the infrahyoid muscles serve to depress the hyoid bone and the larynx.

Fig. 7.10 Boundaries and roofs of both anterior triangles of the neck. The midline is the division between the two triangles.

Fig. 7.11 Contents of the anterior triangle. The right omohyoid and sternohyoid muscles have been removed to show the deeper thyrohyoid and sternothyroid muscles.

Ansa cervicalis

Under cover of sternocleidomastoid two nerves, called the roots of the ansa, unite to form a loop, the ansa cervicalis (Fig. 7.12), which provides the motor supply to the strap muscles. The superior root (descending limb) from the hypoglossal nerve consists solely of C1 fibres and descends to joint the inferior root, C2 and C3 fibres from the cervical plexus, to form the ansa.

Thyroid gland

The thyroid gland (Fig. 7.13) is a vascular endocrine gland enclosed by the pretracheal fascia and closely applied to the anterior and lateral surfaces of the trachea. The fascia links the gland to the larynx so that during swallowing both structures are elevated simultaneously. The two lateral lobes of the gland are joined across the midline by a narrow isthmus at the level of the third tracheal ring. A single pyramidal lobe is often present and projects upwards from the isthmus. Each lateral lobe is pear-shaped with its superior extremity reaching the oblique line on the thyroid cartilage whilst its lower pole lies at the level of the fifth tracheal ring.

Lying anterior to the isthmus of the gland are the sternothyroid muscles and the anterior jugular veins. The lateral lobes are covered anterolaterally by the other infrahyoid muscles and the anterior borders of the sternocleidomastoid muscles. Posterolaterally lie the carotid sheaths whilst posteromedially are the trachea, larynx and oesophagus. In the interval between the oesophagus and trachea the recurrent laryngeal nerves course upwards towards the larynx. A superior and an inferior parathyroid gland are embedded in the posterior surface of each lateral lobe.

The thyroid gland is a highly vascular organ and is supplied on each side by a superior and an inferior thyroid artery. The superior thyroid artery, a branch of the external carotid artery, descends to the upper pole of the gland. The inferior thyroid artery, from the thyrocervical trunk of the subclavian artery, ascends to enter the posterolateral aspect of the gland from behind the carotid sheath. A venous plexus on the surface of the gland drains via superior and middle thyroid veins into the internal jugular veins and via inferior thyroid veins that descend to the left brachiocephalic vein. Lymph drains from the gland into the jugular chain of nodes.

Root of neck

The root of the neck is the region immediately above the superior thoracic aperture (see page 284). In the midline are

Fig. 7.12 Ansa cervicalis, lying on the internal jugular vein, and its branches to the strap muscles.

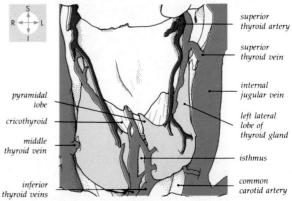

Fig. 7.13 Thyroid gland and its immediate blood supply, revealed by removal of the pretracheal fascia.

the trachea and oesophagus, descending into the superior mediastinum (Fig. 7.14) between the apices of the lungs covered with pleura and suprapleural membrane (Fig. 7.15). The other major structures in the root of the neck are vessels and nerves, which will be described in relation to scalenus anterior and its attachment to the scalene tubercle of the first rib (see page 29).

Veins

Each subclavian vein (Fig. 7.14) begins at the outer border of the first rib as the continuation of the axillary vein (see page 78). The vessel passes over the rib in front of the attachment of scalenus anterior and receives the external jugular vein from above. The subclavian and internal jugular veins unite at the medial border of scalenus anterior to form the brachiocephalic vein, which enters the thorax anteriorly alongside the trachea. On each side of the neck a major lymphatic trunk terminates by drainage into the angle where the subclavian and internal jugular veins unite. On the left, this lymphatic vessel is the thoracic duct, which arches laterally over the apex of the lung from its position alongside the oesophagus. The duct passes between the carotid sheath and the vertebral vessels, crossing in front of the phrenic nerve and the subclavian artery. The thoracic duct is the ultimate drainage channel for lymph from the lower limbs, pelvis, abdomen, left upper limb and the left side of the thorax, head and neck. On the right side of the neck the smaller right lymphatic trunk terminates in the veins in a manner similar to the thoracic duct. However, it drains lymph only from the right upper limb and the right side of the thorax, head and neck.

Arteries

The left common carotid and left subclavian arteries emerge from the thorax on the left of the trachea and oesophagus (Fig. 7.14). On the right, the brachiocephalic trunk divides at the level of the superior thoracic aperture to form the right common carotid and right subclavian arteries (Fig. 7.14). Each common carotid artery ascends into the neck within its sheath and gives no branches before its termination. Each subclavian artery passes laterally over

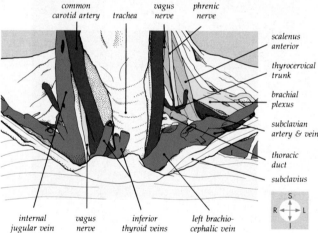

Fig. 7.14   Root of the neck after removal of the clavicles, pretracheal fascia, thyroid gland, carotid sheaths and left internal jugular vein.

the upper surface of the first rib posterior to scalenus anterior and continues into the axilla as the axillary artery (see page 77).

Three branches of the subclavian artery, namely internal thoracic, thyrocervical and vertebral arteries (Figs 7.14 & 7.15), arise medial to scalenus anterior. The internal thoracic artery (see page 36) descends into the thorax to supply the anterior thoracic and abdominal walls. The thyrocervical trunk is short and divides into three branches, the inferior thyroid (see page 291), suprascapular and transverse cervical arteries. The latter two vessels cross the posterior triangle of the neck. The suprascapular artery supplies the scapula and related structures and the transverse cervical artery supplies superficial structures in the posterior part of the neck. The vertebral artery (Fig. 7.15) inclines upwards and backwards medial to scalenus anterior and crosses in front of the transverse process of the seventh cervical vertebra. Continuing superiorly through the foramina transversaria of the upper six cervical vertebrae, it eventually enters the skull through the foramen magnum (see page 330).

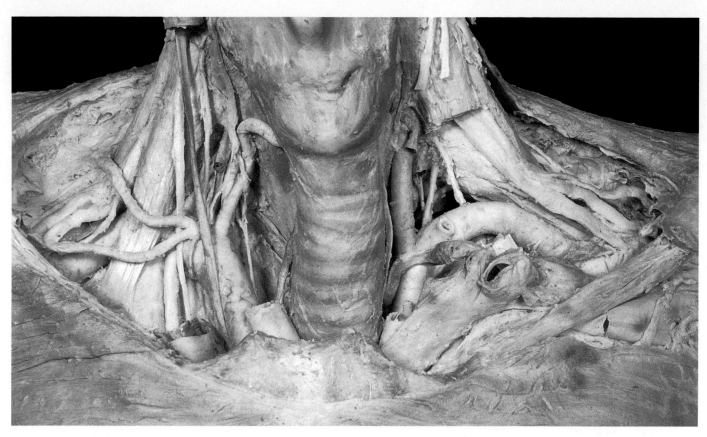

The costocervical trunk (Fig. 7.15) arises from the subclavian artery behind scalenus anterior and arches backwards over the suprapleural membrane as far as the neck of the first rib, where it divides to form the superior intercostal artery supplying the upper two intercostal spaces (see page 35) and the deep cervical artery, which supplies the muscles of the back of the neck.

Nerves

The vagus (X) and phrenic nerves, both sympathetic chains and parts of both brachial plexuses all traverse the root of the neck. Each vagus nerve (Fig. 7.14) descends within the carotid sheath and enters the superior mediastinum between the main arterial and venous structures medial to the phrenic nerve. On the right side of the neck the recurrent laryngeal nerve arises from the vagus, hooking under the subclavian artery to ascend in the groove formed by the lateral surfaces of the trachea and oesophagus. On the left, the recurrent laryngeal nerve follows a similar course but arises from the vagus in the thorax (see page 61).

The phrenic nerve (Fig. 7.15), formed from the anterior rami of the third, fourth and fifth cervical spinal nerves, passes inferiorly on the anterior surface of scalenus anterior beneath the prevertebral fascia and leaves the medial side of the muscle near its lower end. It then enters the thorax between the main arterial and venous structures lateral to the vagus nerve.

The sympathetic trunks (Fig. 7.15), covered by the prevertebral fascia, lie alongside the bodies of the cervical vertebrae. In the neck each trunk bears only three sympathetic ganglia, the superior, middle and inferior. The lowest ganglion fuses frequently with the first thoracic ganglion to form the stellate (cervicothoracic) ganglion. The trunk continues into the thorax in front of the neck of the first rib. The middle and inferior cervical sympathetic ganglia are often linked by a nerve, the ansa subclavia, which curves around the subclavian artery.

The brachial plexus (Fig. 7.14) originates from the anterior rami of the lowest four cervical and first thoracic spinal nerves. These nerves, partly covered by scalenus anterior, constitute the roots of the plexus. They combine to form the trunks of the plexus, which emerge from behind the lateral border of the muscle. The

Fig. 7.15 Deeper structures of the root of neck, revealed by removal of most of the left vagus and phrenic nerves, the left scalenus anterior, both common carotid arteries and the large veins.

plexus continues into the upper limb enclosed with the axillary artery in a prolongation of the prevertebral fascia called the axillary sheath. (A detailed account of the brachial plexus is given on page 78.)

Scalene muscles

Scalenus anterior (Fig. 7.15) is the most anterior of the prevertebral group of muscles. Superiorly it is attached to the transverse processes of the third, fourth, fifth and sixth cervical vertebrae. Inferiorly it gains attachment to the scalene tubercle on the first rib (see page 29). Behind it lie scalenus medius (Fig. 7.15) and scalenus posterior, which arise from the transverse processes of the lower six cervical vertebrae and attach inferiorly to the upper surfaces of the first and second ribs respectively. These prevertebral muscles are supplied segmentally by cervical spinal nerves. They elevate the first and second ribs and laterally flex the neck.

CONTENTS OF CAROTID SHEATH

The carotid sheaths form part of the fascial layers of the neck (see pages 286 & 287) and extend from the base of the skull into the superior mediastinum. Each sheath contains the common, the internal and part of the external carotid arteries, the internal jugular vein and parts of the glossopharyngeal (IX), vagus (X) and accessory (XI) nerves.

Carotid arteries

The common carotid artery arises on the left from the aortic arch and on the right from the brachiocephalic artery, then ascends within its sheath into the neck. At the upper border of the thyroid cartilage it divides into internal and external carotid arteries (Fig. 7.17). At its origin the internal carotid artery is dilated to form the carotid sinus. The vessel ascends within the carotid sheath without branching and, in company with its sympathetic nerve plexus, enters the carotid canal. In the cranial cavity the internal carotid artery terminates as the anterior and middle cerebral arteries (see page 331), having given rise to the ophthalmic artery, which supplies the contents of the orbit.

The external carotid artery leaves the carotid sheath, inclines superolaterally and enters the deepest part of the parotid gland, where it divides into terminal branches at the level of the neck of the mandible. Separating the external and internal carotid arteries are the styloid process, stylopharyngeus, the glossopharyngeal (IX) nerve and the pharyngeal branch of the vagus (X) nerve.

The external carotid artery has eight branches (Fig. 7.17), supplying much of the extracranial portion of the head and upper part of the neck. The first branch, the ascending pharyngeal artery, arises on the medial aspect of the external carotid artery and ascends on the lateral surface of the pharynx. The next branch, the superior thyroid artery, inclines downwards and forwards from the anterior surface of the external carotid to supply the thyroid gland and the larynx. The lingual artery passes forwards from the anterior surface of the external carotid artery into the base of the tongue (see page 311). The facial artery, another anterior branch, supplies the tonsil and descends under the body of the mandible, grooving the submandibular gland and emerging from beneath the mandible at the anterior border of masseter to supply the face (see Fig. 7.35).

Arising from the posterior surface of the external carotid artery, the occipital artery passes upwards and backwards deep to sternocleidomastoid (Fig. 7.17; see Fig. 7.24). The vessel crosses the apex of the posterior triangle of the neck to supply the posterior part of the scalp. The posterior auricular artery arises below the pinna and passes upwards and backwards to supply the pinna and the scalp.

The terminal branches of the external carotid artery arise within the parotid gland

Fig. 7.16 Internal jugular vein and some cervical lymph nodes, revealed after removal of sternocleidomastoid and part of the parotid gland.

and are named the superficial temporal and maxillary arteries. The former supplies the lateral part of the scalp while the maxillary artery supplies the infratemporal fossa, pterygopalatine fossa and lateral wall of the nose. Postganglionic sympathetic nerve fibres accompany the external carotid artery and its branches.

Internal jugular vein

The internal jugular vein (Figs 7.16 & 7.17) is formed within the jugular foramen by the union of the sigmoid and inferior petrosal dural venous sinuses. The vein descends through the neck within the carotid sheath and receives the facial, lingual, pharyngeal, and superior and middle thyroid veins. The internal jugular vein also communicates with the external jugular system via the anterior branch of the retromandibular vein. It terminates by uniting with the subclavian vein to form the brachiocephalic vein.

Nerves

Within the carotid sheath lie the glossopharyngeal (IX), vagus (X) and accessory (XI) nerves, which leave the skull via the jugular foramen. The glossopharyngeal nerve passes inferiorly and leaves the carotid sheath. It winds around the posterolateral surface of stylopharyngeus and enters the posterior third of the tongue. The nerve supplies stylopharyngeus and gives a sensory branch which descends to innervate the carotid sinus (see page 311).

The vagus (X) nerve (Fig. 7.17) bears two sensory ganglia, one lying superiorly in the jugular foramen and one below the base of the skull, between which the nerve receives the cranial part of the accessory nerve. The vagus nerve descends in the posterior part of the carotid sheath between the carotid artery and internal jugular vein and gives rise to pharyngeal, superior laryngeal and cardiac branches before traversing the superior thoracic aperture. The pharyngeal branch passes forwards between the internal and external carotid arteries to gain the outer surface of the pharynx, where it contributes to the pharyngeal plexus. The superior laryngeal nerve accompanies the superior thyroid artery and vein supplying the larynx. The cardiac branches of the vagus join those from the sympathetic trunk and descend into the thorax. The right vagus gives a recurrent laryngeal branch in the neck which curves around the right subclavian artery and passes superiorly to reach the larynx (see page 293). The left recurrent laryngeal nerve arises from the left vagus nerve in the thorax and passes around the aortic arch before ascending into the neck.

The accessory (XI) nerve (Fig. 7.17) is formed by the fusion of cranial and spinal roots in the posterior cranial fossa. In the jugular foramen the nerve divides into a cranial part joining the vagus nerve and a spinal part which leaves the carotid sheath to supply sternocleidomastoid and trapezius.

Lymphatics

Lymphatic vessels from structures in the head and neck accompany the vascular supply and drain into superficial or deep groups of lymph nodes.

Superficial lymph nodes

Several groups of superficial nodes form an incomplete ring around the lower part of the head. The submental nodes lie between the anterior bellies of the two digastric muscles, draining lymph from the tip of the tongue and the mental region. The submandibular group (Fig. 7.16) lies on the superficial surface of the submandibular gland and receives lymph from the submental nodes, from the remainder of the anterior two-thirds of the tongue, from the floor of the mouth (including the gums and teeth), and from the nose, face and anterior part of the scalp. The parotid nodes lie on or within the parotid gland, the mastoid group (Fig. 7.16) on the lateral surface of the mastoid process, and the occipital

Fig. 7.17 Branches of the external carotid artery and the vagus, accessory and hypoglossal nerves, after removal of part of the internal jugular vein, carotid sheath and posterior belly of digastric.

lymph nodes at the apex of the posterior triangle of the neck. The parotid, mastoid and occipital nodes drain the remainder of the face and scalp, including the external ear. Lymph from all the superficial nodes drains into the deep cervical nodes.

Deep cervical lymph nodes

The deep cervical or jugular lymph nodes

(Fig. 7.16) form a chain in and around the carotid sheath. Two of the deep cervical nodes are of particular clinical significance. The jugulodigastric node receives lymph mainly from the tongue and tonsil and the jugulo-omohyoid node drains the tongue. From the deep cervical nodes lymph drains inferiorly, via the jugular lymphatic trunk, usually into the thoracic duct on the left and into the right lymphatic duct on the right.

SUPERFICIAL STRUCTURES OF FACE AND SCALP

The subcutaneous tissue of the face and scalp is highly vascular and is traversed by several nerves. Most of the nerves are sensory to the skin of the region and include branches of the trigeminal (V) and upper cervical spinal nerves. In addition, there are branches that are motor from the facial (VII) nerve to a group of muscles in the subcutaneous tissues of the face, scalp and front of the neck, known collectively as the muscles of facial expression.

Muscles of facial expression

In general, these muscles are arranged as sphincters or dilators around the orifices of the face (Fig. 7.18). Most are anchored to bone at one end and attached to skin at the other.

Palpebral fissure

The sphincter of the palpebral fissure (the gap between the eyelids) is orbicularis oculi, which is divided into inner palpebral and outer orbital parts. The palpebral part lies within the eyelids and is attached to the medial and lateral palpebral ligaments. The orbital portion is attached only to the medial palpebral ligament and its fibres lie around the orbital margin. Both parts close the palpebral fissure, the palpebral part gently and the orbital part forcefully as when 'screwing up the eyes'. The dilator components are provided by levator palpebrae superioris within the orbit (see page 334), and by occipitofrontalis in the scalp. The latter muscle has two bellies, occipital and frontal, linked by an extensive intermediate tendon, the epicranial aponeurosis. This aponeurosis forms a mobile layer over the vault of the skull. From its posterior extremity the occipital belly (occipitalis) descends to its attachment

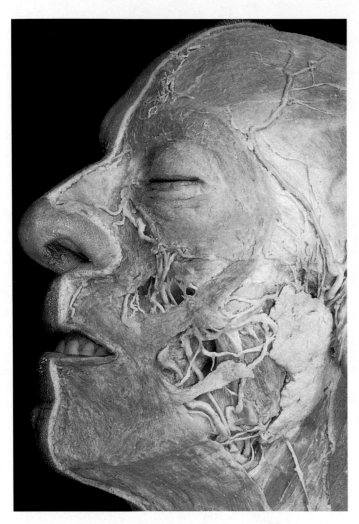

Labels (top to bottom, left): frontalis; orbital & palpebral parts of orbicularis oculi; levator labii superioris alaeque nasi; levator anguli oris; orbicularis oris; depressor labii inferioris; mentalis

Labels (right): epicranial aponeurosis; transverse part of nasalis; levator labii superioris; zygomaticus major & minor; buccinator; risorius; depressor anguli oris

Fig. 7.18 Muscles of facial expression. The skin and subcutaneous fat have been removed.

Labels: epicranial aponeurosis; occipitalis; sternocleidomastoid; highest nuchal line; trapezius

Fig. 7.19 Posterior view to show occipitalis and part of the epicranial aponeurosis.

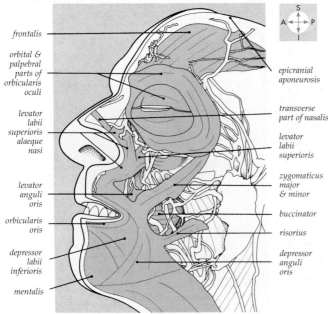

on the highest nuchal line of the occipital bone (Fig. 7.19); from its anterior end the frontal belly (frontalis) descends in the forehead and its fibres interdigitate with those of orbicularis oculi and attach to skin near the eyebrow. Occipitalis fixes the epicranial aponeurosis allowing frontalis to raise the eyebrows.

Nostril

Around each nostril is nasalis with two feeble parts, alar and transverse, which dilate and compress the nostrils respectively.

Mouth

Orbicularis oris, the sphincter of the mouth, is embedded in the lips and attaches near the midline to the mandible and maxilla. In addition there are dilators around the mouth whose fibres continue into orbicularis oris. The most medial dilator of the upper lip is levator labii superioris alaeque nasi. This muscle attaches near the medial margin of the orbit and runs to the alar cartilage of the nose and to the upper lip. Levator labii superioris is attached to bone beneath the orbital margin, whereas levator anguli oris lies slightly deeper and its fibres incline towards the angle of the mouth. Two of the dilator muscles take attachment from the zygoma: zygomaticus major and minor. Attached to the mandible are three muscles, called, from lateral to medial, depressor anguli oris, depressor labii inferioris and mentalis.

The buccinator muscle (Figs 7.18 & 7.20) lies deep to the other dilator muscles in the wall of the cheek. Anteriorly it blends with the deep surface of orbicularis oris. Posteriorly it gains attachment to the outer surface of the mandible from the level of the first to the third molar teeth. Passing behind the third molar tooth, buccinator is attached to the pterygomandibular raphe and the pterygoid hamulus. The muscle attachment continues forwards along the outer surface of the maxilla as far as the first upper molar tooth. Buccinator controls the size of the vestibule of the mouth (that part of the buccal cavity lying between the cheek and the teeth).

The platysma (Fig. 7.21), the most extensive muscle of facial expression, descends in the subcutaneous tissue of the neck from the inferior border of the mandible and fades out on the anterior surface of the thorax. A few fibres may run horizontally from the angle of the mouth as risorius. Platysma is most easily seen in action during respiratory distress when the skin of the neck is pulled taut.

Ear

In the human the auricular muscles are almost vestigial.

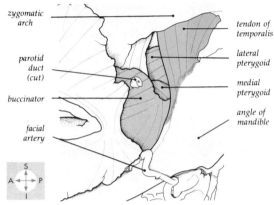

Fig. 7.20 Buccinator seen after removal of some superficial facial muscles, the parotid gland and most of its duct, and masseter.

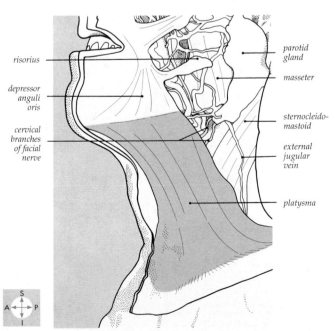

Fig. 7.21 Platysma, the largest muscle of facial expression, and its nerve supply.

Facial nerve

All the muscles of facial expression derive their motor nerve supply from the facial (VII) nerve. Occipitalis and some of the auricular muscles are innervated by the posterior auricular branch of the nerve (see page 301); the remaining muscles are supplied by the five sets of branches (Fig. 7.22) that emerge from the anterior border of the parotid gland (see page 301). The temporal branch of the facial nerve ascends to supply the remaining auricular muscles and frontalis. The zygomatic branch is directed towards the eye and supplies muscles above and below the palpebral fissure. The third branch, the buccal, runs horizontally forwards to innervate buccinator and the muscles of the upper lip. The mandibular branch supplies the muscles of the lower lip, dipping below the mandible in its course. The cervical branch descends to supply platysma.

Blood supply of face

Most of the superficial structures of the face obtain their blood supply from the facial artery (Fig. 7.22), a branch of the external carotid artery. The facial artery enters the face by hooking under the inferior border of the mandible where it is easily palpated. The vessel then pursues a tortuous course across the face towards the inner angle of the orbit. The area of the face in front of the ear is supplied by the transverse facial artery, an anterior branch of the superficial temporal artery. Emerging from the orbit to supply the forehead are the supraorbital and supratrochlear branches of the ophthalmic artery.

Blood from the face drains into the facial vein (Fig. 7.22), which accompanies the facial artery. The vein also receives the supratrochlear and supraorbital veins and thus communicates with ophthalmic veins in the orbit. Blood from the lateral part of the face drains into the superficial temporal vein.

Sensory supply

The sensory nerve supply of the face is conveyed in branches of the three divisions of the trigeminal (V) nerve (Fig. 7.23).

Scalp

The scalp (Fig. 7.24) extends from the superior nuchal line posteriorly to the superior orbital margin anteriorly, and to the external acoustic meatus and zygomatic arch laterally. It comprises

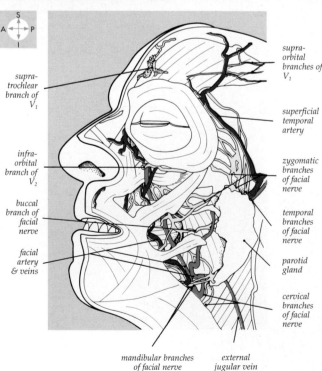

Fig. 7.22 Neurovascular structures of the face. In this specimen the facial vein is duplicated, a common variation.

Fig. 7.23 Dermatomes of the face. Areas of the face are supplied with sensory fibres from the different divisions of the trigeminal nerve.

two functional layers applied to the outer surface of the vault of the skull. Close to the bones lies the pericranium, which forms the periosteum of the skull. This is loosely attached over each constituent bone but is firmly bound to the sutures so that subperiosteal bleeding is limited to the area of the bones involved. Superficial to the pericranium, but separated from it by a layer of loose connective tissue, lie the epicranial aponeurosis (intermediate tendon of occipitofrontalis) and the skin of the scalp, firmly bound to each other so that they move as one over the underlying pericranium and skull.

The arteries and nerves that supply the scalp enter at its circumference and because they accompany each other they will be described together, starting anteriorly. Near the midline are the supratrochlear and supraorbital nerves, arteries and veins. The nerves are derived from the ophthalmic division of the trigeminal (V) nerve. The vessels communicate with their ophthalmic counterparts within the orbit.

Lateral to the orbit the zygomaticotemporal nerve from the maxillary division of the trigeminal nerve, accompanied by its vessels, ascends a short distance into the scalp. Just in front of the ear the auriculotemporal nerve from the mandibular division of the fifth cranial nerve passes into the scalp. The superficial temporal artery and vein follow a similar course.

The area of the scalp behind the ear is supplied by the lesser occipital nerve (C2 anterior ramus) accompanied by the posterior auricular artery and vein. Posteriorly near the midline the scalp receives the greater occipital nerve (C2 posterior ramus) and the occipital artery and vein.

In addition, venous blood may drain via the diploic veins of the skull into the intracranial venous sinuses.

Fig. 7.24 Vessels and nerves of the scalp lying on the epicranial aponeurosis.

PAROTID GLAND

The parotid is the largest of the salivary glands and is pyramidal in shape (Fig. 7.25). Its base faces laterally between the anterior border of sternocleidomastoid and the ramus of the mandible, while its apex lies deeply against the styloid process. The gland extends upwards between the external acoustic meatus and the temporomandibular joint, movements of which may be painful when the parotid is inflamed.

The parotid gland is deeply indented in front by the mandible, masseter and medial pterygoid. Deep to the gland are the infratemporal fossa and the styloid apparatus, the latter separating it from the carotid sheath and the pharyngeal wall.

The investing fascia of the neck splits into two layers to enclose the gland (see page 286). The superficial layer attaches above to the zygomatic arch whilst anteriorly it merges with the tissues of the cheek. The deep layer is attached to the

tympanic part of the temporal bone and is thickened between the styloid process and the angle of the mandible to form the stylomandibular ligament.

The parotid duct (Fig. 7.26) passes forwards across the surface of masseter, turns medially and pierces buccinator to open obliquely into the vestibule of the mouth opposite the upper second molar tooth. When masseter contracts, the duct may be palpated over the anterior edge of the muscle. An accessory part of the gland may lie alongside the duct.

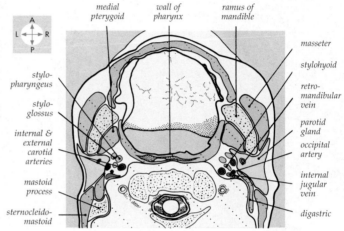

Fig. 7.25 Transverse section of the head through the parotid glands. Superior aspect. Compare Fig. 7.93.

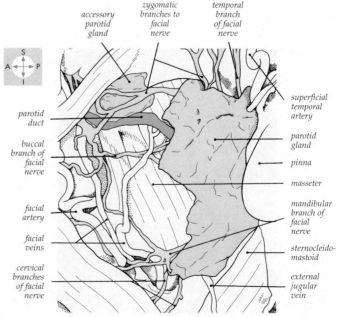

Fig. 7.26 Parotid gland and branches of the facial nerve, exposed by the removal of the superficial layer of parotid fascia.

Structures traversing parotid gland

Of these, the most superficial are branches of the facial (VII) nerve that run forwards to the face and pass superficial to the retromandibular vein and its tributaries. The deepest is the termination of the external carotid artery.

Facial (VII) nerve

The facial nerve emerges from the skull through the stylomastoid foramen and turns forwards to enter the posterior surface of the parotid gland. Before penetrating the gland it gives two branches. The posterior auricular branch passes behind the external acoustic meatus to supply occipitalis and the auricular muscles. The other supplies the posterior belly of digastric and stylohyoid. Within the gland the facial nerve forms a plexus from which five groups of branches (Fig. 7.26) emerge at the periphery of the gland to supply the muscles of facial expression (see page 298).

Retromandibular vein

Within the parotid gland the superficial temporal and maxillary veins unite to form the retromandibular vein (Fig. 7.27). Inferiorly this short vein terminates as anterior and posterior divisions which escape from the gland. The anterior division joins the facial vein, which drains into the internal jugular vein. The posterior division unites with the posterior auricular vein to form the external jugular vein (see page 288).

Termination of external carotid artery

Entering the parotid from below, the external carotid artery ascends through the gland and at the level of the neck of the mandible divides into the maxillary and superficial temporal arteries (Fig. 7.28). The former runs anterosuperiorly to leave the gland and enter the infratemporal fossa. The superficial temporal artery continues upwards between the external acoustic meatus and the temporomandibular joint to supply the temple. Its pulsation can be felt just above the joint.

Several lymph nodes lie just under the fascia covering the parotid gland or within the gland itself.

Neurovascular supply

The gland receives its vascular supply from the vessels traversing it. Parasympathetic secretomotor fibres follow a tortuous route to the gland. The preganglionic fibres arise from the inferior salivatory nucleus in the brain stem and pass in the tympanic branch of the glossopharyngeal (IX) nerve to the tympanic plexus in the middle ear, leaving the skull in the lesser petrosal nerve to synapse in the otic ganglion (see page 304). Postganglionic parasympathetic fibres travel to the gland in the auriculotemporal branch of the mandibular (V$_3$) division. By contrast, postganglionic sympathetic nerves are conveyed in the plexus accompanying the external carotid artery.

Fig. 7.27 Retromandibular vein and its communications, seen after removal of the superficial portion of the parotid gland.

Fig. 7.28 External carotid artery and its terminal branches, revealed by complete excision of the parotid gland.

MASSETER, TEMPORALIS AND INFRATEMPORAL FOSSA

Masseter

Masseter (Fig. 7.29) attaches along the length of the zygomatic arch and its fibres slope downwards and backwards to the lateral surface of the ramus of the mandible adjacent to the angle (Fig. 7.31). This muscle is a powerful elevator of the mandible and is easily palpated when the teeth are clenched. It is supplied by the masseteric branch of the mandibular (V_3) division of the trigeminal nerve.

Temporalis

Temporalis (Fig. 7.30) is a large fan-shaped muscle occupying the temporal fossa and taking attachment from the area of bone bounded by the inferior temporal line. The more superficial fibres arise from the temporal fascia that covers the muscle and is attached to the superior temporal line. All the fibres descend deep to the zygomatic arch to attach to the coronoid process and anteromedial aspect of the ramus of the mandible (Fig. 7.31). Temporalis elevates the mandible, as in closing the mouth, and its posterior fibres retract the mandible. The deep temporal branches of the mandibular (V_3) division of the trigeminal nerve supply the muscle from its deep surface.

Infratemporal fossa

This fossa lies deep to the ramus of the mandible and is limited on its medial aspect by the lateral wall of the pharynx and the medial pterygoid plate of the sphenoid bone. The fossa is bounded by the posterior surface of the maxilla in front and by the styloid process and its attached muscles behind. The roof is provided by the temporal and sphenoid bones in the base of the skull whilst inferiorly the fossa is continuous with the neck.

Within the fossa are the two pterygoid muscles, the mandibular (V_3) division of the trigeminal nerve and its branches, and the maxillary vessels and their branches. Adjacent to the fossa is the temporomandibular joint.

Pterygoid muscles

Each of the lateral and medial pterygoid muscles (see Figs 7.32–7.34) has two attachments to the skull. The upper head of the lateral pterygoid attaches to the inferior surface of the greater wing of the sphenoid. The lower head attaches to the lateral surface of the lateral pterygoid plate. Both heads converge on the neck of the mandible and the capsule of the temporomandibular joint. The lateral pterygoid pulls forward both the neck of the mandible and the articular disc, thus depressing the mandible and opening the mouth.

The lower head of the lateral pterygoid is clasped by the two heads of the medial pterygoid. The deep head of the latter is larger and attaches to the medial surface of the lateral pterygoid plate. The superficial head is attached to the tuberosity of the maxilla. The fibres of both heads incline obliquely downwards and backwards to attach to the medial surface of the angle of the mandible. The muscle is a powerful elevator of the mandible.

Temporomandibular joint

The temporomandibular joint (see Fig. 7.32) is a synovial joint. The head of the mandible articulates with the articular fossa and eminence of the temporal bone. Fibrocartilage covers the articular surfaces and also forms an articular disc which divides the joint into two separate cavities. Within these cavities the non-cartilaginous surfaces are lined with synovial membrane.

The fibrous capsule surrounding the joint is attached to the margin of the articular cartilage and to the neck of the mandible. Anteriorly it receives the attachment of the lateral pterygoid while its deep surface is firmly adherent to the periphery of the articular disc.

Fig. 7.29 Masseter, showing its attachment to the zygomatic arch and the angle of the mandible, after removal of the parotid gland.

Fig. 7.30 Temporalis, seen after removal of masseter, part of the zygomatic arch and the temporal fascia.

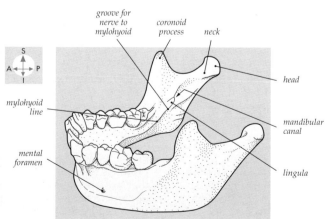

Fig. 7.31 Mandible. The right wisdom tooth is partially erupted.

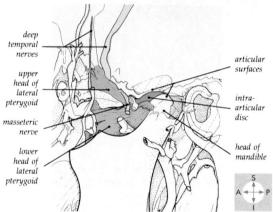

Fig. 7.32   Temporomandibular joint opened by excision of the lateral part of its capsule.

Fig. 7.33   Contents of the infratemporal fossa seen after excision of part of the mandible.

Laterally the capsule (see Fig. 7.30) is thickened to form the lateral ligament, which inclines posteroinferiorly from the root of the zygomatic arch to the neck of the mandible. Two accessory ligaments lie medial to the joint, although not in contact with the capsule. The sphenomandibular ligament extends from the spine of the sphenoid to the lingula adjacent to the mandibular foramen. The stylomandibular ligament, a thickening of the parotid fascia, passes from the styloid process to the angle of the mandible.

The joint receives its nerve supply from the auriculotemporal and masseteric branches of the mandibular (V_3) division of the trigeminal nerve.

Movements at the joint include elevation, depression, protraction and retraction of the mandible. The head of the mandible does not merely rotate in the articular fossa but also moves forwards onto the articular eminence of the temporal bone, taking the articular disc with it. The alternate protraction and retraction of right and left sides produces the grinding movements used in chewing. The muscles responsible for these movements are known collectively as the muscles of mastication. The mouth is closed by contraction of masseter, temporalis and medial pterygoid. The lateral pterygoid protracts the mandible and, assisted by digastric and mylohyoid (see page 307), also opens the mouth. Retraction is produced by the posterior fibres of temporalis. When the mandible is fully depressed the joint is relatively unstable and dislocation may occur, the head of the mandible moving in front of the articular eminence and resulting in an inability to close the mouth.

Mandibular (V_3) division of trigeminal nerve

The mandibular division of the trigeminal nerve (Figs 7.33 & 7.34) contains sensory and motor fibres and enters the infratemporal fossa through the foramen ovale in the sphenoid. Two small branches arise from the short main trunk of the nerve. The first branch ascends through the foramen spinosum to receive sensation from the meninges of the middle cranial fossa. The other branch is motor, supplying the medial pterygoid and giving a small

deep temporal nerve

nerve to upper head of lateral pterygoid

buccal nerve

lingual nerve

inferior alveolar nerve & artery

middle meningeal artery

auriculo-temporal nerve

medial pterygoid

chorda tympani

Fig. 7.34 Branches of the mandibular division of the trigeminal nerve and the maxillary artery, revealed by removal of the mandibular head and lateral pterygoid.

branch that passes through the otic ganglion (lying just medial to the main trunk of the mandibular division) to supply tensor tympani and tensor veli palatini.

The main trunk descends between the lateral pterygoid and tensor palati muscles, dividing into anterior and posterior divisions. The anterior division is mainly motor and gives masseteric, deep temporal, lateral pterygoid and buccal branches. The masseteric nerve (Fig. 7.32) curves laterally above the lateral pterygoid to enter the deep surface of masseter. Two or three deep temporal nerves (Fig. 7.33) ascend deep to temporalis, which they supply, and further branches enter the deep surface of the lateral pterygoid. The buccal nerve (Figs 7.33 & 7.34) is a sensory branch that passes forwards between the two heads of the lateral pterygoid to supply the skin over the cheek and the mucosa lining the cheek, which it reaches by piercing, but not supplying, buccinator.

The posterior division of the main trunk is mainly sensory and has three branches, the auriculotemporal, lingual and inferior alveolar nerves. The auriculotemporal nerve (Fig. 7.34) arises by two roots, which clasp the origin of the middle meningeal artery. The nerve passes backwards before turning superiorly behind the temporomandibular joint to ascend in company with the superficial temporal vessels. It gives secretomotor branches to the parotid gland (see page 301) and conveys sensation from the temporal region, the upper half of the pinna and most of the external acoustic meatus.

The lingual nerve (Figs 7.33 & 7.34) inclines downwards and forwards between the pterygoids, deviating medially to pass below the superior constrictor of the pharynx. In the floor of the mouth it runs forwards lateral to the hyoglossus muscle, at whose anterior border it again turns medially to pass inferior to the submandibular duct and enter the base of the tongue. It conveys general sensation from the anterior two-thirds of the tongue. Near the lower border of the lateral pterygoid the lingual nerve is joined by the chorda tympani (a branch of the facial nerve). Arising within the temporal bone, the chorda tympani emerges from the petrotympanic fissure. It carries taste fibres, which have travelled in the lingual nerve from the anterior two-thirds of the tongue and preganglionic parasympathetic fibres destined for the submandibular ganglion (see page 311).

The inferior alveolar nerve (Figs 7.33 & 7.34) descends medial to the lateral pterygoid and gives rise to a motor branch that curves downwards to supply mylohyoid and the anterior belly of digastric. The inferior alveolar nerve then enters the mandibular foramen in the ramus of the mandible and runs forwards in the mandibular canal, supplying the lower teeth. Its mental branch emerges from the mental foramen to supply skin overlying the chin.

Maxillary artery

This artery (Figs 7.33 & 7.34) arises in the parotid gland (see page 301) as a terminal branch of the external carotid artery, passes anterosuperiorly across the infratemporal fossa, usually lateral to the lateral pterygoid, and traverses the pterygomaxillary fissure to enter the pterygopalatine fossa where terminal branches arise. These correspond to branches of the maxillary nerve (see page 312).

In the infratemporal fossa the maxillary artery gives branches to supply masseter, temporalis and the pterygoid muscles. In addition, the middle meningeal artery arises deep to the lateral pterygoid, embraced by the two roots of the auriculotemporal nerve. It traverses the foramen spinosum and within the cranium supplies the meninges of the middle cranial fossa and the cranial vault.

The maxillary artery also gives rise to the inferior alveolar artery which accompanies the nerve into the mandibular canal. Further small branches supply the middle ear and the lining of the external acoustic meatus.

Pterygoid venous plexus

Veins within the pterygopalatine fossa form a plexus that extends through the pterygomaxillary fissure into the infratemporal fossa, where the plexus is related to the pterygoid muscles. This pterygoid plexus has important connections to the cavernous sinus in the skull and infraorbital and ophthalmic veins. The plexus drains by the maxillary vein into the retromandibular vein (see page 301).

DIGASTRIC AND STYLOID MUSCLES

inferior
alveolar
nerve

lingual
nerve

nerve to
mylohyoid

styloglossus

stylohyoid

anterior
belly of
digastric

nerve to
thyrohyoid

maxillary artery (cut)

styloid
process

posterior
belly of
digastric

external carotid
artery (cut)

sternocleido-
mastoid

facial artery

hypoglossal nerve

lingual artery

Fig. 7.35 Digastric and stylohyoid seen after removal of part of the mandible. The superficial part of the submandibular gland has also been excised.

Digastric

The digastric muscle (Fig. 7.35) consists of anterior and posterior bellies united by an intermediate tendon. The posterior belly attaches to the medial surface of the mastoid process and inclines forwards and downwards, becoming continuous with the intermediate tendon close to the hyoid bone. This tendon pierces stylohyoid and is anchored by a fascial sling to the hyoid bone. The anterior belly continues forwards from the intermediate tendon to attach to the inferior border of the mandible near the midline. Digastric elevates the hyoid bone during swallowing and assists mylohyoid and the lateral pterygoid in depressing the mandible when opening the mouth. The posterior belly is innervated by the facial (VII) nerve (see page 301). The anterior belly receives its motor supply from the mandibular (V_3) division of the trigeminal nerve via the mylohyoid branch of the inferior alveolar nerve (see page 305).

Muscles of styloid process

Three muscles, stylohyoid, stylopharyngeus and styloglossus, attach to the styloid process but diverge to reach the hyoid bone, the pharynx and the tongue respectively.

Stylohyoid (Fig. 7.35) inclines downwards and forwards from the posterior surface of the styloid process to attach to the body of the hyoid bone alongside the lesser horn. The muscle or its tendon is pierced by the intermediate tendon of digastric near the hyoid bone. Stylohyoid elevates the hyoid and is innervated by the facial (VII) nerve.

Stylopharyngeus (Fig. 7.36) is attached to the medial side of the root of the styloid process and passes inferomedially on the lateral surface of the superior pharyngeal constrictor. It enters the wall of the pharynx between the superior and middle constrictors and blends with the other longitudinal muscles of the pharynx. The muscle elevates the pharynx and larynx during swallowing and is the only muscle innervated by the glossopharyngeal (IX) nerve.

Styloglossus (Fig. 7.36) inclines anteromedially from the tip of the styloid process and upper end of the stylohyoid ligament and passes between the superior and middle constrictors of the pharynx to enter the tongue. It elevates and retracts the tongue and, in common with other muscles of the tongue, is supplied by the hypoglossal (XII) nerve.

styloid process

occipital artery

stylo-pharyngeus

glosso-pharyngeal nerve

ascending palatine artery

sternocleido-mastoid

stylohyoid ligament (cut)

styloglossus

mylohyoid

Fig. 7.36 Stylopharyngeus and styloglossus seen after excision of digastric, stylohyoid and the middle portion of the stylohyoid ligament.

MYLOHYOID AND RELATED STRUCTURES

Fig. 7.37 Mylohyoid, revealed by removal of the right anterior belly of digastric and superficial part of the submandibular gland.

Fig. 7.38 The hypoglossal nerve, lingual nerve and submandibular duct passing above mylohyoid.

Suspended from the body of the mandible is a thin sheet of muscle formed by the two mylohyoid muscles. The fibres of each muscle incline downwards and medially, meeting each other in the midline to form a shallow gutter. This gutter slopes downwards and backwards and ends at the free posterior borders of the two muscles on either side of the hyoid bone.

Each mylohyoid separates the superficial tissues in the upper part of the neck from the tongue and related structures within the mouth. Below the muscle lie the anterior belly of digastric (see page 307), part of the platysma (see page 297), the facial artery and vein, and the superficial part (the bulk) of the submandibular salivary gland (Fig. 7.37). This gland curves around the posterior border of mylohyoid so that its

deep part and the submandibular duct lie above the muscle. Also located on the superior aspect of mylohyoid are the sublingual glands, the tongue with its vessels and nerves and the geniohyoid muscles.

Mylohyoid

This muscle (Figs 7.37 & 7.38) takes attachment from the mylohyoid line on the inner aspect of the body of the mandible. Most of its fibres reach a midline raphe, where they interdigitate with those from the opposite side. However, the fibres close to the posterior edge of the muscle descend to the body of the hyoid bone. The mylohyoid muscles raise the hyoid bone and the tongue during swallowing; they

also help to depress the mandible when the hyoid bone is fixed from below. The muscle is innervated by the mylohyoid nerve, a branch of the inferior alveolar nerve from the mandibular division of the trigeminal nerve (V_3).

Geniohyoid

Above mylohyoid a small muscle, geniohyoid (Fig. 7.39), lies close to the midline, passing from the inferior mental spine (inferior genial tubercle) on the mandible to the body of the hyoid bone. Innervated by C1 spinal nerve fibres that are conveyed in the hypoglossal nerve, geniohyoid either elevates the hyoid or depresses the mandible.

lingual nerve
styloglossus
sublingual gland
sub-mandibular duct (cut)
geniohyoid
mylohyoid (cut)
position of hyoid bone

stylohyoid ligament
hypoglossal nerve
submandibular ganglion
hyoglossus

Fig. 7.39 Structures deep to mylohyoid, seen after partial removal of the mylohyoid and the mandible. The submandibular ganglion is elongated in this specimen.

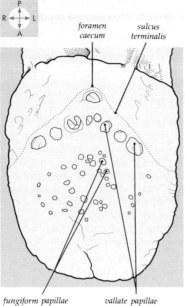

foramen   sulcus
caecum   terminalis

fungiform papillae   vallate papillae

Fig. 7.40 Surface features of the tongue.

Tongue

The tongue is a muscular organ and lies mostly within the oral cavity although its posterior part projects into the oropharynx.

Surface features

The tongue is covered by mucosa, which is reflected anteriorly and laterally onto the inferior surface of the organ. Under the tip of the tongue the mucous membrane forms a midline fold, the frenulum. The upper surface of the tongue (Fig. 7.40) is divided into anterior two-thirds and posterior one-third by a V-shaped groove, the sulcus terminalis. A midline depression, the foramen caecum, lies at the apex of the sulcus terminalis. A row of round elevations, the vallate papillae, lie just in front of the sulcus. From the mucosa of the tongue, somatic sensory and taste fibres pass centrally to reach the brain. From the anterior two-thirds of the tongue (and adjacent oral mucosa) these fibres travel in the lingual nerve (see page 304). Somatic sensory fibres continue to the brain in the mandibular (V_3) division of the trigeminal nerve. However, taste fibres leave the lingual nerve and are conveyed via the chorda tympani nerve to the facial (VII) nerve (see pages 304 & 305). Both taste and somatic sensory nerve fibres from the posterior third of the tongue (including the vallate papillae) are conveyed in the glossopharyngeal (IX) nerve.

Muscles

The musculature of the tongue, divided into two functional halves by a fibrous septum, consists of both extrinsic and intrinsic muscles. In general, the extrinsic muscles alter the position of the tongue and the intrinsic muscles alter its shape.

The extrinsic muscles comprise styloglossus (see page 307), hyoglossus and genioglossus. Hyoglossus (see Fig. 7.39) is attached to the body and greater horn of the hyoid bone and its fibres pass upwards and forwards to reach the side of the tongue. Hyoglossus depresses the tongue, particularly at the sides. Genioglossus (Figs 7.41 & 7.42) forms much of the bulk of the tongue, its fibres radiating from the superior mental spine (superior genial tubercle) close to the midline to most parts of the tongue. The superior fibres reach the tip whilst the inferior fibres pass into the posteroinferior part of the organ. Genioglossus draws the tongue forwards and downwards and its anterior fibres retract the tip.

lingual nerve

submandibular duct

genioglossus

mandible

geniohyoid

hypoglossal nerve (cut)

hyoglossus (cut)

stylopharyngeus

ascending palatine artery

glossopharyngeal nerve

tonsillar artery

facial artery

lingual artery

Fig. 7.41 Deeper structures in the base of the tongue, revealed after removal of the sublingual gland and part of hyoglossus.

Palatoglossus descends from the soft palate and enters the side of the tongue posteriorly. Although it helps to elevate the tongue it is usually considered to be a muscle of the palate (see page 318).

The intrinsic muscles comprise interlacing longitudinal, transverse and vertical groups of fibres on either side of the midline fibrous septum. The shape of the tongue is changed by integrated contractions of the various groups.

The hypoglossal (XII) nerve (see Fig. 7.39) supplies all the muscles of the tongue, both intrinsic and extrinsic. (The nerve supply to palatoglossus is described with the other muscles of the palate; see page 318.)

Blood supply

Arising from the front of the external carotid artery, the lingual artery (Fig. 7.41) loops upwards above the greater horn of the hyoid bone and continues forwards into the base of the tongue deep to hyoglossus. Having supplied structures in the tongue, the lingual artery terminates in the tip. Venous drainage follows a reciprocal course into the internal jugular vein.

Submandibular and sublingual glands

The superficial part of the submandibular salivary gland (see Fig. 7.37) lies inferior to mylohyoid and extends below the medial surface of the mandible. It is continuous around the posterior border of mylohyoid with the smaller deep part (see Fig. 7.38) of the gland that lies above the muscle. The lateral surface of the superficial part of the gland is indented by the facial artery as the vessel arches forwards to reach the inferior border of the mandible (see page 298). From the deep part of the gland the submandibular duct passes forwards and medially to open close to the midline at the base of the frenulum of the tongue. A number of small sublingual glands (see Fig. 7.39) lie beneath the mucosa adjacent to the submandibular duct. These glands are drained by ducts that open either into the submandibular duct or directly into the mouth. Both the sublingual and submandibular glands receive postganglionic parasympathetic secretomotor fibres from the submandibular ganglion (see Fig. 7.39). Preganglionic fibres reach the submandibular ganglion from the facial nerve by way of the chorda tympani and lingual nerves.

Hypoglossal (XII) nerve

The twelfth cranial nerve (see Fig. 7.38) leaves the skull through the hypoglossal canal and descends between the internal jugular vein and internal carotid artery to turn forwards close to the origin of the occipital artery from the external carotid artery, where the superior root of the ansa cervicalis (see page 291) arises. The

Fig. 7.42 Sagittal section through the tongue and surrounding structures.

hypoglossal nerve then continues forwards across the loop of the lingual artery and passes between mylohyoid and hyoglossus to enter the tongue whose muscles it supplies. The branches given to thyrohyoid and geniohyoid are composed of C1 fibres which are distributed via the hypoglossal nerve.

Glossopharyngeal (IX) nerve

The glossopharyngeal nerve (Fig. 7.41) emerges from the skull through the jugular foramen. Initially contained within the carotid sheath, the nerve curves forwards around the stylopharyngeus muscle (which it also supplies) and passes between the superior and middle constrictors of the pharynx to enter the posterior part of the tongue. The glossopharyngeal nerve conveys both somatic and taste sensation from the posterior third of the tongue, oropharynx and lateral parts of the soft palate. The nerve has an autonomic sensory branch, the carotid sinus nerve, which ascends from the carotid sinus and carotid body. In addition, a tympanic branch passes to the tympanic plexus in the middle ear. The lesser petrosal nerve arises from this plexus.

PALATE

The palate consists of hard and soft parts covered by mucous membrane (Fig. 7.54). The hard palate separates the oral and nasal cavities whilst posteriorly the soft palate separates the nasopharynx from the oropharynx.

Hard palate

The bones that comprise the hard palate are the palatine processes of the maxillae anteriorly and the horizontal plates of the palatine bones posteriorly (see Fig. 7.81). The hard palate is bounded in front and laterally by the superior alveolar ridge. The soft palate is attached to the free posterior border of the hard palate. Sensory fibres reach the palate in branches of the maxillary (V_2) division of the trigeminal nerve. The nasopalatine nerve emerges from the incisive foramen and supplies the anterior part of the hard palate. The greater palatine nerve gains the hard palate via the greater palatine foramen and innervates its posterior portion.

Soft palate

The soft palate projects into the cavity of the pharynx from its attachment to the posterior edge of the hard palate. When elevated it separates the oropharynx from the nasopharynx. Five paired muscles attach to the soft palate and contribute to its structure. In the midline the uvula projects downwards from its posterior free border.

Fig. 7.54 Sagittal section through palate and pharynx showing communications with the nasal, oral and laryngeal cavities.

Fig. 7.55 Further dissection of Fig. 7.54 to show some of the muscles of the soft palate.

Muscles

Tensor veli palatini (Fig. 7.56) attaches to the scaphoid fossa and spine of the sphenoid and to the lateral surface of the cartilaginous portion of the auditory (eustachian) tube. Its fibres descend between the lateral and medial pterygoid plates on the lateral aspect of the pharyngeal wall and give way to a tendon just above the pterygoid hamulus. The tendon hooks under the hamulus and turns medially to enter the soft palate, where it forms the palatine aponeurosis by fanning out and attaching to the posterior border of the hard palate. The palatine aponeurosis forms the basic structure of the soft palate to which other muscles gain attachment. Tensor veli palatini is supplied by the mandibular (V$_3$) division of the trigeminal nerve and tenses the soft palate.

Levator veli palatini (Figs 7.55 & 7.56) attaches to the inferior surface of the petrous temporal bone just medial to the opening of the auditory tube and to the adjacent part of the tube. Its fibres descend medial to the medial pterygoid plate within the pharynx and attach to the upper surface of the palatine aponeurosis. The muscle is innervated by the pharyngeal plexus (see page 320). Levator veli palatini elevates the soft palate during swallowing, preventing regurgitation of food into the nasal cavities.

Palatoglossus (Fig. 7.55) descends from the inferior surface of the palatine aponeurosis and inclines slightly forwards to enter the posterolateral part of the tongue. The position of palatoglossus is evident on the inner surface of the oral cavity as a mucosal elevation, the palatoglossal ridge (anterior pillar of the fauces; Fig. 7.54). The two palatoglossal ridges form the oropharyngeal isthmus, which marks the posterior boundary of the oral cavity. Innervated by fibres from the pharyngeal plexus, palatoglossus lowers the soft palate, raises the posterior part of the tongue and moves the palatoglossal ridge towards the midline, thus narrowing the isthmus.

Palatopharyngeus (Figs 7.55 & 7.56) attaches to the undersurface of the soft palate. Most of its fibres run posteroinferiorly as part of the longitudinal layer of muscle inside the pharynx and form the palatopharyngeal ridge (posterior pillar of the fauces). On contraction these fibres depress the soft palate. Other fibres pass horizontally backwards, raising the mucosa into a ridge against which the soft palate is elevated. Palatopharyngeus receives its motor supply from the pharyngeal plexus.

The uvular muscle (Figs 7.55 & 7.56), also supplied by the pharyngeal plexus, lies entirely within the soft palate and elevates the uvula. In cases of unilateral paralysis of the soft palate the uvula rises asymmetrically, being pulled away from the paralysed side.

Sensory and secretomotor innervation to the soft palate is from the lesser palatine nerves of the maxillary (V$_2$) division of the trigeminal nerve, supplemented laterally on the undersurface of the palate by the glossopharyngeal (IX) nerve.

Fig. 7.56 Posterior view of soft palate after removal of cervical vertebral column and posterior wall of pharynx. On the left side the medial pterygoid and the mucosa of the soft palate have been removed to reveal the muscles.

LARYNX

The larynx acts as a sphincter guarding the lower respiratory tract and is responsible for phonation. It lies in the neck and its inlet is continuous with the laryngopharynx (Figs 7.60 & 7.61). Inferiorly the larynx is continuous with the trachea. It consists of a framework of cartilages and bone, which supports the vocal and vestibular folds and the muscles that move them. Anteriorly lie the infrahyoid strap muscles.

Skeleton

The skeleton of the larynx comprises the thyroid, cricoid and arytenoid cartilages, the epiglottis and the hyoid bone.

The thyroid cartilage (see Figs 7.66 & 7.67) has two flat laminae joined anteriorly to form the midline laryngeal prominence ('Adam's apple'). The posterior margin of each lamina is free and bears a superior and an inferior horn. The tips of the inferior horns articulate by tiny synovial joints with the lateral surfaces of the cricoid cartilage.

The cricoid cartilage (see Figs 7.66 & 7.70) lies below the thyroid cartilage and is shaped like a signet ring, with a narrow anterior arch and a wide posterior lamina. Its inferior border lies horizontally whilst the superior border slopes upwards posteriorly. Movement at the cricothyroid joints allows the arch of the cricoid to tip upwards whilst the lamina tips backwards.

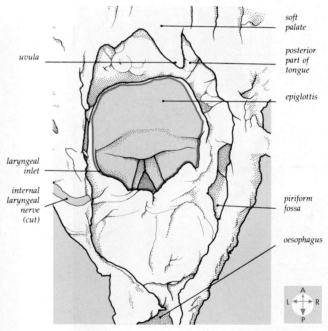

Fig. 7.60 Posterosuperior view of the larynx, seen through the opened laryngopharynx. The lumen of the larynx is visible through the laryngeal inlet.

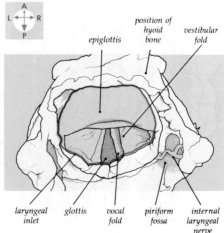

Fig. 7.61 Superior view into the larynx. The mucosa lining the laryngopharynx has been removed to reveal the internal laryngeal nerve.

In addition to its articulations with the thyroid cartilage, the upper border of the cricoid lamina bears articular surfaces, one on each side of the midline, for synovial joints with the two arytenoid cartilages. Each arytenoid (Figs 7.63, 7.66 & 7.70) is pyramidal in shape, with its base on the cricoid lamina and its apex superiorly. It has four surfaces (medial, posterior, anterolateral and inferior) and two processes. Anteriorly lies the vocal process, to which the vocal fold is attached, whilst its muscular process projects laterally. Each arytenoid is able to rotate around its own vertical axis. In addition, the arytenoids can slide laterally and downwards away from the midline on the slope of the articular surface on the cricoid.

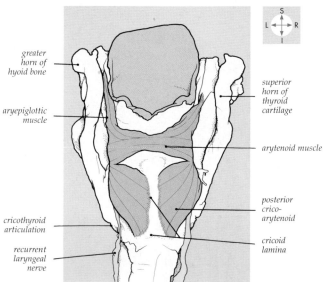

Fig. 7.62 Some of the intrinsic muscles of the larynx, seen after removal of the mucosa of the laryngopharynx.

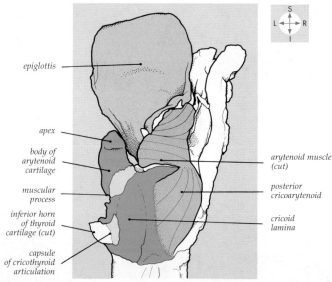

Fig. 7.63 Cricoid and arytenoid cartilages, exposed by removal of most of the soft tissues on the left of the larynx.

The epiglottis (Figs 7.63 & 7.66) is attached in the midline to the inner surface of the thyroid cartilage, just below the laryngeal prominence. It extends upwards and backwards behind the tongue. During swallowing it overlies the laryngeal inlet when the larynx is raised against the tongue.

The hyoid bone (Figs 7.61 & 7.66) is the uppermost skeletal element of the larynx. It consists of a body bearing greater and lesser pairs of horns.

Membranes and ligaments

Several membranes are attached to the laryngeal framework and fill the gaps between the skeletal structures. The conus elasticus (cricovocal membrane) (Fig. 7.65) is elastic and attaches inferiorly to the upper border of the cricoid cartilage. In the midline anteriorly, it reaches the inferior border of the thyroid cartilage, forming the inelastic cricothyroid ligament. Posteriorly it is attached to the vocal processes of the arytenoids. The membrane has a free upper border, which runs between the arytenoids and the thyroid cartilage and forms the basis of the vocal folds (true vocal cords).

The inelastic quadrangular (aryepiglottic) membrane (Fig. 7.65) attaches posteriorly to the body and apex of the arytenoid and anteriorly to the lower part of the lateral edge of the epiglottis. It has a lower free border which forms the vestibular fold (false vocal cord) whilst the upper free edge forms the aryepiglottic fold (part of the laryngeal inlet).

The thyrohyoid membrane (see Fig. 7.67) fills the gap between the thyroid cartilage and the hyoid bone. Its posterior free edges are thickened to form the lateral thyrohyoid ligaments whilst the midline thickening is the median thyrohyoid ligament.

Mucous membrane (Fig. 7.64) lines the interior of the larynx. The epithelium is of the respiratory type, except over the vocal and aryepiglottic folds where it is stratified and squamous. A pouch of mucous membrane protrudes laterally between the vocal and vestibular folds, forming the saccule. It contains numerous mucous glands whose secretions moisten the vocal folds.

Intrinsic muscles

The intrinsic laryngeal muscles control the position and tension of the vocal and aryepiglottic folds, therefore modifying the shape of the airway through the larynx, acting both at the glottis (rima glottidis), the gap between the vocal folds, and at the inlet (see Fig. 7.61). During swallowing both openings narrow, but in coughing and phonation only the glottis narrows. The glottis widens during inspiration, especially when deep. The muscles are symmetrical in their arrangement.

The cricothyroid muscle (see Fig. 7.67) attaches to the anterolateral surface of the cricoid cartilage and to the inferior edge of the thyroid cartilage and adjacent part of the inferior horn. It raises the arch of the cricoid cartilage, tipping the lamina backwards and thereby increasing the tension and length of the vocal folds. This has the effect of raising the pitch of the voice and narrowing the glottis.

The thyroarytenoid muscle (see Fig. 7.69) attaches to the posterior surface of the thyroid cartilage adjacent to the conus elasticus. Its fibres pass posteriorly to gain the vocal process and adjacent body of the arytenoid cartilage. The muscle opposes the action of cricothyroid, drawing the arytenoids forwards and relaxing the vocal folds. Part of the muscle (vocalis) lies in the free edge of the vocal fold. The vocalis gives rigidity to the edge of the fold and also modifies tension differentially along its length.

Two muscles attach to the muscular process of each arytenoid. The lateral cricoarytenoid (see Fig. 7.68) attaches to the lateral surface of the cricoid, its fibres passing posterosuperiorly to gain the muscular process of the arytenoid. The muscle rotates the arytenoid around its vertical axis, adducting the vocal folds and thereby closing the glottis. The posterior

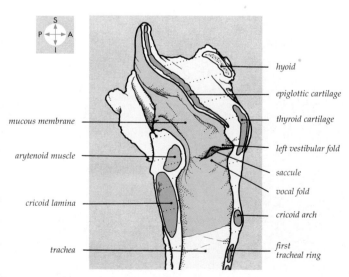

Fig. 7.64 Median sagittal section showing the lumen and mucous membrane of the larynx.

hyoid

epiglottic cartilage

thyroid cartilage

mucous membrane

arytenoid muscle

left vestibular fold

saccule

vocal fold

cricoid lamina

cricoid arch

trachea

first tracheal ring

cricoarytenoid (Figs 7.62 & 7.68) inclines anterosuperiorly from the lamina of the cricoid to the muscular process of the arytenoid. Its action opposes that of the lateral cricoarytenoid, rotating the arytenoid so that the folds are abducted and the glottis opened. Simultaneous contraction of the lateral and posterior cricoarytenoid muscles separates the arytenoids by sliding them down the cricoid lamina.

The arytenoid muscle (Figs 7.62 & 7.64) spans the gap between the bodies of the arytenoid cartilages and has transverse and oblique parts. The muscle approximates the arytenoids, closing the glottis. The oblique arytenoids continue anterosuperiorly in the aryepiglottic fold as the aryepiglottic musclea (see Fig. 7.68). These assist in closing the laryngeal inlet and are important during swallowing.

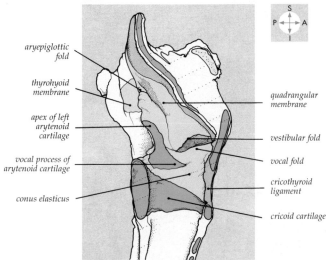

Fig. 7.65 Membranes and folds of the larynx, revealed by removal of most of the mucosa.

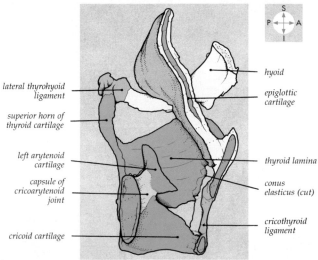

Fig. 7.66 Bisected skeleton of the larynx, revealed by removal of membranes.

Nerve supply

The larynx is supplied by the right and left superior and recurrent laryngeal branches of the vagus (X) nerves. Each recurrent laryngeal nerve (Figs 7.67 & 7.68) ascends from the root of the neck (see page 293) in the groove between the trachea and oesophagus. Passing beneath the lower border of the inferior constrictor, the nerve enters the larynx behind the cricothyroid joint.

It supplies motor fibres to all of the intrinsic muscles (except cricothyroid) and carries sensory fibres from all of the structures within the larynx and laryngopharynx below the level of the vocal folds.

Fig. 7.67   Anterolateral view of the larynx.

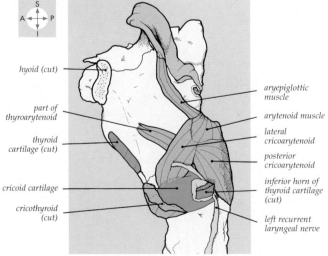

Fig. 7.68   Deeper intrinsic muscles seen after removal of half of the thyroid cartilage and the hyoid bone.

The superior laryngeal nerve (Figs 7.57 & 7.67) arises from the vagus nerve just below the skull and descends to the thyrohyoid membrane where it divides, forming a motor external laryngeal branch and a sensory internal laryngeal branch. The external laryngeal nerve (Fig. 7.67) descends on the outer surface of the larynx to supply the cricothyroid muscle. The internal laryngeal branch (Figs 7.61 & 7.67) pierces the thyrohyoid membrane and provides sensory fibres to the larynx and laryngopharynx above the vocal folds.

Blood supply

The laryngeal branches of the superior and inferior thyroid arteries (see Figs 7.13 & 7.15) supply the larynx whilst venous blood drains via superior and middle thyroid vessels into the internal jugular vein.

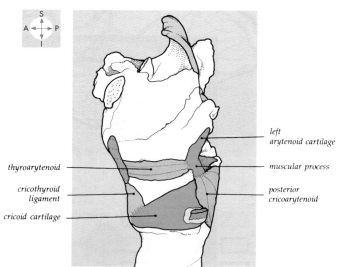

Fig. 7.69 Thryoarytenoid and the arytenoid cartilage after excision of the lateral cricoarytenoid, interarytenoid and aryepiglottic muscles.

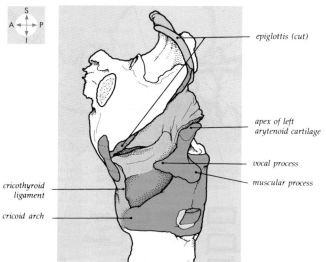

Fig. 7.70 Cartilages of the larynx, revealed by removal of muscles and membranes on the left side.

Nerves

Several nerves reach the orbit from the middle cranial and pterygopalatine fossae. The optic (II) nerve (Fig. 7.88), which conveys visual sensation, traverses the optic canal with the ophthalmic artery. Enveloped by meninges and cerebrospinal fluid, the nerve passes forwards and laterally within the cone of rectus muscles and enters the eyeball just medial to its posterior pole. Other nerves gain the orbit through the orbital fissures.

The oculomotor (III) nerve (Figs 7.88 & 7.90) enters the cone of muscles via the superior orbital fissure. It has superior and inferior divisions, which are often formed before entering the orbit. The superior division supplies the superior rectus and levator palpebrae superioris while the inferior division gives branches to inferior rectus, inferior oblique, medial rectus and the ciliary ganglion. Sympathetic fibres to the smooth muscle in levator palpebrae superioris and inferior rectus enter the oculomotor (III) nerve in the cavernous sinus and travel with its branches to these muscles.

The trochlear (IV) nerve (Fig. 7.88) enters the orbit via the superior orbital fissure, passing above the muscle cone to supply superior oblique.

The abducens (VI) nerve (Figs 7.89 & 7.90) gains the orbit via the superior orbital fissure and passes forwards on the inner surface of lateral rectus, which it supplies.

The ophthalmic (V₁) division of the trigeminal nerve divides into lacrimal, frontal and nasociliary nerves, each of which enters the orbit through the superior orbital fissure. The lacrimal nerve (see Fig. 7.87) passes forwards, outside the muscle cone, along the angle between the roof and lateral wall of the orbit. It is joined by parasympathetic secretomotor fibres from the zygomatic nerve (see page 312), which are destined for the lacrimal gland. In addition, the lacrimal nerve conveys sensation from the lacrimal gland and the lateral part of the upper eyelid.

The frontal nerve (see Fig. 7.87) lies on the upper surface of levator palpebrae superioris and divides into supraorbital and supratrochlear nerves. The supraorbital nerve (see Figs 7.85 & 7.87) curves around the upper part of the orbital margin, occupying the supraorbital notch, and conveys sensation from the upper eyelid, forehead, scalp and frontal air sinus. The supratrochlear nerve (see Figs 7.85 & 7.87) lies more medially, leaving the orbit just above the trochlea to supply sensory fibres to the medial part of the upper eyelid, forehead and scalp.

The nasociliary nerve (Fig. 7.88), lying within the muscle cone, crosses above the optic (II) nerve and continues forwards along the medial wall of the orbit to terminate below the trochlea. Its branches include one to the ciliary ganglion, two long ciliary nerves, posterior and anterior ethmoidal nerves and the infratrochlear nerve. The long ciliary nerves, which carry sympathetic vasoconstrictor fibres that join the nasociliary nerve in the cavernous sinus, pass forwards to supply vessels within the eyeball. The posterior and anterior ethmoidal nerves leave through their respective foramina, supplying ethmoidal air cells. The anterior ethmoidal nerve passes between the frontal and ethmoid bones and emerges on the upper surface of the cribriform plate. Leaving the anterior fossa, the nerve penetrates the plate to run on the inner surface of the nasal bone as the external nasal nerve and eventually reaches the tip of the nose. It conveys sensation from a strip of nasal skin close to the midline and from the nasal septum. The infratrochlear nerve supplies the medial part of the upper eyelid (see Fig. 7.85).

Autonomic nerves

The ciliary ganglion lies just behind the eyeball, lateral to the optic (II) nerve. It receives sensory fibres from the nasociliary nerve, sympathetic fibres from the internal carotid plexus in the cavernous sinus and parasympathetic fibres from the oculomotor (III) nerve. Only the last synapse in the ganglion. From the anterior part of the ganglion, short ciliary nerves (Fig. 7.88) pass forwards into the eyeball, conveying general sensory fibres from the eyeball (including the cornea), parasympathetic fibres to the ciliary muscle and sphincter pupillae and sympathetic fibres to dilator pupillae.

Vasoconstrictor sympathetic fibres reach the eyeball in the long ciliary branches of the nasociliary nerve. Other intraorbital sympathetic fibres travel in the oculomotor (III) nerve to the smooth muscle component of levator palpebrae superioris and inferior rectus. Parasympathetic fibres reach the lacrimal gland via the lacrimal nerve, which communicates with the zygomatic branch of the maxillary (V₂) division of the trigeminal nerve. The cell bodies of these fibres lie in the pterygopalatine ganglion (see page 313).

trochlea

superior oblique

ophthalmic artery

optic (II) nerve

posterior ethmoidal nerve

nasociliary nerve

trochlear (IV) nerve

levator palpebrae superioris (cut)

optic (II) nerve

frontal nerve (cut)

levator palpebrae superioris (cut)

superior oblique tendon

superior rectus (cut)

lacrimal gland

long ciliary nerve

short ciliary nerves

superior division of oculomotor (III) nerve (cut)

superior rectus (cut)

Fig. 7.88 Structures of the orbit seen following excision of superior rectus, levator palpebrae superioris and the superior division of the oculomotor nerve along with a quantity of orbital fat.

Vessels

The ophthalmic artery (Figs 7.88 & 7.89), a branch of the internal carotid artery in the middle cranial fossa, enters the orbit through the optic canal inferior to the optic (II) nerve. The artery then accompanies the nasociliary nerve, passing above the optic nerve and continuing forwards along the medial wall of the orbit. Its first branch, the central retinal artery, enters the optic nerve and passes into the eyeball to supply the retina. Occlusion of this artery results in blindness. Other branches of the ophthalmic artery accompany those of the ophthalmic (V_1) division of the trigeminal nerve. In addition, there are posterior and anterior ciliary branches to the eyeball, and branches to the extraocular muscles.

Venous blood from the eyeball and adjacent structures drains into inferior and superior ophthalmic veins. The superior ophthalmic vein terminates posteriorly in the cavernous venous sinus while the inferior vein passes through the inferior orbital fissure into the pterygoid venous plexus in the pterygopalatine fossa. Both superior and inferior ophthalmic veins communicate with veins on the face.

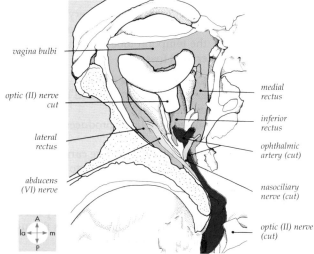

Fig. 7.89 Muscles of the orbit seen after removal of the upper eyelid, part of the optic nerve, and superior oblique.

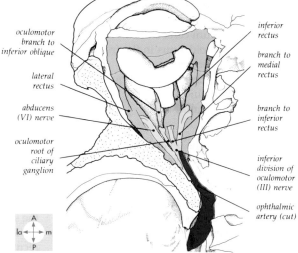

Fig. 7.90 Inferior division of the oculomotor nerve, revealed by excision of the distal part of the ophthalmic artery and the nasociliary nerve.

Identify the structures indicated. The answers are supplied at the foot of the page.

Fig. 7.99   Transverse section showing the orbits and posterior cranial fossa. Inferior aspect. Compare Fig. 7.92.

Fig. 7.100   Transverse section showing the maxillary sinuses and nasal cavities. Inferior aspect.

Answers

Fig. 7.99   1 = nasal septum, 2 = eyeball, 3 = temporalis, 4 = temporal lobe, 5 = carotid canal, 6 = inner ear, 7 = pons, 8 = fourth ventricle, 9 = falx cerebelli, 10 = cerebellum, 11 = sigmoid sinus, 12 = pinna, 13 = basilar artery, 14 = sphenoid sinus, 15 = ethmoid air cells, 16 = lens.

Fig. 7.100   1 = nasal cavity, 2 = ethmoid air cells, 3 = maxillary sinus, 4 = nasopharynx, 5 = mandible, 6 = internal carotid artery, 7 = parotid gland, 8 mastoid process, 9 = pinna, 10 = sternocleidomastoid, 11 = trapezius, 12 = cervical spinal cord, 13 = internal jugular vein, 14 = lateral pterygoid, 15 = masseter, 16 = temporalis.

Identify the structures indicated. The answers are supplied at the foot of the page.

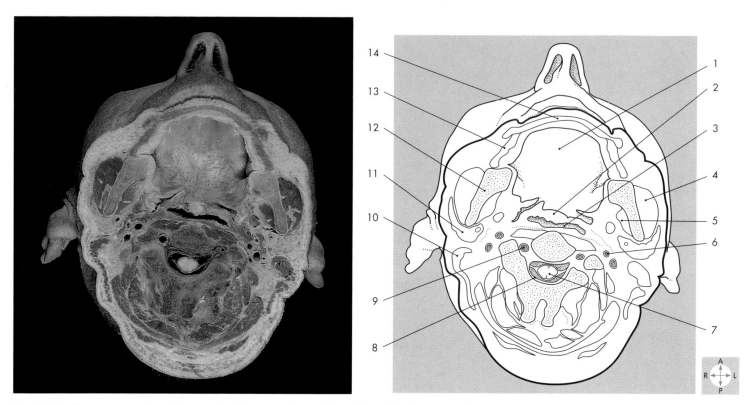

Fig. 7.101 Transverse section at the level of the second cervical vertebra. Inferior aspect. Compare Fig. 7.93.

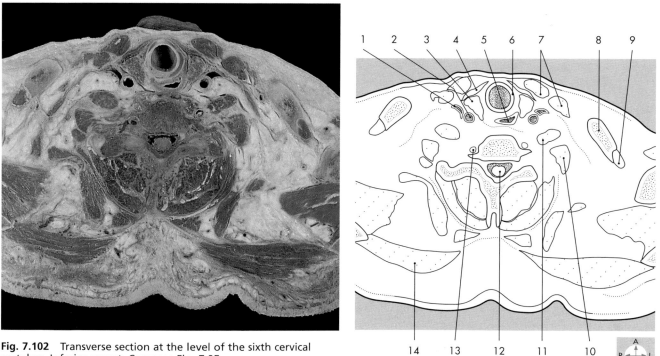

Fig. 7.102 Transverse section at the level of the sixth cervical vertebra. Inferior aspect. Compare Fig. 7.95.

Answers

Fig. 7.101 1 = hard palate, 2 = soft palate, 3 = oropharynx, 4 = masseter, 5 = medial pterygoid, 6 = internal carotid artery, 7 = cervical spinal cord, 8 = dura mater, 9 = vertebral artery, 10 = sternocleidomastoid, 11 = parotid gland, 12 = mandible, 13 = buccinator, 14 = orbicularis oris in lower lip.

Fig. 7.102 1 = internal jugular vein, 2 = common carotid artery, 3 = thyroid gland, 4 = strap muscle, 5 = laryngopharynx, 6 = cricoid cartilage, 7 = sternocleidomastoid, 8 = clavicle, 9 = subclavius, 10 = scalenus medius, 11 = scalenus anterior, 12 = spinal cord, 13 = vertebral artery, 14 = trapezius.

INTRODUCTION

The back consists of the vertebrae, the intervertebral joints and ligaments, and the muscles that clothe their posterior and lateral aspects (Fig. 8.1). The vertebral column encloses the spinal cord and its meninges.

The vertebral column comprises vertebrae which are classified regionally as cervical (7), thoracic (12), lumbar (5), sacral (5 vertebrae fused to form the sacrum) and coccygeal (3–5) (Fig. 8.2). Typically, a vertebra consists of a body, two pedicles, two laminae, two transverse processes and a single spinous process (Fig. 8.3). The body and vertebral arch, formed by the pedicles and laminae, surround the vertebral canal which encloses the meninges and spinal cord (Fig. 8.5). Pairs of superior and inferior articular processes form synovial joints with corresponding processes on adjacent vertebrae. The vertebral bodies are united by fibrocartilagenous discs (Fig. 8.2). Each vertebra usually possesses features characteristic of its region.

The vertebral column is curved anteroposteriorly. In the adult, the thoracic and sacral/coccygeal vertebrae form curves that are concave anteriorly (primary or kyphotic curves), whereas in the cervical and lumbar regions the curves are concave posteriorly (secondary or lordotic curves) (Fig. 8.2).

The movements between adjacent vertebrae are relatively limited although summation enables the vertebral column as a whole to achieve a wide range of motion. Both flexion and extension occur throughout the length of the vertebral column, particularly in the cervical region. Lateral flexion is greatest in the cervical and lumbar regions and rotation occurs mainly in the upper thoracic region.

The muscles of the back (Fig. 8.4) may be classified into superficial, intermediate and deep groups. The superficial muscles

occipital bone

seventh cervical vertebra

clavicle

scapula

humerus

first thoracic vertebra

twelfth rib

fourth lumbar vertebra

sacrum

coccyx

hip bone

☐ **extent of cutaneous innervation by posterior rami of spinal nerves**

☐ **extent of deep back muscles**

Fig. 8.1   Posterior aspect of the back.

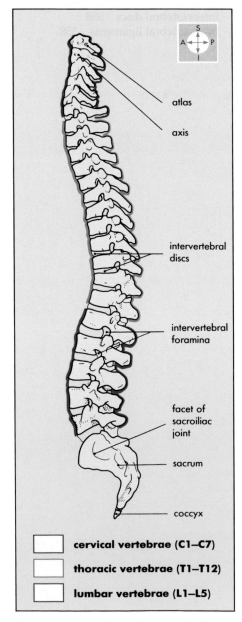

atlas

axis

intervertebral discs

intervertebral foramina

facet of sacroiliac joint

sacrum

coccyx

☐ **cervical vertebrae (C1–C7)**

☐ **thoracic vertebrae (T1–T12)**

☐ **lumbar vertebrae (L1–L5)**

Fig. 8.2   Lateral view of the vertebral column.

(trapezius, latissimus dorsi, levator scapulae, rhomboid major and minor) act on the upper limb (see pages 97 & 98). The intermediate group (the two serratus posterior muscles) are respiratory.

The deep muscles (see page 360), including splenius, erector spinae and transversospinalis, interconnect the base of the skull, the sacrum and the intervening vertebrae. Erector spinae is subdivided into named components, including iliocostalis, longissimus and spinalis, which usually span several vertebrae. Deep to erector spinae is the transversospinalis, whose components usually run obliquely, attaching adjacent vertebrae (Fig. 8.4). Transversospinalis comprises semispinalis,

multifidus and rotatores. The deep muscles are all supplied by the posterior rami of the spinal nerves (Fig. 8.5).

Within the vertebral canal three meningeal layers, the dura mater, the arachnoid mater and the pia mater, invest the spinal cord (see Fig. 8.29). The dura mater is the outer layer and attaches to the foramen magnum where it is continuous with the cranial dura. Inferiorly the dura attaches to the second sacral vertebra. The arachnoid mater is applied to the inner aspect of the dura. The pia is a vascular layer which closely invests the spinal cord and spinal nerve roots. Between the arachnoid and the pia is the subarachnoid space containing cerebrospinal fluid.

The spinal cord, within its meningeal coverings, is continuous above with the medulla oblongata. In the adult it extends inferiorly to the level of the second lumbar vertebra. The cord gives rise to paired spinal nerves: 8 cervical, 12 thoracic, 5 lumbar, 5 sacral and 3 coccygeal. The leash of lumbar, sacral and coccygeal nerve roots descends beyond the lower end of the cord and is known as the cauda equina (see Fig. 8.30). The spinal nerves emerge from the vertebral canal through the intervertebral foramina, and divide into posterior and anterior rami (Fig. 8.5). The posterior rami supply the deep muscles of the back and the overlying skin (Fig. 8.1).

Fig. 8.3   Oblique view of a lumbar vertebra to show its processes, vertebral foramen and intervertebral notches.

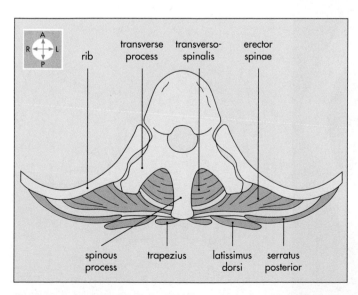

Fig. 8.4   A thoracic vertebra with the main groups of back muscles. Inferior aspect.

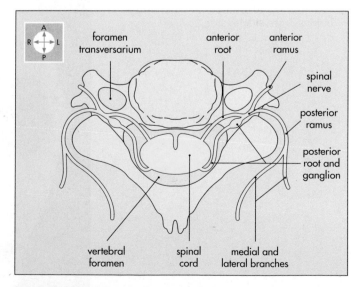

Fig. 8.5   A cervical vertebra with the spinal cord and a pair of spinal nerves. Inferior aspect.

VERTEBRAE AND JOINTS

Cervical vertebrae

The seven cervical vertebrae are relatively small and enclose a wide vertebral canal with adequate space for the cervical part of the spinal cord. Each transverse process is perforated by a foramen transversarium transmitting the vertebral vessels. The spinous processes all give attachment to a strong midline elastic ligament, the ligamentum nuchae.

Four of the cervical vertebrae have a typical appearance whereas the first, second and seventh are modified. The typical vertebrae (Fig. 8.6) possess short bifid spines and their transverse processes have anterior and posterior tubercles. The facets on the superior articular processes face obliquely backwards and upwards and therefore rotation and lateral flexion always occur together.

The first cervical vertebra, the atlas (Fig. 8.7), has anterior and posterior arches, relatively large transverse processes and two lateral masses. The atlas has no body and its spinous process is represented by a tubercle. On the superior surface of each lateral mass is a concave facet which articulates with the convex occipital condyle of the skull. The atlanto-occipital joints permit flexion and extension (nodding movements).

The second cervical vertebra, the axis (Fig. 8.8), possesses some of the features of a typical cervical vertebra but it has a unique vertical projection, the dens (odontoid process). This projects superiorly from the upper surface of its body and represents the body of the atlas. The dens articulates by a synovial joint with a facet on the posterior surface of the anterior arch of the atlas, where it is retained by the alar, apical and transverse ligaments (see Figs 8.10 & 8.11). The planes of the lateral atlantoaxial joints and the pivot joint of the dens (Fig. 8.9) allow rotation of the head as in looking from side to side.

Fig. 8.6 Lateral and superior views of a typical (fourth) cervical vertebra.

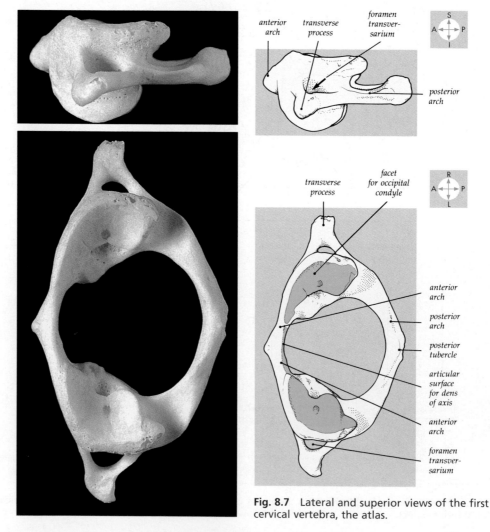

Fig. 8.7 Lateral and superior views of the first cervical vertebra, the atlas.

Fig. 8.8 Lateral and superior views of the second cervical vertebra, the axis.

Fig. 8.9 Base of the skull, atlas and axis, seen in an expanded posterior view.

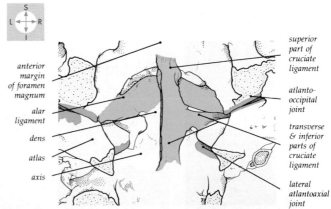

Fig. 8.10 Ligaments of the atlantoaxial joint. The posterior longitudinal ligament, spinal cord and meninges, vertebral arches and the posterior part of the skull have been removed. On the left side part of the cruciate ligament has been excised.

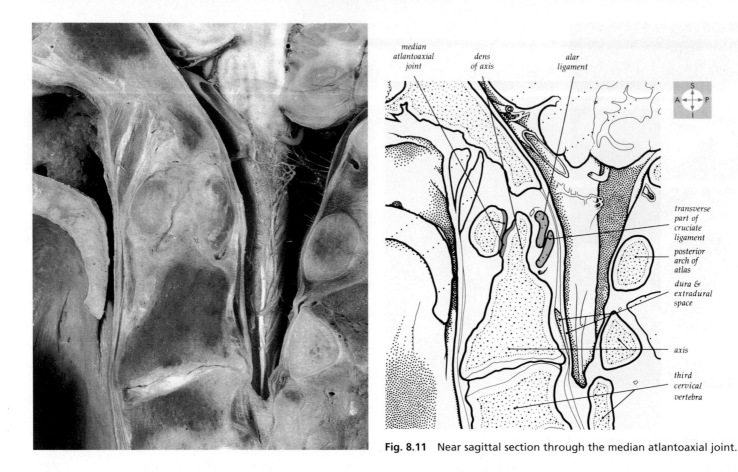

median
atlantoaxial
joint

dens
of axis

alar
ligament

transverse
part of
cruciate
ligament

posterior
arch of
atlas

dura &
extradural
space

axis

third
cervical
vertebra

Fig. 8.11   Near sagittal section through the median atlantoaxial joint.

body

transverse
process

spinous
process

body

superior articular
facet

spinous
process

lamina

pedicle

transverse
process

Fig. 8.12   Lateral and superior views of the seventh
cervical vertebra, the vertebra prominens.

The seventh cervical vertebra (Fig. 8.12)
possesses a long, non-bifid spine, which
provides the inferior attachment for the
ligamentum nuchae. The spinous process is
easily palpable and hence the vertebra is
called the vertebra prominens. The
foramina transversaria of this vertebra are
traversed by the vertebral veins but not by
the arteries.

The joints of the whole cervical column
allow movements of flexion, extension,
rotation and lateral flexion. These
movements are brought about by the
prevertebral and postvertebral muscles
(Fig. 8.13), assisted by sternocleidomastoid
and trapezius. The prevertebral muscles
comprise the scalene group (see page 293)
and the longus colli group. The latter passes
from the base of the skull down the anterior
surface of the vertebral column into the
thorax.

Injuries to the cervical column,
particularly involving fracture or
dislocation of vertebrae, may result in
spinal cord injury leading to quadriplegia
or death. The atlantoaxial joint is
particularly liable to disruption in
hyperextension injuries.

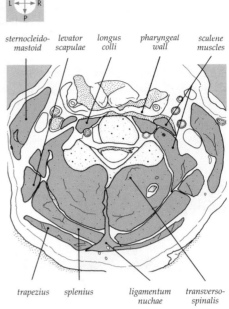

Fig. 8.13 Transverse section at the level of the fourth cervical vertebra, showing the muscles of the neck. Superior aspect. Compare Fig. 7.94.

Thoracic vertebrae

The bodies of the twelve thoracic vertebrae increase in size from above downwards. The bodies bear characteristic costal facets (Fig. 8.14), which form synovial joints with the heads of the ribs. Typically a vertebral body possesses one pair of facets on each side adjacent to the attachment of the pedicle. The upper facet receives the rib whose number corresponds to the vertebra. However the first, tenth, eleventh and twelfth vertebrae possess single facets on each side, which are for articulation with their own ribs. The vertebral canal is smaller than in any other region of the spine.

The transverse processes project laterally and backwards and typically each bears near its tip a facet for the tubercle of the corresponding rib. The spinous processes are long and slope steeply downwards. The plane of the joints between the facets on the articular processes is almost vertical and permits rotation. However, all movements in the thoracic region are restricted by the rib cage.

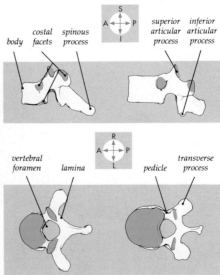

Fig. 8.14 Lateral and superior views of the second and tenth thoracic vertebrae.

Lumbar vertebrae

The upper four lumbar vertebrae are very similar. The vertebral foramina are moderate in size (Fig. 8.15) but the bodies are comparatively large, with concave sides. The transverse processes taper and are directed laterally and backwards. The spinous processes are deep and rectangular. Facets on the superior articular processes face medially and 'grasp' the laterally directed inferior facets of the vertebra above, permitting wide ranges of flexion, extension and lateral flexion but severely restricting rotation.

The fifth lumbar vertebra has shorter transverse processes and a less angular spinous process. Its inferior articular facets are widely separated and face anteriorly. They articulate with the sacrum (Fig. 8.16) and prevent forward displacement of the vertebra. One or both transverse processes may be fused with the upper part of the sacrum (sacralization of the fifth lumbar vertebra), which can cause difficulty in the interpretation of radiographs.

Sacral and coccygeal vertebrae

The sacrum is a triangular bone formed by the fusion of five vertebrae (Figs 8.17 & 8.18). The upper surface of the sacrum resembles that of a lumbar vertebra and carries the lumbosacral disc. Below the apex of the sacrum lies the coccyx (Fig. 8.18), which may be a small single bone or up to four rudimentary vertebrae. The coccyx and the sacrum usually articulate via a small intervertebral disc, although they may be fused. The sacrum slopes backwards and downwards and is concave anteriorly. The fused pedicles and laminae enclose the sacral canal, triangular in cross-section, which opens posteroinferiorly at the V-shaped sacral hiatus. The canal contains the lower part of the cauda equina, comprising the roots of the sacral and coccygeal nerves. The anterior rami of the upper four sacral

Fig. 8.15 Lateral and superior views of a typical (third) lumbar vertebra.

Fig. 8.16 Fifth lumbar vertebra and the upper part of the sacrum, seen in an expanded anterior view.

nerves pass into the pelvis via the anterior sacral foramina and contribute to the sacral plexus. The posterior rami traverse the posterior sacral foramina (Fig. 8.17). Lateral to the foramina are the lateral masses, each of which bears an auricular surface for articulation with the ilium (Fig. 8.18).

The sacroiliac joint is synovial but allows very little movement because of the irregularity of the articulating surfaces and the thick posterior interosseous ligament. Each joint is further supported by the anterior and posterior sacroiliac ligaments and the iliolumbar, sacrospinous and

sacrotuberous ligaments. Body weight, acting downwards through the lumbosacral disc, tends to rotate the lower part of the sacrum backwards, a movement prevented by the sacrospinous and sacrotuberous ligaments (see Fig. 8.20).

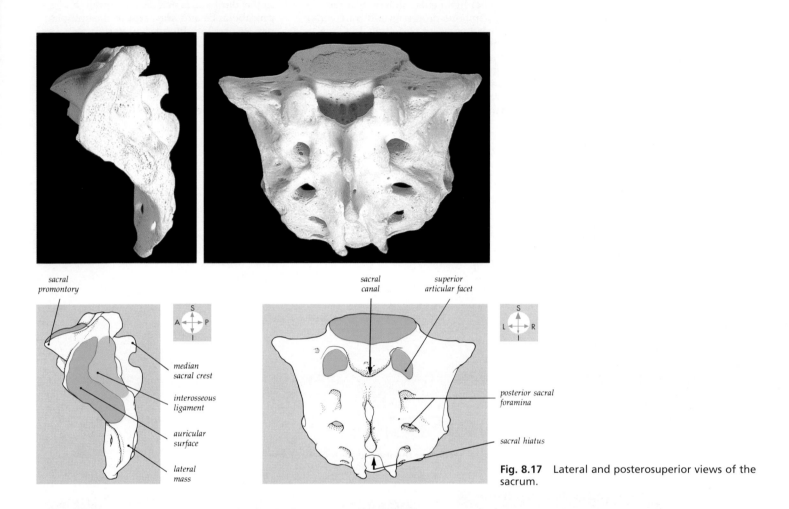

Fig. 8.17 Lateral and posterosuperior views of the sacrum.

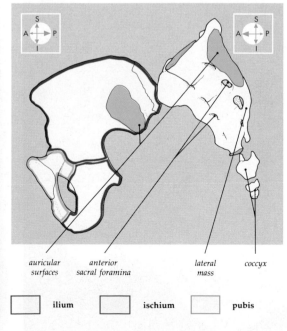

Fig. 8.18 Oblique view of the sacrum, coccyx and right hip bone.

Intervertebral discs

Intervertebral discs connect adjacent vertebral bodies (Fig. 8.19) and act as fibrocartilagenous joints along the whole length of the vertebral column. Like the vertebral bodies, the discs gradually increase in size from above downwards, the largest being the lumbosacral disc between the fifth lumbar vertebra and the sacrum (Fig. 8.20). Each disc consists of a laminated anulus fibrosus surrounding a gelatinous nucleus pulposus (Fig. 8.23). The nucleus pulposus lies closer to the posterior surface of the disc and thus is more liable to posterior herniation when the disc is damaged.

Intervertebral ligaments

The intervertebral discs are reinforced by posterior and anterior longitudinal ligaments (Figs 8.21 & 8.22). These ligaments attach to vertebral bodies and intervertebral discs and anchor inferiorly to the sacrum and superiorly to the cervical vertebrae or skull. Other ligaments interconnect the laminae, spinous processes and transverse processes of adjacent vertebrae. Ligamenta flava interconnect the laminae within the vertebral canal. The high content of elastic tissue gives these ligaments their yellow appearance and they assist return of the vertebral column to the erect position following flexion. Supraspinous and interspinous ligaments connect adjacent spinous processes of thoracic and lumbar vertebrae. It is through these ligaments that a needle is inserted to withdraw cerebrospinal fluid during lumbar puncture.

The supraspinous and interspinous ligaments are replaced in the cervical region by the ligamentum nuchae, which attaches to the skull at the external occipital protuberance and crest and to the spinous processes of all the cervical vertebrae. Intertransverse ligaments connect the transverse processes of adjacent vertebrae. The lumbosacral joint is reinforced by the iliolumbar ligament which attaches the transverse process of the fifth lumbar vertebra to the iliac crest (Fig. 8.23).

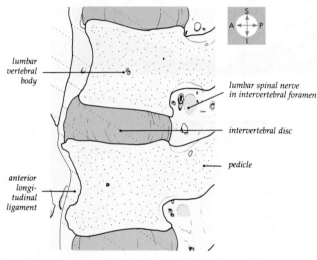

Fig. 8.19   Sagittal section of the lumbar vertebral column.

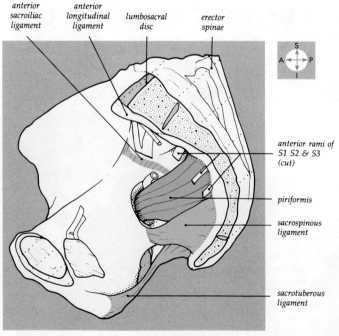

Fig. 8.20   Right hemipelvis, showing the sacrum and coccyx in sagittal section.

anterior
longitudinal
ligament

intervertebral
discs

fourth
lumbar
vertebral
body

cut
edge

Fig. 8.22 Oblique view of anterior longitudinal
ligament of the lumbar spine.

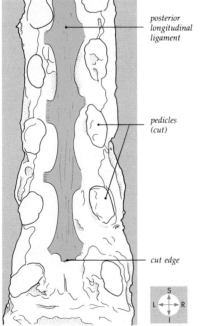

posterior
longitudinal
ligament

pedicles
(cut)

cut edge

Fig. 8.21 Posterior longitudinal ligament,
exposed by removal of the vertebral arches,
meninges and spinal cord.

quadratus lumborum

psoas major

transversus abdominis

iliolumbar ligament
& iliac crest

lumbar vessels

erector spinae

thoracolumbar fascia

spinous process of
L3 vertebra

nucleus pulposus

Fig. 8.23 Oblique view of a transverse section of the lumbar spine and muscles at the
level of the disc between the third and fourth lumbar vertebrae.

MUSCLES

The muscles of the erector spinae group are covered in the lumbar region by the thoracolumbar fascia, in the thoracic region by the serratus posterior muscles and in the neck by the splenius muscles.

In the lumbar region the thoracolumbar fascia is trilaminar and encloses erector spinae posteriorly and quadratus lumborum anteriorly (see Fig. 8.23). At the lateral margins of both muscles the laminae of the fascia fuse and give attachment to the transversus abdominis (see Fig. 8.23).

Serratus posterior superior and inferior (Figs 8.24 & 8.25) are weak respiratory muscles which connect lower cervical and upper thoracic spines with upper ribs, and lower thoracic and upper lumbar spines with lower ribs respectively. They are supplied by branches of anterior rami of thoracic spinal nerves (intercostal nerves).

Splenius muscles

Splenius (Fig. 8.26) attaches medially to the lower part of the ligamentum nuchae and to the upper thoracic spinous processes. The superior part, splenius capitis, attaches laterally to the mastoid process and superior nuchal line. The inferior part, splenius cervicis, attaches laterally to the transverse processes of the upper cervical vertebrae.

Erector spinae

On each side erector spinae (see Fig. 8.28) occupies the groove between the spinous and transverse processes of vertebrae. The muscle attaches inferiorly to the posterior surface of the sacrum and the posterior part of the iliac crest. In the lumbar region it forms a prominent vertical muscle mass

pinna

splenius

levator scapulae (cut)

serratus posterior superior

erector spinae

Fig. 8.24   Serratus posterior superior. The upper limb girdle and its muscles have been removed.

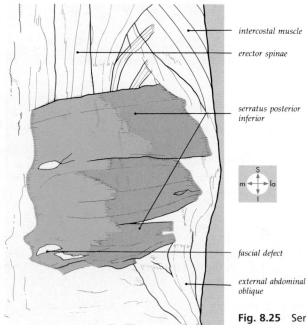

intercostal muscle

erector spinae

serratus posterior inferior

fascial defect

external abdominal oblique

Fig. 8.25   Serratus posterior inferior revealed by removal of latissimus dorsi.

(see Fig. 8.32) and attaches to the spinous and transverse processes of the lumbar vertebrae. In the upper lumbar region the muscle divides into three columns. The lateral column forms iliocostalis, which attaches to the angles of the ribs and transverse processes of the lower cervical vertebrae. The intermediate column forms the longissimus, which attaches to the ribs and the transverse processes of the thoracic and cervical vertebrae. The medial part of the erector spinae forms the spinalis, which attaches to the spinous processes of the upper lumbar, thoracic and lower cervical vertebrae.

Erector spinae is innervated by branches from the posterior rami of spinal nerves.

Transversospinalis

The muscles of this group lie obliquely (Fig. 8.27), covered by erector spinae (see Fig. 8.4). They interconnect transverse processes and spinous processes of vertebrae at higher levels. Semispinalis forms the longest and most superficial member of this group and interconnects lower thoracic transverse processes and upper thoracic and cervical spinous processes. Multifidus lies deep to semispinalis. Its fibres attach the transverse process of each vertebra to the spinous processes of one to three vertebrae above. The deepest fibres of transversospinalis form the rotatores, which connect the lamina of one vertebra to the transverse

process of the vertebra below. The rotatores are best developed in the thoracic region.

The transversospinalis muscles are supplied by the posterior rami of the spinal nerves.

Actions

Simultaneous contraction of the deep muscles of both sides extends the vertebral column and regulates or prevents flexion. Unilateral contraction produces lateral flexion and rotation, assisted by the abdominal oblique muscles. The short muscles are important in the maintenance of posture.

splenius capitis

splenius cervicis

erector spinae

Fig. 8.26 Splenius cervicis and capitis after excision of serratus posterior superior.

Fig. 8.27 Transverse section at the level of the sixth thoracic vertebra to show the back muscles and the vertebral foramen. Inferior aspect.

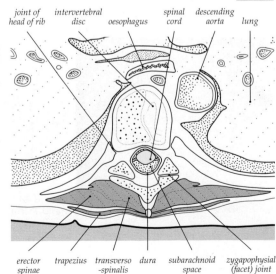

joint of head of rib   intervertebral disc   oesophagus   spinal cord   descending aorta   lung

erector spinae   trapezius   transverso-spinalis   dura   subarachnoid space   zygapophysial (facet) joint

Fig. 8.28   Splenius and erector spinae exposed by removal of overlying muscles and fasciae.

MENINGES

The spinal cord is surrounded by three membranes (dura mater, arachnoid mater and pia mater; Fig. 8.29), which are continuous through the foramen magnum with the cranial meninges.

Dura mater

The dura mater surrounding the spinal cord forms a sheath that corresponds to the inner (meningeal) layer of the cranial dura (see page 330). The spinal dura is separated from the periosteum of the vertebral canal by the extradural (epidural) space (see Figs 8.11 & 8.27), which contains fat, vessels and loose connective tissue. Anaesthetic agents are instilled into this space to produce epidural anaesthesia. Spinal dura is attached to the margins of the foramen magnum and via fibrous slips to the posterior longitudinal ligament within the vertebral canal. Inferiorly the dura covers the filum terminale (Fig. 8.30). At the level of the second sacral vertebra the dura attaches to the filum terminale and these continue onto the back of the coccyx to fuse with the periosteum.

Each spinal nerve root is surrounded by a sleeve of dura mater which extends through the intervertebral foramen before fusing with the epineurium of the spinal nerve.

Arachnoid mater

The arachnoid mater is a delicate membrane that surrounds the spinal cord and the nerves within the vertebral canal. Above it is continuous with the cranial arachnoid through the foramen magnum and below it ends at the level of the second sacral vertebra. The arachnoid is connected to the pia mater by numerous delicate strands that cross the subarachnoid space between the two meninges. This space is filled with cerebrospinal fluid and also contains blood vessels, which

supply the spinal cord. Cerebrospinal fluid is usually sampled by inserting a needle between the arches of the third and fourth or fourth and fifth lumbar vertebrae. The needle will thus enter the subarachnoid space below the termination of the spinal cord.

Pia mater

The pia mater is a highly vascular layer that closely invests the spinal cord and nerves. On each side the pia mater is attached to the dura by the ligamentum denticulatum between the anterior and posterior spinal roots. The pia surrounds the

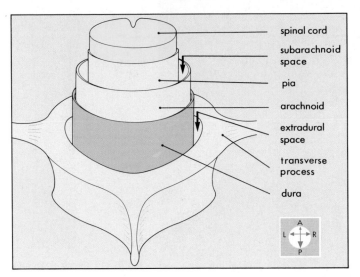

spinal cord
subarachnoid space
pia
arachnoid
extradural space
transverse process
dura

Fig. 8.29 Spinal meninges.

lumbar enlargement

spinal dura (cut and reflected)

conus medullaris

posterior nerve roots

cauda equina

filum terminale

Fig. 8.30 Spinal dura and arachnoid opened posteriorly and reflected laterally, exposing the lumbar enlargement, conus medullaris and cauda equina.

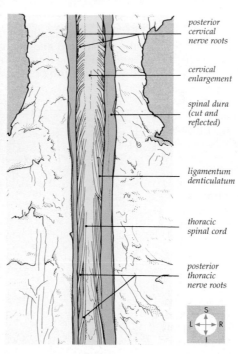

posterior
cervical
nerve roots

cervical
enlargement

spinal dura
(cut and
reflected)

ligamentum
denticulatum

thoracic
spinal cord

posterior
thoracic
nerve roots

Fig. 8.31 Cervical spinal cord and dorsal nerve roots. The spinal dura has been reflected laterally.

liver

psoas major

kidney

quadratus
lumborum

cauda
equina

spinous
process

crus of
diaphragm

descending
colon

transversospinalis

abdominal wall
muscles

erector
spinae

thoracolumbar
fascia

Fig. 8.32 Transverse section at the level of the first lumbar vertebra to show the back muscles and the contents of the vertebral foramen. Inferior aspect.

termination of the spinal cord (conus medullaris) and continues as the filum terminale as far as the posterior surface of the coccyx.

SPINAL CORD

Surface features

At the level of the upper border of the atlas the spinal cord is directly continuous with the medulla oblongata. Inferiorly the cord usually extends as far as the first lumbar intervertebral disc, where it terminates as the conus medullaris. In transverse section the spinal cord is oval, with its smaller diameter anteroposteriorly. The cord is especially wide at the cervical and lumbar enlargements due to increased numbers of nerve cell bodies within the spinal cord which innervate the upper and lower limbs.

On the anterior aspect of the cord lies the anterior median fissure, whereas posteriorly there is a relatively shallow posterior median sulcus. On each side a posterolateral sulcus marks the site of attachment of the posterior nerve roots.

Spinal nerve roots

The spinal nerves are attached to the spinal cord by anterior and posterior nerve roots (Fig. 8.31). The region of the spinal cord to which one pair of anterior and posterior nerve roots attaches is called a spinal segment.

Each anterior spinal root emerges from the cord as a series of small rootlets while similar branches from each posterior spinal root sink into the posterolateral sulcus. The anterior and posterior roots cross the subarachnoid space and unite in the appropriate intervertebral foramen to form a spinal nerve. Each posterior root is characterized by a ganglion just proximal to the union of anterior and posterior roots.

Because the spinal cord is shorter than the vertebral column the lower spinal nerve roots descend within the vertebral canal before leaving through their intervertebral foramina. These lumbar, sacral and coccygeal nerve roots are clustered around the conus medullaris and filum terminale to form the cauda equina (Fig. 8.32).

Blood supply

The spinal cord receives its arterial supply from anterior and posterior spinal arteries that arise from vertebral arteries and are reinforced by branches of the deep cervical, intercostal and lumbar arteries. These vessels form a longitudinal anastomosis that runs the length of the spinal cord. The venous return from the spinal cord drains into a series of longitudinal anastomosing channels, which empty into veins corresponding to the arteries.

Exam Skills

Each of the incomplete statements below is followed by five suggested answers or completions.
Decide which are true and which are false. The answers are supplied on page 367.

1. **During walking and/or running the following normally occur:**
   a) lateral flexion at the lumbar intervertebral joints.
   b) movement at the hip joints.
   c) contraction of the gluteal muscles.
   d) movement at the sacroiliac joints.
   e) rotation of the thoracic vertebral column.

2. **Concerning the joints between the atlas and the axis:**
   a) they are all synovial.
   b) they allow rotation of the head.
   c) they are supported by the alar ligaments.
   d) dislocation is usually fatal.
   e) they are closely related to the first cervical nerves.

3. **The sacroiliac joint:**
   a) is a fibrous joint.
   b) allows rotation in which the lower part of the sacrum moves anteriorly.
   c) is stabilized by the sacrotuberous ligament.
   d) is a posterior relation of the common iliac artery.
   e) is stabilized by the iliolumbar ligament.

4. **The lumbar region of the vertebral column:**
   a) is the least mobile region of the spinal column.
   b) has vertebrae which possess mamillary processes.
   c) is flexed by the rectus abdominis.
   d) has a secondary curvature.
   e) has spinous processes which overlap the body of the adjacent vertebra below.

5. **The spinal cord:**
   a) gives rise to eight pairs of cervical spinal nerves.
   b) is continuous above with the medulla oblongata.
   c) is intimately related to the pia mater.
   d) extends throughout the length of the vertebral canal.
   e) is separated from CSF by the arachnoid mater.

6. **The intervertebral disc between vertebrae L3 and L4:**
   a) is the smallest intervertebral disc.
   b) is related anteriorly to the abdominal aorta.
   c) provides attachment for psoas major.
   d) is related posteriorly to the cauda equina.
   e) is closely related to the second lumbar nerves.

7. **The atlas vertebra:**
   a) has no spinous process.
   b) possesses no foramina transversaria.
   c) has a vertebral body.
   d) permits nodding movements at its joints with the cranium.
   e) has large transverse processes.

8. **Intervertebral discs:**
   a) occur between the bodies of adjacent vertebrae.
   b) are intimately related to the anterior and posterior longitudinal ligaments.
   c) are secondary cartilaginous joints.
   d) form part of the borders of the intervertebral foramina.
   e) contribute to the curvatures of the vertebral column.

9. **The sacrum:**
   a) usually consists of fused components of five vertebrae.
   b) is concave anteriorly.
   c) is attached by ligaments to the ilium and ischium.
   d) forms synovial joints with the articular processes of the fifth lumbar vertebra.
   e) possesses on each side an ala which is crossed by the anterior ramus of the fifth lumbar nerve.

10. **The thoracic vertebral column:**
    a) has a primary curvature which is concave anteriorly.
    b) includes 12 vertebrae.
    c) articulates with the heads of ribs.
    d) throughout its length is related anteriorly to the oesophagus.
    e) permits lateral flexion which is restricted by the ribs.

11. **The thoracolumbar fascia:**
    a) provides attachment for transversus abdominis.
    b) encloses psoas major muscle.
    c) has no attachment to bone.
    d) provides attachment for external abdominal oblique muscle.
    e) provides attachment for latissimus dorsi.

12. **The spinal dura mater:**
    a) is attached to the vertebral periosteum.
    b) lies deep to the spinal arteries.
    c) lies superficial to the vertebral venous plexus.
    d) terminates at the level of vertebra L2.
    e) attaches to the margins of the foramen magnum.

13. **A typical cervical vertebra possesses:**
    a) two pairs of synovial joints.
    b) a bifid spinous process.
    c) a relatively wide vertebral foramen.
    d) a relatively small body.
    e) foramina transversaria.

14. **The vertebral canal:**
    a) transmits the vertebral artery.
    b) contains ligamenta flava.
    c) contains a venous plexus.
    d) is narrowed by rotation of the head.
    e) lies anterolateral to the cervical vertebral discs.

15. **The following relate to lumbar puncture at vertebral level L4/L5:**
    a) the spinal cord terminates at a higher vertebral level.
    b) at this level the ligaments are thinner and easier to penetrate.
    c) there is no overlap of the spinous processes.
    d) the spinal nerves that exit from the vertebral column below this level are of little importance.
    e) the subarachnoid space extends inferiorly to below vertebral level L5.

16. **The joints between vertebrae C4 and C5 allow:**
    a) rotation.
    b) flexion with rotation.
    c) pure extension.
    d) lateral flexion.
    e) lateral flexion with rotation.